P9-BUI-654

MEGA-NUTRIENTS
FOR YOUR NERVES

MEGA

H. L. Newbold, M. D.

NUTRIENTS FOR YOUR NERVES

PETER H. WYDEN/ Publisher/ New York

MEGA-NUTRIENTS FOR YOUR NERVES

COPYRIGHT © 1975 BY H. L. Newbold, M.D.

All rights reserved, including the right to reproduce this book, or parts thereof, in any form, except for the inclusion of brief quotations in a review.

Library of Congress Cataloging in Publication Data

Newbold, Herbert Leon, 1921–
    Mega-nutrients for your nerves.

    Includes bibliographical references and index.
    1. Nervous system—Diseases—Nutritional aspects. 2. Vitamins in human nutrition. 3. Nutrition. I. Title. [DNLM: 1 Diet—Popular works. 2. Nutrition—Popular works. QU145 W978m]
RC351.N53   616.8   75-22360
ISBN 0-88326-095-6

MANUFACTURED IN THE United States of America

Design by Bob Antler

9 8 7 6 5

For
Margot Norton
and
Rebecca Watson

All our provisional ideas in psychology will some day be based on organic structure. This makes it probable that special substances and special chemicals control the operation.

—SIGMUND FREUD

CONTENTS

AUTHOR'S NOTE

I urge each reader to consult his or her physician before embarking upon any change in diet.

H.L.N.

MEGA-NUTRIENTS
FOR YOUR NERVES

HOW I ENTERED
NUTRITIONAL PSYCHIATRY

CHAPTER ONE

Since you do not know me, let me take a few moments to introduce myself, sketch my background, and tell you how I came to enter the field of nutritional psychiatry, which is the subject of this book. This will, I hope, give you some basis for judging the validity of the rather unorthodox views I champion.

First let me say that I consider myself very much a part of the medical establishment. After receiving my B.S. and M.D. degrees at Duke University, I completed a rotating internship at the University of Chicago and an internship in obstetrics and gynecology at the University of Minnesota. This was followed by a residency in internal medicine at the Veterans Administration Hospital associated with Vanderbilt University, and then a three-year psychiatric residency at the University of Illinois and its affiliated V.A. hospital. To complete my training, I also underwent a nine-hundred-hour, five-year analysis by a graduate of the Chicago Analytical Institute.

I taught neurology and psychiatry at Northwestern University Medical School, published a number of scientific papers in medical journals, and am the author of a textbook on psychology which is used in medical schools around the world. I am a member of the American Medical Association, the New York State and New York County medical societies and the American Psychiatric Association, as well as a fellow of the Academy of Psychosomatic Medicine, the Society for Clinical Ecology, the Royal Society of Health, and the International College of Applied Nutrition.

That's about as steeped in traditional medicine as one can get. If a particular event had not happened to me a few years ago, I might have gone on practicing "cookbook" medicine the way most physicians do and, indeed, the way I myself practiced it until then.

The particular event was an unusually severe attack of hypoglycemia, low blood sugar, though it was only much later that this correct diagnosis surfaced.

Now, you may be certain that when a physician becomes ill, he selects his attending physician with some care. The man I selected was a graduate of the prestigious Johns Hopkins University, who had taken his postgraduate training at the equally prestigious Columbia University Presbyterian Medical Center. I respected him as a person and as a thoroughly competent specialist. But I soon learned that, in common with almost all other physicians, he had certain limitations. This was not his fault, nor perhaps even the fault of the institutions where he had studied. These institutions merely reflected the universal neglect heaped on the science of nutrition in this country. I still respect my physician as a kind, generous, and learned man.

While in the hospital, I began awakening each morning at about 4:30 and, as is so often the custom, the nurse would give me a glass of sweetened orange juice. Each morning after drinking the orange juice I dropped off again immediately to sleep soundly until 7:30, when we were all roused for the taking of morning temperatures.

When I returned home to recuperate I put myself on a medium-carbohydrate, low-protein, low-fat diet in order to reduce my high blood cholesterol level. Since my weight was a bit out of hand, too, I restricted my total calorie intake in the hope of losing ten or fifteen pounds.

I had been on this diet for about two days when suddenly I felt weak, began sweating, and experienced a feeling of impending doom. I returned to the hospital where my physician checked me over, did further tests, found no cause for my symptoms, and discharged me. After several days on my home regimen the same symptoms returned, and I went back to the hospital once more. This time I was checked by both my physician and his associate. Neither could find anything amiss, and I was discharged once more—no doubt with *sotto voce* muttering about the hypochondriasis of psychiatrists.

As if on cue, the symptoms of weakness, perspiration, and anxiety returned the next day. At that point I decided that I had exhausted my physician's diagnostic abilities. If anything was to be done for me, I would either have to sign myself into some medical center for a complete work-up—or find out for myself what was wrong.

Perhaps none of us really thinks until forced to do so. I decided to begin using my own head to solve my problems, since it was not likely that anyone else would solve them for me. As I lay sweating in bed, turning possibilities over in my mind, it struck me that each time I had awakened early at the hospital I had been given sweetened orange juice and promptly gone back to sleep. I asked myself whether I could be having hypoglycemic attacks—attacks of low blood sugar.

The more I thought about it, the more possible this seemed, though in my then ignorant state I had never made such a diagnosis in anyone except the diabetic who had taken too much insulin. Still, my symptoms fitted. I knew there was such a thing as functional hypoglycemia, a condition existing for no apparent reason, though I had only heard the term and knew almost nothing about it. Well, proof would not be hard to come by.

I sent for a wedge of apple pie garnished with three scoops of ice cream, propped my weak and sweaty self upright in bed, and broke my diet. Within five minutes, all symptoms had disappeared: the sweating, the weakness, the feeling of impending doom, the fear that I was about to die—all vanished as if by magic. The first step toward the diagnosis of hypoglycemia had been taken.

I was disturbed to realize that my two knowledgeable doctors had failed even to consider hypoglycemia during a total of three hospital stays. These men represented the ultimate in the medical establishment. If they were not able to diagnose hypoglycemia, how could I be certain that they were correct in any sphere?

Questions now poured in on me. What diet should I follow? If I ate a high-protein, high-fat, low-carbohydrate diet, as would be indicated for hypoglycemia, would it raise my cholesterol level? Would this predispose me to a heart attack? Who knew? Evidently not the medical establishment. And so I began to think seriously, perhaps for the first time, about the connection between nutritional disorder and mental unrest.

My attacks of hypoglycemia, if that's what they were, had made me feel weak, anxious and miserable. Certainly in my psychiatric practice I had had a full load of patients who also felt weak, anxious, and miserable; how many of them might have hypoglycemia too? For that matter, how many other kinds of nutritional imbalance might be at the root of emotional problems that most psychotherapists treat with words or drugs?

I thought back to a schizophrenic patient who had consulted me a few months earlier and demanded niacin (vitamin B_3) therapy. Like any card-carrying member of the medical establishment, I had told the boy's family that niacin was not yet a proven aid in the treatment of schizophrenia, and had declined to carry it out. The truth was that I had heard of this treatment (as well as the usefulness of niacin for hypoglycemia), but I knew no details, and lacked time and motivation to investigate a new form of therapy. I had a busy practice and seemed to be helping as many patients as the average psychiatrist. Why embark on a new therapy which had not yet received the medical community's approval? Besides, the new megavitamin approach to psychiatric illness did not fit in with any of my previous training and theory concerning the treatment of schizophrenia.

Then, some months later a second family had requested niacin therapy for their daughter. Since I had tried every other approach with this patient to no avail, I was a shade more receptive. The girl's mother was good enough to secure some basic information for me. Lying in bed, recuperating and thinking, I decided to look at these article reprints.

To my amazement I learned that niacin has many interesting side-effects; one of them is the lowering of blood cholesterol, which could be used to prevent a recurrence of heart attacks. Edwin Boyle, M.D., the director of research at the Miami Heart Institute, had written an article strongly endorsing the use of niacin for post-coronary patients.

At this point, even though the psychiatrist in me might have rolled over and gone back to sleep, Dr. Newbold, the patient, was sitting bolt upright in bed reading further. I learned that niacin decreases the clotting time of blood. It also puts a negative electrical charge on each of the red blood cells, so that they repel each other and travel through the blood vessels individually, instead of clumping together like a bunch of grapes. Each red blood cell could therefore carry more oxygen.

Niacin in megavitamin doses also raises the blood sugar, a very important action for anyone with hypoglycemia.

I made an appointment at a laboratory for a six-hour glucose tolerance test. This test was to be the final clincher in my self-diagnosis of hypoglycemia. It also pointed me in the direction my future career would take.

I appeared at the laboratory at 9 A.M., already slightly weak from not eating breakfast. The fasting blood specimen was drawn, and then I was given a drink of flavored sugar water. After half an hour my blood sugar test was repeated. Another blood sugar test was done half an hour later. By the time of my second-hour test, my sense of well-being was evaporating rapidly, along with my equanimity. I began to feel weak, started to perspire, and had a feeling of impending doom. In short, I reproduced all my earlier hypoglycemic symptoms. Because I considered it dangerous to continue, I stopped the test after the drawing of the third-hour blood sample and ate breakfast, even though it had been scheduled to be a six-hour test (my health is excellent now; all this occurred several years ago).

An abbreviated test is not proper for the diagnosis of hypoglycemia, in most cases. Generally a five- or preferably a six-hour glucose tolerance test is preferred. If the test produces dramatic symptoms, it may be wise to discontinue it. For example, a patient may become psychotic during the test or unconscious, or may develop a severe attack of asthma. These marked symptoms are rare, but should they occur, the test should not be continued since it is clear that the patient does not handle sugar well.

Later in this book, I shall discuss hypoglycemia's emotional symptoms and the entire complex problem of blood sugar and nerves. Here let me say only that at the time when I first took the test my faith in the medical establishment was shaken to about number eight on the Richter scale and I realized that much of my own knowledge of medicine lay in shambles. I was greatly impressed by my own ignorance and that of the medical profession generally. As a devoted physician, my response was to dive in and learn all there was to know about the nutritional aspects of medicine.

I returned to practice, and began to employ some of my newly acquired knowledge of nutrition, vitamin, and mineral supplements for patients with emotional disorders. From that moment on I have helped more people within a few years than in all my preceding years of practice. And from each patient, in turn, I have learned more and more about my chosen sub-specialty, and have gained more and more satisfaction as I watched my knowledge—and my therapeutic instincts— grow.

I should explain that, for me, every person has a particular texture. I have sat across the desk from so many emotionally ill people that by now I have developed a feel for them, much as a cloth merchant must develop a feel for the textures of his stock in trade. A glance at a patient's face, his manner, and a few words from his lips usually tell me much about his level of adjustment—whether he is operating at ninety percent of his potential, at fifty percent, or barely hanging on at a twenty percent level.

It is this texture, this level of well-being, that I find so often changed by nutritional therapy. My main reason for writing this book, therefore, is to bring the possibility of such enhanced well-being within the reach of many more people than I can directly treat in my practice. I want you to know about the role of vitamins in regulating your well-being, the importance of minerals and hormones, and about how hidden, unsuspected food allergies can cause nervous symptoms ranging all the way from mild anxiety and depression to insanity.

This book is about people: about Anne, who turned schizophrenic whenever she ate pasta; about Frank, who needs a vitamin B_{12} injection every four days to stay out of the hospital; and an anxiety-ridden housewife who saw a psychiatrist for therapy when all she needed was to avoid the gas fumes of her kitchen stove.

I think you get the message: If you've ever suffered from a nervous or allergic condition, or a sense of illness that defied classification and cure—read on. There's a pretty good chance that you (*and* your doctor!) may have looked for the explanation in the wrong direction, just by pigeonholing your complaint in a traditional (but not necessarily relevant) slot.

My professional experience has taught me what Edward de Bono calls "lateral think," which means that even though a problem is apparently insoluble, at least by the usual mode of attack, it may practically solve itself when you free yourself from preconceived notions.

So when a patient named Sybil came to see me about her steak allergy, which occurred only when she sat under fluorescent lights at the office, I didn't smile benignly and murmur soothingly about taking it easy. I did some lateral looking around and there, staring me in the face and just waiting to be discovered, was the explanation. Distorted light wave patterns may bring on allergic reactions in certain people.

Such simple "thought lib" can do wonders for clearing up mysterious afflictions, and by means of it, hundreds of my patients have helped me to help them. Now I'm settling accounts by recording my experiences with them to serve as your guidelines toward helping yourself. The last two words are meant to be taken literally because in the coming chapters you will learn how to establish your own best vitamin and mineral regimen; how to test yourself for food allergies; how to perform your own preliminary tests for sugar-related metabolic diseases; and how best to work with a doctor of your own on these and many other problems that have taken on epidemic proportions.

WHAT A "NORMAL" DIET CAN DO TO YOU

CHAPTER TWO

"An Apple a Day Keeps the Doctor Away." Right? Wrong.

We live in an age of elaborate controls, supervision, and specialization. Practically everything in life has become a specialty, requiring expert advice. You need a hospital, two doctors, and a brace of nurses to have a baby. You need a lawyer, $400, and seven pages of single-spaced typing to write a will that says, "I leave everything to my wife." You need an examination, a test, and a license to drive a car or to practice your profession; you even need a license to go fishing. Certainly everything that can affect your health or well-being, or that of the community at large is subject to scrutiny and control by the government and/or by the profession or industry that has made a particular field its special province.

One of the few things left to the discretion of the individual is what to eat. You don't need a license, a prescription, or a Ph.D. degree to go to the grocery store; therefore, most people assume that there can't be anything very complicated about nutrition. We have absorbed a few hoary clichés about the subject from those noted scientific experts, our

8

grandmothers. We certainly spend enough time and money on making our food taste good: So what could be wrong?

Plenty.

In many ways, it sometimes seems to me that the study of medicine, and particularly of psychiatry, is still in the Dark Ages. And the least illuminated of all the medical disciplines is the study of nutrition.

The human body is a fantastically complicated collection of cells and chemical reactions. The more we learn about the diagnosis and cure of that system when something goes wrong, the more we understand how extraordinarily complicated it is. And yet most of us assume that it is a relatively simple matter to nourish the human system properly.

Can that be right?

No, it can't, and it isn't.

The "minimum daily requirement" of vitamins and minerals is a travesty and a good example of what I'm saying.

The American Medical Association and the Food and Drug Administration hold center stage in the medical establishment. They have assumed the responsibility of setting standards and maintaining some controls over the foods we eat and the medicines we take. And they persistently leave Americans with the impression that there is an average daily requirement of carbohydrates, fats, proteins, vitamins, and minerals that suits *all* adults perfectly well no matter what their age, medical history, size, sex, or genetic make-up. They assure us that we can meet all our nutritional needs by eating a "normal, well-balanced American diet" without any nutritional supplements whatever.

This recommendation perpetuates four major fallacies:

1. That the American diet is normal, well-balanced, and nutritionally adequate. It is in fact inadequate on all these counts.
2. That there is some clear-cut, black-or-white difference between having a deficiency and not having one. It may be true that an average diet prevents scurvy or beri-beri, but that does not mean that a deficiency does not exist.
3. That there is an "average" person with "average" nutritional needs.
4. That medical science has adequate information to establish nutritional standards, average or otherwise. It does not.

Because these notions are some of the most strongly held in the current myth of American nutrition, and because I believe them to be exceedingly misleading and potentially dangerous, let's examine them each in turn.

THE FIRST FALLACY OF THE AMERICAN DIET: THAT THE AMERICAN DIET IS NORMAL, WELL-BALANCED, AND NUTRITIONALLY ADEQUATE

CHAPTER THREE

We are said to have one of the highest standards of living in the world. Americans hold on hard to that thesis; it seems to comfort us in the face of social and political confusion and disillusion, racial and sexual unrest, inflation, pollution, crime, terror, depression, frustration, and ennui. No matter how tough things seem sometimes, it improves our perspective to remember that so many people are worse off than we.

Shouldn't a high standard of living mean that we eat well? In fact, with more Americans concerned about overweight than any other aspect of nutrition, don't we eat *too* well?

Of course not. There is no such thing as eating too well. If you eat well, you are trim, fit and healthy, not obese. A great many of us eat too *much*, but that is definitely not the same thing as being well-nourished.

Most people in America assume that malnutrition is confined to the ghettoes and poverty pockets in Appalachia, but the fact is that malnutrition, mild or acute, exists in all levels of our society. America is the only country in the world where the average dog is better fed than the average person. It is literally true that the nutritional requirements established for packaged dog food are far more stringent than those for the food we eat ourselves, *especially* processed convenience foods.

If you doubt this, try comparing the labels of a can of Alpo with a can of ravioli. Processors of human foods are not required to guarantee that the food contains *any* nutrients, nor do they have to list the quantities of protein, fat, or carbohydrates, or the vitamins or minerals. To be competitive, they simply have to try to keep it clean and make it taste good.

Keeping food clean and making it taste good; that's the half-staff of life

To take a single example of the ways our attitudes about food are confused and manipulated, consider the case of "refined" wheat and wheat products. For centuries, wheat has been so central to the Western diet that bread is referred to as the staff of life. Taking into account bread, cakes, cookies, snacks, crackers, pasta, and cereal, Americans eat an enormous quantity of wheat; it forms a percentage of the diet that is by no means "balanced" for an animal with the basic enzyme system of a carnivore.

Up to the last century, most wheat products contained the whole grain, including the wheat germ which is a rich source of protein, B vitamins, and certain essential minerals. Today, nearly all wheat flour and wheat products have been "refined." According to the dictionary, "refined" means "free of worthless matter and impurities." But refined wheat flour is so free of any nutrients, of the germ with all its vitamins and minerals and amino acids, that the white flour that is left will not support even a weevil.

This is of great value to the manufacturer; it means that a product will last in the bin or on the shelf for weeks or perhaps months without growing rancid or buggy, because there is nothing in the flour for a bug or bacterium to live on. We have learned to like this stuff, even to prefer it, and not the least of the reasons is that it's called "refined," sounding pure and modern and classy.

In actuality it ought to be called "stripped."

As for "enriched" refined wheat products (sound delicious, don't they?) the enriching consists of taking out some twenty-three essential nutrients, and putting back six of the least expensive ones. That's like saying a mugger enriched you when he stole everything in your wallet and then gave you back enough change for bus fare.

The same holds true for the refining of other grains. White rice is produced by removing the brown husk that surrounds the rice kernels. The husk is the very part that contains the nutrients that sustain life, including large amounts of B vitamins and minerals. Chickens fed a diet of white rice develop beri-beri. The disease is cured by adding to the meal the rice polish removed by "refining."

The problem of the long storage of "refined" food

Some of my colleagues and I who are interested in the interrelationships between food allergies and emotional illness have made a special study of bread and found its main constituent—wheat—to be highly allergenic. In all probability this is due not only to its relative newness in human nutrition but also to the particles of rat feces and cockroaches that it acquires during storage. Quite possibly, man's genetic makeup has not evolved sufficiently to handle grains efficiently and he is not able to detoxify wheat quickly and metabolize it as he can foods that his ancestors have eaten for millions of years like meat, nuts, roots, berries, and fruits.

Filth and contaminants form a normal part of many mass-produced foods

Next time you feel like munching a chocolate bar, remember the following story told me at a recent meeting of the Society for Clinical Ecology. Food allergies are almost an obsession with members of the society, and they are forever tracking down the sources of allergenic substances. One member recently visited a South American country to study the cocoa bean from which chocolate is made. He began at the site where it was grown, and traced it all the way through the manufacturing process. At one point he went down to the docks where the beans stood on open wharves awaiting shipment. On opening one of the crates he found it alive with cockroaches. He estimates that about one-fourth of chocolate consists of dead, ground-up, melted-down cockroach, and that this is one of the factors that makes it such a common allergen.

*Even unprocessed foods may not provide the nourishment
you think they do*

In the process of drying, storing, refining, freezing, and canning foods, many valuable nutrients are lost. In addition, most processed foods contain colorings, flavorings, and preservatives that can be dangerously allergenic. The additives may cause serious disorders, including cancer.

Even if you eat mainly fresh foods from the supermarket you are by no means assured of getting adequate vitamins and minerals from your diet alone. Fresh fruits and vegetables lose vitamins on the shelf, and you rarely know how long a tomato has been sitting in a crate or on a truck between the time it gets from the vine to you; furthermore, minerals and many vitamins in fruits and vegetables come from the soil, and many of the elements have long since been depleted in farmlands that have been in constant production decade after decade.

Many more nutrients are lost during cooking, either literally going up in steam, or, most often, thrown out in the cooking water. So the charts you can get from the government assuring you that there are x number of milligrams of vitamin A in a serving of something or other are virtually useless unless you grow and harvest your produce yourself and eat most of it raw—and even then you will lose nutrients if you smoke, have alcoholic drinks, or lack hydrochloric acid in your stomach.

In sum, it is extraordinary that a nation so obsessed with food knows so little about nourishment. Many people dismiss the notion that our diets are inadequate, saying that if we are so ill-nourished, why aren't people suffering from it all around us?

The answer is: they are.

We're too fat, too thin, depressed, angry, anxious, sickly. We have a million illnesses—from colds to a world record for heart attacks undreamed of a century ago. Does that sound like a society that is well-nourished? If we were to stop people on the street and test them at random for proteins, fats, carbohydrates, vitamins, hormones, and minerals, we would find an astounding number of deficiencies; and most (if not all) of these people could improve their health and well-being immeasurably by simply having their deficiencies corrected.

The American diet may be average, but it is not normal for a human being

Even if none of the recent and dubious inventions of the food processors had come about, even if you forget for a moment about all the preservatives and additives and freeze-drying and refining that has changed the nutritional value of the food we eat, one other enormous change in eating habits has occurred in the last hundred years. The terrible significance of this one change for our mental and physical health is only beginning to be guessed at; the change is our yearly consumption of sugar.

Man first learned to produce a crude sort of sugar from the sap of sugar cane roughly 2,500 years ago. But between that time and the nineteenth century it was available only in tiny amounts and only to the very rich. During the reign of Queen Elizabeth I, an Englishman would buy sugar by the ounce from the apothecary. Queen Elizabeth herself was said to have been as fond of it as any modern teenage candy addict, and contemporary reports say that her teeth were quite black with decay.

When slave labor came to the Caribbean in the middle of the eighteenth century, the production of sugar increased greatly; but refined sugar has been commonly available for only a little over a hundred years. As in the case of grains, "refined" here means that what few trace vitamins and minerals occur naturally in sugar are removed, leaving a pure white powder that even bugs won't eat. Even with the recent rise in the price of sugar, it is one of today's least expensive foods—if, indeed, you can call it a food. When I say inexpensive, I refer to the purchase price per calorie. Its purchase price in terms of vitamins, minerals, and proteins is higher than the price of gold, considering the infinitesimal quantities of any useful nutrients it contains. And if we take into consideration the incidence of diabetes and hypoglycemia, the obesity, malnutrition, rotted teeth, shortened lives, hardened arteries, depressions, and all the other medical liabilities for which it is wholly or partly responsible, sugar is the most expensive substance on earth.

In 1850, world production of sugar was only about one and one half million tons per year. By 1890, it had risen to five million tons, and by the beginning of this century it stood at eleven million tons. In 1950 it reached thirty-five million tons, and is now well above seventy million tons. So there has been a nearly fifty-fold increase in the total production of sugar over the past 125 years. The use of sugar has jumped from 3 pounds per person per year in 1850 to almost 45 pounds a year at present. But this average was arrived at by including the entire world population, including the inhabitants of underdeveloped countries. Taking the so-called civilized countries alone, the consumption of sugar averages about *100 pounds* per citizen per year—or about one-sixth of a person's total caloric intake! The United States has the highest per capita consumption of sugar—120 pounds a year.

Tragically, the very highest consumption of sugar is to be found among children and adolescents. Youngsters are more at the mercy of their appetites than older people, who have learned some elements of nutrition. Also, it is only natural that mothers try to please their children and make them happy by giving in to their demands for sweets. In addition, the sugar industry has assiduously advertised its product as a source of quick energy; so mother has it in back of her mind that she may be doing her child a favor by "giving him some quick energy." What she forgets or doesn't know is that she is also giving him a good start toward a long list of diseases.

One-sixth of our calorie intake is not even food

Americans are obsessed with the idea of calories. Too many can make them fat, too few leave them listless and thin. But calories are not nourishment in themselves; a calorie is simply a unit of energy. For your body to be nourished you must provide it with proteins and fats and vitamins and minerals as well as calories. Your enzyme systems have evolved over millions of years to process (metabolize) certain kinds of nutrients. You can imagine, for example, that if you fed your dog nothing but pears, he would not thrive. Pears are food of a kind, and they provide plenty of calories, but they would not provide the protein and vitamins and minerals the dog's meat-oriented system calls for. Nor do sugars and massive amounts of starches constitute an adequate diet for a human body.

If it's so bad for us, why do we like it so much?

I believe the answer lies in the story of our evolution. About 65 million years ago, man's ancestors lost the ability to manufacture their own vitamin C. Most animals have an enzyme in the liver that enables them to convert glucose into the ascorbic acid their bodies need. At some point in his evolution, man's ancestor began eating large quantities of fresh fruit, which supplied him with all the vitamin C he needed. When an enzyme is no longer necessary, nature eliminates it, since it is more efficient to use the chemical energy in other, more productive ways. Man's forebears lost the enzyme L-gulonolactone oxidase that helped them manufacture vitamin C, and became *dependent* on a steady intake of fruit to provide it instead.

Gradually they developed a craving for the sweetness of fruit, which is, of course, full of fructose, or fruit sugar. This craving was a very positive development, since our ancestors who ate plenty of vitamin C were more energetic, more efficient at hunting and fighting, and threw off disease more easily and healed more quickly than their cousins who craved sweets less and thus ate less fruit.

In the past hundred years, the positive genetic trait, the craving for sweet fruit, has been perverted into an addiction to sugar which is little short of grotesque. Fructose, or fruit sugar, is easily metabolized by the human system without the use of insulin. Sucrose or table sugar, on the other hand, *is* regulated by insulin. Our enzyme systems have not had the evolutionary time needed to evolve an efficient way to handle sugar.

Our current body chemistry systems are makeshift at best, easily overstrained and driven haywire, leading to hypoglycemia and diabetes and numerous other diseases a great deal more serious than children's tooth decay. Recent studies strongly implicate sugar as the real killer behind heart disease and strokes.

Refined sugar does not simply fail to provide nutrients: it actually robs your system of nutrients vitally needed elsewhere, since the chemical systems mobilized to metabolize it have to take ingredients from somewhere.

Viewed in a historical context, in terms of what kind of animal man is, what his enzyme systems are designed to do, and what we ask them to do instead, it is clear that the average American diet is not normal, well-balanced or nutritionally adequate. But if that is the case, why does the FDA and the medical establishment continue to insist that it *is* adequate?

THE SECOND FALLACY OF THE AMERICAN DIET: THAT YOU HAVE A DEFICIENCY OR YOU DON'T HAVE A DEFICIENCY

CHAPTER FOUR

Physicians tend to think of their patients' conditions in all-or-nothing terms. You have pneumonia or you don't. You are pregnant or you're not. Your appendix is inflamed or it isn't. This is appropriate when dealing with infectious diseases, but distinctly not when dealing with nutrition.

When the medical establishment says your diet is adequate, it generally means that it is adequate to prevent scurvy, bery-beri, kwashiorkor, or rickets. Preoccupied with acute clinical syndromes, very few doctors have even begun to consider the possible shades of the nutritional gray area between someone being definitely well or definitely ill.

Consider the case of anemia. This condition is caused by a shortage of hemoglobin, the special protein in the bloodstream that carries oxygen to the cells. Physicians encounter anemia frequently, and it is often caused by a nutritional deficiency. But the condition often remains undiagnosed and untreated because a patient is rarely clearly anemic or clearly not anemic. As his hemoglobin drops he may simply tire more easily, feeling neither completely well nor definitely ill. Such a state can continue for many years. The sufferer may never know that anemia is affecting the way he feels—unless he is given a nutritional supplement that wipes it out.

Nutritional problems are different from infectious diseases because they tend to develop slowly

The patient ignores them, gets used to them, forgets what it was like to feel really well, if he ever knew. The doctor in turn tends to dismiss the complaints as "psychosomatic," by which he means that you must feel sick because you're neurotic, and he may never even consider that you may have become listless, depressed, angry, paranoid, or whatever *because* you are suffering from a nutritional disorder.

Physicians like to regard themselves as exact scientists, capable of quickly and accurately diagnosing an illness and prescribing medication that will cure it, or at least keep it within manageable bounds. The fact that so few doctors know much about nutrition tempts them to dismiss the whole subject as "unscientific." Which amounts to saying, "I don't know for sure what's wrong with you, so it must be something else I *do* know about."

The disturbing truth is that most physicians don't even recognize a case of acute nutritional deficiency when they see it. H. R. Follis, Jr., M.D., and his colleagues at Johns Hopkins University hospital reported that out of sixty-nine cases of scurvy discovered at autopsy, the attending physicians had diagnosed that disease before death *in only six cases.* If the gifted and superbly trained physicians at Johns Hopkins miss this rather elementary diagnosis 91 percent of the time, how often must the disease go unrecognized in less sophisticated hospitals? And how much more often are milder deficiencies undiagnosed?

Nutritional deficiencies often exhibit themselves through emotional symptoms long before physical signs of acute deficiencies appear

The average physician, indoctrinated at medical school with the belief that nutritional deficiences only occur among alcoholics, on the dirt farms of Appalachia, or in Uganda, tends to assume that emotional symptoms have little to do with physical health. It will probably never occur to him that his own son's mood swings and bad grades might be caused by a nutritional disorder associated with a diet of potato chips and soda pop.

If the family doctor resists this notion, the psychiatrist resists it even harder. In one of my scientific publications,[1] I once pointed out that one-third of my psychiatric patients from the New York area had low serum vitamin B_{12} levels, and that their conditions usually improved substantially when the deficiency was corrected. The paper was brought to the attention of the psychiatric departments of the National Institutes of Health, the Harvard University School of Medicine, St. Luke's Hospital, Lenox Hill Hospital, and Gracie Square Hospital. So far as I have been able to discover, not one of these institutions has begun the routine testing of psychiatric patients for serum B_{12} levels.

Why do physicians neglect this test? When asked, they say, "Well, yours is only one study." Or, "It's too expensive." But I doubt that these are the real reasons. A more personal factor prevents physicians (particularly psychiatrists) from adopting the test: Psychiatrists (as well as psychologists and psychiatric social workers and marriage counselors) tend to assume that anyone they see suffers, almost by definition, from an "emotional" problem, by which they usually mean a disorder brought about by a reaction to a traumatic environmental event. These experts seem to have blocked out Freud's statement that "all our provisional ideas in psychology will some day be based on an organic structure. This makes it probable that special substances and special chemicals control the operation." In this instance, Freud's prediction was certainly correct. And when the day finally comes that his prediction is generally accepted, a principal key to psychological health will be found in the currently neglected chemistry of nutrition.

After the body chemistry is normalized, I find that some of my patients require psychotherapy. Others are so sick that they may require some supportive psychotherapy while the chemistry is being normalized. There is no reason not to use any psychiatric or medical technique along with proper nutrition. For example, a patient with tuberculosis may be treated with surgery on the diseased lung or with chemotherapy to kill the tuberculous lesion; but this does not preclude the use of a proper diet and nutritional supplements.

NOTES

1. H. L. Newbold. "The Use of Vitamin B$_{12b}$ in Psychiatric Practice," *Orthomolecular Psychiatry*, Vol. 1, No. 1, 1972, p. 27.

THE THIRD FALLACY OF THE AMERICAN DIET: THAT THERE IS AN "AVERAGE" PERSON WITH "AVERAGE" NUTRITIONAL NEEDS

CHAPTER FIVE

If we hadn't been brought up with the idea of a "minimum daily requirement" of vitamins that the government and the manufacturers of grossly inadequate "fortified" cereals drum into our heads, we would see at once that the idea of an average person with average nutritional needs is irrational. People come in different sizes and shapes and with a vast range of different genetic characteristics. They can't possibly all be properly nourished by a single standard amount of anything.

Larger bodies require more nutrients, and very active people require more vitamins and minerals, just as they require a larger total amount of calories.

As we will see in more detail later, many people are born with physiological characteristics that cause them to need vastly more of some nutrients than the government presumes to standardize. Some people are missing crucial enzymes in their systems that prevent their metabolizing the vitamins they eat. Others may lack a particular protein needed to carry the vitamin or mineral to the cells where they are needed. Such a person will require massive doses of the vitamin in order to finally get an adequate supply into the tissues. Some people's cell walls cannot be penetrated easily by certain substances. They too will need vastly more of that particular nutrient. Some have systems that "dump" or destroy certain vitamins and minerals. This appears to be particularly true of many people with mental illness.

Most people's need for vitamins and minerals increases as they get older

Our human ancestors of fifty thousand years ago lived to age thirty, so our own chemistry was designed to last only about thirty years. Hence old age, the failure of our body chemistry, actually starts at about age thirty. This is why after that age it is especially important that you get the best nutrition possible, the individual nutrition that is correct for you and you alone.

Some people acquire greater needs for particular vitamins and minerals during their lifetime

There is growing evidence that a period of malnutrition may cause a *permanent* enzyme change, so that the person who has been temporarily malnourished will require larger doses of certain vitamins for the rest of his life. The most acute, clear-cut cases of this occur in prisoners of war, who have been forced to live on a severely inadequate diet for months or years. When they return to society, their condition does not improve even when they are given fairly large doses of vitamins. They only feel well if they take what would be monstrous amounts of vitamins for a person with a more normal nutritional history.

I believe that this syndrome occurs in milder forms throughout our society. Now that I am familiar with the symptoms of vitamin deficiencies, I believe I can pick out in retrospect several occasions in my life when I was suffering a deficiency of one or more vitamins, even though I was raised on a perfectly "normal" American diet. Perhaps that explains why my system thrives on a quantity of vitamins that will no doubt seem very large to you (more of that in Chapter 11).

I suspect the same thing is true of anyone who has lived for any length of time on an inadequate diet, be it an unwise reducing diet or a student's menu of potato chips and beer, a teenager's sugar binges or a young couple's early years on kisses and cheese. You may have felt fine on such a diet at the time, particularly if you were young, but when essential nutrients are missing, your elaborate system of enzymes and chemical responses has to compensate somehow, and the effects of those changes eventually show up in the form of altered nutritional needs.

Many environmental stresses elevate your vitamin needs

In addition to its many other dangers, tobacco destroys vitamin A, some of the B vitamins, and especially vitamin C. Alcohol imposes stresses on the body, increasing your need for vitamins. Like sugar and refined grains, alcohol contains calories but virtually no nutrients, so it drains the body of vitamins and minerals in the course of being metabolized. The connection between nutrition and alcohol consumption is so important that Dr. Roger Williams of the University of Texas believes that it is impossible for a properly nourished person to become an alcoholic.

Certain drugs and medicines, including birth control pills, either rob the system of vitamins or create an elevated need for them

Your environment imposes other stresses as well, particularly air pollution and noise pollution. We all talk about these pressures but have you considered that these are not abstract emotional elements but concrete physiological strains on the chemistry of your body? The same applies to emotional stress. Your emotions are not abstract, disembodied feelings; they possess chemical and physical components. When you feel a rush of fear or rage or anxiety, chemicals, minerals and electrical impulses undergo changes in your nervous system. If you are under emotional stress you must replenish the nutrients you need to keep the nervous system functioning properly. If you don't supply these nutrients the deficiency can *cause* further emotional symptoms of all kinds.

THE FOURTH FALLACY OF THE AMERICAN DIET: THAT MEDICAL SCIENCE HAS ADEQUATE INFORMATION TO ESTABLISH NUTRITIONAL STANDARDS

CHAPTER SIX

Compared with other branches of medicine, the study of infectious diseases, or even of surgery, our knowledge of the chemistry of nutrition is in its infancy. The word vitamin was not even coined until 1911, and even then it was a misnomer. Although scurvy had been a dread disease since the time of Hippocrates and decimated the ranks of the Crusaders and of seamen all over the world, it was not until 1753 that the Scottish physician James Lind discovered that it could be cured by adding fresh fruit to the diet.

It took forty years for the medical establishment to accept his findings. In 1795 the British navy for the first time ordered all ships to carry a supply of citrus fruit, which gave rise to the British nickname, Limey. In 1886 it was discovered that beri-beri occurred when chickens were fed polished rice, and could be cured when unpolished rice was returned to the diet. But even then, people did not believe that there were special nutrients in the rice husk, but that there was poison in the germ or kernel of the rice, and that the husk contained some unknown natural antidote.

25

In 1911 Casimir Funk, a Polish chemist who worked at the Lister Institute in London, succeeded in isolating the nutrient in the rice polish that prevented beri-beri (it was thiamine, or vitamin B_1). He called it a "vital amine" because he believed that it was an amine, the generic name of the compound ammonia, which was incorrect. The great significance of his discovery was that he had proved at last that beri-beri was caused not by a germ, nor by a poison, but by the absence of an *essential nutrient* that must be present in every healthy human body but cannot be manufactured by the body itself. It must come from the diet. Funk suspected, correctly, that if there was one such nutrient there must be more.

In the next twenty years vitamins A, D, and C were recognized. Research has continued through the century. Vitamin B_{12} was first synthesized shortly after World War II, and vitamin E, so significant in its interaction with hormone levels and its ability to decrease blood clotting and blood cholesterol levels was not recognized by the FDA as essential to human nutrition until 1973.

Without doubt, there are more discoveries to come. Vitamin K, a clotting agent, has been recognized, but little is known about it, and research is being done on substances called vitamins P and Q (though they may or may not turn out to be vitamins).

In short, we are far from knowing everything there is to know about nutrition. More important, what we do know is far from being widely taught, accepted, or even understood in the medical establishment or by the public. Thousands of doctors who practice now went to medical school before vitamin B_{12} was even heard of, and in many cases these established, illustrious figures are precisely the ones undertaking to declare what is and is not essential for optimum human nutrition.

Not long ago I learned that only twenty-four percent of America's medical schools currently offer *any* courses on nutrition to their students. Although I was aware that the establishment neglects this subject, I was startled. My own school, Duke University, had given at least some instruction in nutrition. Perhaps southern medical schools, aware of the nutritional problems around them, stress nutrition more than northern schools.

Since I often walk past Cornell University Medical School, I decided to drop in one day and check their curriculum. When I looked through this prestigious school's catalogue I could hardly believe what I saw: not a single required *or* elective course on nutrition! I studied the subheadings under biochemistry, physiology, and medicine, thinking the subject must be tucked away in another department. Still nothing. As a final check, I crossed the street and made inquiries at the bookstore run for medical students. It stocked exactly one book on nutrition—a rather naive volume written for nurses.

What a sad situation! Here we have a collection of modern medical skyscrapers, shiny with wealth and prestige, seemingly ignoring that most basic of life's realities—the fact that cells require proper nutrition to live.

There are many excellent scientific books and journals devoted to the field of nutrition. These publications could and should interest physicians, but are usually ignored. And they are likely to continue being ignored unless you put pressure not only on your physician but also on your political representative to learn the importance of nutrition. The Food and Drug Administration does a great deal of harm with its false and often contradictory pronouncements on human nutrition. Public money, whether paid directly or in taxes, supports the FDA, physicians, and medical institutions. The public has a right to *demand* that these people have the knowledge to advise the public correctly on nutritional matters. This is no trivial issue; we are dealing with the welfare of individual cells that add up the most valuable thing in the universe—life.

A twenty-five-year-old actress I know of suffered from a slipped vertebral disk, a very painful back disorder. A surgeon operated to remove the disk at Columbia Presbyterian Hospital in New York. Because she remained in great pain, a second operation—a spinal fusion—was undertaken, but the bones did not knit properly and the pain continued. She returned to the hospital for a body cast and electrical stimulation to encourage the bones to fuse. When these measures failed, an anesthesiologist tried acupuncture. This, too, failed. She still remains in pain.

In this instance, a competent surgeon at one of the country's great hospitals apparently forgot that bone tissue, in order to thrive, requires generous quantities of calcium, magnesium, vitamin D, and especially vitamin C. In fact, Houston neurosurgeon J. Greenwood, Jr., M.D.[1] found massive doses of vitamin C of great benefit to patients suffering from pain caused by slipped disks. The New York surgeon, not thinking in nutritional terms, forgot that many actresses subsist on wretched diets.

He made no tests to determine her vitamin levels, or the calcium or magnesium levels of her tissues. Only hardware was considered: the scalpel, a cast, acupuncture needles.

I don't mean to imply that all back pain—or even *her* back pain—can be cured by proper nutrition. I do suggest that nutrition should have been among the first considerations in this as in any other therapy. No matter how skillfully an orthopedic surgeon sets a broken bone, that bone will not heal if its cells are not given proper nutrition. Even the healing of fractures rests upon cellular chemistry, which in turn rests upon nutrition.

Had her surgeons been confronted with the question of nutritional supplements, they would most likely have fallen back on the hoary, often disproved, but apparently ineradicable cliché that the average American diet is nutritionally adequate.

Emotional symptoms are even more rarely considered as nutritional in origin than are physical ones

Psychiatrists continue to think of emotions as separate from the human body, unconnected with the chemistry of the brain cells. Freud, misinterpreted, has so captured our imaginations that even physicians forget that the brain is an organ in the body.

Unfortunately, a physical malfunction in the brain often does not signal its presence as obviously as do dysfunctions in other organs. If your liver fails to clear the bile from your bloodstream you become jaundiced. Your yellow skin is there for all to see. Your physician takes one look and orders liver function tests. Neither he nor your friends consider your ochre complexion a moral, spiritual, or marital problem, an interpersonal relationship problem, or an unresolved childhood conflict brought about by Great-aunt Sara's spanking you for pulling the cat's tail.

When the cells of your central nervous system malfunction, there may be no such telltale sign. The cause may be just as physical, though the resulting disorder may manifest itself in depression or elation, misinterpretation of other people's motives, perceptual distortions, or inability to concentrate.

But nervous symptoms of this kind continue to be regarded as mere results of environmental influences. When a patient tells his doctor that he is depressed, the doctor automatically asks what has been troubling him, and the patient will promptly recite a list of difficulties: His wife doesn't understand him, his colleagues are unfriendly, his boss expects too much, and life generally disagrees with him. Some or all of these grievances may even be founded in fact. But think a moment: Aren't we all subject to such irritants? Life is hardly a bowl of cherries and each of us suffers losses, setbacks, and frustrations. The healthy person is able to push his way through these difficulties without undue discomfort. The depressed individual who reacts in inappropriate ways is unable to cope with ordinary jolts of life. Since the patient, his family, and the doctor all need to explain his condition, they have a built-in propensity to think in conventional terms and to blame the depression and maladaptation on the patient's unhappy circumstances. In reality, the cause is usually some chemical disorder which affects the central nervous system—one that can often be traced to faulty nutrition.

Vitamin deficiency is not the only serious nutritional disorder

Recently I saw a man in his twenties who suffers from schizophrenia. He spent many months at one of the most prestigious private psychiatric centers in the east, where his parents invested $22,000 in the most advanced psychotherapy, sophisticated tranquilizers, and even electrical shock treatments. Instead of improving, his emotional state grew worse, and in addition he gained 120 pounds. I asked how this incredible weight gain had come about, and learned that he was in the habit of eating large quantities of cake and candy at the institute. When I tested the patient, he turned out to be allergic to wheat, milk, and sugar, the basic ingredients of candy and cake. This is a very prevalent finding, especially among schizophrenics, as we'll discuss in a later chapter.

Allergies and emotions are far more closely interconnected than most people realize

I tested the above mentioned patient's allergies by having him fast for five days and then fed him one food at a time as a so-called "challenge feeding" to see what foods he could not tolerate. During the fast, his mental symptoms cleared up entirely. After the challenge feedings of wheat, milk, and sugar, his psychotic symptoms bloomed again.

Further tests also indicated deficiencies in the male hormone testosterone and in the B vitamin folic acid. Decreased levels of folic acid have been shown to cause brain damage.

This patient would not stay on the diet that we gave him, and the last I heard he was still psychotic. His father was too lenient with him. He did not get testosterone as I suggested. If he had, it might have cut down the seriousness of his allergic condition, and made it easier for him to follow the diet.

Here, then, is a modern institution of high caliber and repute, which not only failed to test for allergies and basic hormonal and nutritional deficiencies, but permitted the patient to gorge himself on the very foods that were demonstrably bad for him. If such gross neglect of basic nutritional values is practiced at so excellent and prestigious an institution, what can be expected of lesser ones?

Dr. F. C. Dohan[2,3] at the University of Pennsylvania demonstrated in a state hospital setting that wheat products are toxic for many patients afflicted with schizophrenia, and showed that those wards in which wheat products were forbidden had a much higher discharge rate than those in which they were permitted.

All this underscores the physician's lack of training in nutrition and nutritional supplements, and brings us back to the fact that each one of us must establish for ourselves our own optimum nutrient intake. This must be done with the advice of a physician, so you should do as much as you can to encourage your doctor to educate himself on the subject. But it is most important also to educate yourself, to know what clinical tests to ask your doctor for (and how to interpret the results better than he may be able to). In the coming chapters I will show you, for instance, not only how to establish your own vitamin and mineral needs but how to recognize deficiencies or overdoses, and how to correct them.

You should not, of course, become your own physician, diagnosing your own symptoms and trying to treat them yourself. It is dangerous for you to ignore persistent symptoms without medical advice, because by the time you discover—to mention only one possibility—that your illness is not related to nutrition, the delay may have done you serious harm.

But if you are one of the millions who are sometimes more nervous, angry, anxious, depressed, tired, or confused than is altogether necessary, then it is time for you to take an interest in your nutrition. To do this you will need to understand something of the general biochemical heritage you share with all mankind. You must discover how your system may differ from everyone else's. Let us count the ways.

NOTES

1. J. Greenwood, Jr.
2. F. C. Dohan. "Cereals and Schizophrenia, Data and Hypothesis," *Acta Psychiatrica Scandinavica*, Vol. 42, 1966, p. 125.
3. Dohan *et al.* "Cereal-Free Diet in Relapsed Schizophrenics," *Federation Proceedings*, Vol. 27, 1968, p. 219.

HOW NUTRITION AFFECTS
THE NERVOUS SYSTEM

CHAPTER SEVEN

We tend to forget that we inherit specific chemical attributes as well as specific physical ones—that, in fact, many physical attributes are based on the chemical ones. We see the color of skin as being, say, either black or white. This observable physical attribute is simply a manifestation of an inherited compound known as melanin. If this chemical substance is present in large quantities, your skin is black; if present in lesser amounts, you appear pinkish white; if totally absent, you are an albino.

Similarly, you inherit your own individual enzyme systems, those unique chemical-action-triggering proteins that enable you to utilize food, to obtain energy, to repair your body tissue, and to remove waste products from the cells. If enough measurements were taken of everyone in the world, it would undoubtedly be discovered that each person is endowed with slightly different enzyme systems. Of course, the environment in which a person lives has some bearing on how he functions; but the different ways people react to their experiences and environments are in turn affected by all kinds of inherited constitutional differences.

In this book we are particularly concerned with the brain and central nervous system, whose physical attributes differ from person to person. The brain is a system of checks and balances, with one part checking as well as stimulating another. Different people have different numbers of cells in different parts of the brain. As a consequence, each person needs a different number of enzyme systems to service each part; more cells require more enzymes to handle cellular metabolism.

The messages which go back and forth between the brain, spinal cord, and nerves do not flow like electricity in the copper wiring of a house. Each nerve cell in the brain and in other parts of the nervous system communicates with another set of nerves by sending out chemical substances called catecholamines, which act as chemical transmitters from cell to cell.

One of the most important of the nervous system transmitters is a chemical called norepinephrine. We know that sometimes this particular transmitter is not produced normally by the nerve cells, and therefore is not available to stimulate other nerve cells. When proteins enter the digestive system, they are broken down by enzymes into amino acids. Norepinephrine has to be made from an amino acid called tyrosine; tyrosine, in turn is made from the amino acid phenylaline. So if the diet lacks the simple protein phenylaline, the nervous system will eventually lack norepinephrine, and transmission will be impaired. A child born with a severe defect in the liver enzyme phenylaline hydroxyglase is doomed to be mentally defective, unless the defect is corrected by proper diet immediately after birth.

Nerve cell defects may come about in a number of ways

For example, not only may a cell fail to form norepinephrine at a normal rate, but the cell membrane may not allow the chemical to pass out of the cell easily, thus preventing the chemical from stimulating the next nerve. The norepinephrine traveling from one nerve to the next may be destroyed too fast or not fast enough, depending upon the supply of an enzyme known as monoamine oxidase. Or the nerve cell which is touched by the chemical after it travels through the neural cleft (the space between the cells) may be relatively impervious to it, and fail to respond properly to its stimulation. All these transmissions of signals in the nervous system depend upon the supply of vitamins and minerals.

Vitamins and minerals are part of the enzyme systems that are in charge of the activity in your nervous system

The way you think and feel about what happens in your life depends very much on whether the proper chemicals, including vitamins and minerals, are present to insure healthy transmission within the system.

Suppose you suffer a disappointment; say you didn't get a promotion you felt you deserved. You may react by saying, "Well, that's a bum deal" and feel mildly annoyed or unhappy for a few days; or you may become wildly angry; or you may conclude that the world is totally mismanaged, that life is intolerably unjust, and that you had better kill yourself. A lot depends on how the information about your disappointment is flashed through your nervous system—whether it proceeds in a normal, orderly way, or is derailed or exploded by a chemical accident along the way.

The enzyme systems that control this operation differ from person to person. First, as I've said, some people have more of them than others. Second, some enzyme systems are more healthy and efficient than others. Third, each person's systems have varying—sometimes enormously different—needs for specific vitamins and minerals.

ARE YOU VITAMIN-DEPENDENT?

Dr. Leon E. Rosenberg of Yale University[1] is devoting much of his time to studying variations in individuals' needs for various vitamins. He refers to people with large requirements for certain vitamins as "vitamin-dependent" rather than "vitamin-deficient." This may sound like the same thing, but actually it isn't. Rosenberg's formulation highlights the important distinction between people whose need for vitamins is normal but who aren't ingesting a "normal" amount (vitamin-deficient), and those who have an above-average need for these nutrients (vitamin-dependent). It is my contention, based on years of clinical experience, that such a condition is far from uncommon, especially among people with emotional problems. (You can also suffer from a *combination* of below-average intake and above-average need. Then you're in real trouble).

One way to test an individual's vitamin needs is by giving a "loading test," in which massive doses of a vitamin are administered. When you give a normal person a huge dose of one of the water-soluble vitamins (C or the Bs, which cannot be stored in the body) his system will take what it needs of the vitamin on that day and will excrete the rest in the urine.

At California's Stanford University Dr. Linus Pauling conducted a series of loading tests financed by the National Institutes of Health.[2] He found that when huge doses of vitamin C—as much as 40 grams—were given to schizophrenics, *little or none* of it was discarded in the urine. In other words, the seriously mentally ill patients needed more than *one thousand* times the amount the FDA recommends as a daily requirement. Similar loading tests with other vitamins produced similar results. Pauling concluded that many people suffering from schizophrenia require many times the normal amount of vitamins in their enzyme systems, and my own clinical experience bears this out.

Absorption counts as much as intake

In addition to considering how much of a particular substance an individual needs and how much he gets, you have to consider how well he is able to use what he gets.

It is a well-known fact, for instance, that some people are constitutionally unable to absorb vitamin B_{12} because their enzyme systems do not produce what we call the "intrinsic factor" in the stomach. Such people eventually develop pernicious anemia, often accompanied by disorders of the nervous system, including emotional disorders such as depression and anxiety. These individuals can't be effectively treated by any amount of orally administered B_{12}. They have to take it by injection, to bypass their gastric malfunction.

In other instances, a person's blood level of vitamin B_{12} may indicate normal absorption, but he lacks a certain protein that is crucial in moving the vitamin B_{12} from the bloodstream into the tissue where it is used.[3] Such people also suffer from vitamin B_{12} deficiency, normal absorption from the stomach notwithstanding. They have to take massive amounts of B_{12} by injection, so that what small amount of protein *is* available can carry a maximum of the vitamin into the tissue. We may assume that similar mechanisms work with other vitamins. The missing protein cannot be supplied in any other way.

Over one thousand enzyme systems exist in the human liver and individual variations are almost infinite. To cite just one example, it has been discovered that the amount of the enzyme phosphatase in a given person's system can vary from four to eighty-three units; obviously eighty-three units of enzyme are going to require more vitamins than four.

What is true of vitamins is equally true of other nutrients. For example, Roger Williams, professor of biochemistry at the University of Texas and former president of the American Chemical Association, has made studies in depth concerning individual chemical differences among both laboratory animals and humans.[4] He has discovered that certain people require five times the amount of calcium and amino acids (simple proteins) that others do.

Your brain structure makes a difference

As I mentioned earlier, from person to person, there are variations in anatomical brain structure which may be crucial in determining a person's nutritive requirements for mental health. Of course, we all have similar brain sections and roughly the same *type* of cells in them, but the *number* of cells in the various parts of the brain differs from person to person, as does the *total number* of brain cells.[5] Obviously, people who have more brain cells than others are likely to have greater nutritive requirements.

By now you can appreciate why it is so difficult to determine—"calibrate" may be an even better word—the "normal" vitamin requirement for any one person.

Not only are we far, far away from knowing all the answers about nutrition; we're not even sure we have all the questions. Yet the FDA blithely sets minimum vitamin requirements that are supposed to apply to all of us, and conventional medicine tends to go along with this naive stand.

In my experience, most physicians avoid facing the more complex facts about nutrition, although they could solve nutritional problems for individual patients *if* they were willing to study the literature and accept the trial-and-error process that is required to practice effective nutritional therapy. No physician likes to work by trial and error, but at the moment it's the only method we have. I admit that the field is extremely intricate and full of unknowns; that may explain the reluctance to enter it, but it is not an excuse for refusal. Many people are sick for lack of proper nutrition, and many more are working at half capacity. They can't be expected to wait until science has unraveled all the threads; they need help now, not twenty-five years from now. With or without the help of their doctors, they need to know now the level of each vitamin at which they function best.

The idea of treating emotional illness with nutritional supplements is still new, but is rapidly unfolding into a fascinating psychiatric subspecialty. I say subspecialty, but it should really be a part of every psychiatrist's knowledge, for the enzyme defects demonstrated in the emotionally ill are so widespread that I feel every patient with an emotional disorder deserves a trial at this form of therapy.

And psychiatric patients are far from the only potential beneficiaries of nutritional therapy. Think of all the overweight people with their sad, unnatural relationship to food; think of the people who drink too much; of all the surly people with hair-trigger tempers; of the insomniacs; the exhausted, depressed, older men and women whose feelings have affected their tempers and their judgment; think of all the anxious souls who live as if balanced on one foot on the rim of disaster, and you will realize that most people don't feel nearly as well as they should. Think of yourself! Much of this life lived in limbo between health and illness can be corrected with proper nutrition and nutritional supplements. It's up to you.

NOTES

1. Leon E. Rosenberg. "Finding and Treating Genetic Diseases," *Science News of the Week*, Vol. 98, August 29, 1970, p. 157.
2. Linus Pauling *et al. Orthomolecular Psychiatry* (San Francisco: Freeman Press, 1973), Chapter II.
3. N. Hakami *et al.* "Neonatal Megoblastic Anemia Due to Inherited Transco-balmin II Deficiency in Two Siblings," *New Eng. Jrnl. of Med.*, Vol. 285, No. 21, November 16, 1971, pp. 1163–1170.
4. R. J. Williams. *Biochemical Individuality: The Basis for the Genotropic Concept* (New York: Wiley, 1956).
5. K. S. Lashley. "Structural Variations in the Nervous System in Relation to Behavior," *Psychological Review*, Vol. 54, 1947, p. 33.

HOW FOOD ALLERGIES AND NUTRITIONAL ADDICTIONS CAN SHATTER YOUR NERVES

CHAPTER EIGHT

ALLERGIES

Suppose you walk into the office of today's more or less typically well-trained doctor and complain of vague symptoms like depression, listlessness, anxiety. (*He's* the one likely to call them "vague"; to you they're quite concrete.) Two centuries ago, he'd have bled you. One century ago, he'd have doled out a laxative. Today, he's more sophisticated: he'll prescribe a tranquilizer or an antidepressant, or both. What he almost certainly will *not* do is test you for allergies.

Although your physician may not be aware of it, the relationship between food allergies and emotional illness has been known for hundreds of years. As early as 1621, the famous English savant Robert Burton, in his classic, *The Anatomy of Melancholy*, flatly declared: "Milk and all that comes from milk increases melancholy." He was neither the first nor the last to recognize this effect. Here, as in so many medical discoveries, Hippocrates—the "Father of Medicine"—led the way in the fourth century before the birth of Christ. Since Burton's day, similar observations have been made by physicians of many nations. In this country, reports of psychological reactions caused by allergies began to proliferate in the 1870s, and they continue to this day. Yet the psychological symptoms produced by allergies are largely ignored by our medical schools. Even the best physicians instantly think of allergies in terms of "pollen" when you sneeze in summer, "dust" when you wheeze, or "shellfish allergy" when they see your face ablaze with hives after a lobster dinner. But not many physicians consider allergies when you slump into a depression or threaten to punch your mate without apparent reason.

I myself knew little about the link between allergies and emotions until a few years ago, when I saw a film produced by Dr. Theron Randolph. It was filmed in a patient's room at Chicago's Wesley Memorial Hospital, one of the teaching hospitals associated with the Northwestern University School of Medicine. Since seeing that film, I have tested every new patient for allergic reactions to establish the role they might be playing in his or her emotional life.

The film that so impressed me opened with a sequence showing Dr. Randolph talking with a young woman who appeared calm, poised, and thoroughly in control of herself. The doctor then inserted a tube through her nose into her stomach so that, standing behind her, he could introduce foods through the tube. This method ruled out any possibility that visual suggestion could influence her reactions to any foods. I watched Dr. Randolph feed her the first food (through the tube) mixed with water. He then returned to the front of the bed and conversed with the patient for a few minutes. She remained her composed self. After enough time had passed to be certain that no reaction had occurred, Dr. Randolph again walked around the bed, out of the patient's sight. This time, he injected a solution of corn into the stomach tube.

Within minutes, the woman began striking at him viciously, threw herself off the bed, and struggled with the nurse and attendants as she tried to force her way out of the room. She shouted and argued and could not be reasoned with. In short, she displayed psychotic behavior. This anger and loss of control continued for four days, then ended as quickly as it began. Suddenly the woman snapped out of her confused state, and had no idea that most of a week had passed since she lost contact with reality.

The woman had consulted Dr. Randolph because she suffered periodic psychotic spells. Now, the doctor told those who were watching the film, she was free of the attacks, and able to live a normal life simply by avoiding those substances to which she had proved allergic.

In another film, Dr. Randolph showed us a patient whom he could throw into convulsions simply by introducing certain common foods into her system.

These films came as a revelation to me. Like all physicians, I had known something about food allergies, but the subject had not particularly interested me. The field of allergy is so complex and so full of controversy that many busy physicians tend to push the subject to the back of their minds. But after seeing Dr. Randolph's films I could no longer ignore or allow my patients to ignore, a factor that might well be a prime catalyst of their emotional symptoms.

To learn more about the connection between allergy and mental illness, I performed a study, along with William H. Philpott, M.D., formerly assistant medical director of Fuller Memorial Sanitarium, South Attleboro, Massachusetts (now practicing in Dana Point, California) and Marshall Mendell, M.D., director of the New England Foundation for Allergic and Environmental Diseases, Norwalk, Connecticut. We reported our findings in a paper presented at the 1972 meeting of the Academy of Orthomolecular Psychiatry in Dallas, Texas. (If you want to pursue this subject with medical assistance, I will cite medical sources throughout this chapter so that you can encourage your doctor to study the literature.)

In our study we examined patients for multiple food and chemical sensitivities by giving provocative tests after a four-day fast. Occasionally we tested non-fasting patients by placing extracts of the test materials under the tongue, where they are rapidly absorbed and produce emotional symptoms in sensitive patients.

The symptoms induced by these tests varied from a slight itching of the skin to fullblown psychotic seizures. One patient cried all afternoon after a test for milk sensitivity. Another, when tested for tobacco sensitivity, suddenly turned on her mother with a savage verbal attack that lasted half an hour. Another patient, known to be sensitive to sugar and wheat, suffered from chronic schizophrenia, but his illness was rather easily controlled unless he ignored his prescribed diet. One afternoon he ate a piece of apple pie à la mode, and shortly he began to hallucinate. He turned delusional and went into an uncontrollable rage. A strong tranquilizer was needed to calm him down. After sleeping for eight hours, he awoke in a state of composure. Another patient, also suffering from schizophrenia, was known to be wheat-sensitive. He ate a meal containing various mixtures of food in a Chinese restaurant, and became psychotic for two days. It turned out, of course, that the food he had eaten had contained wheat products.

Our methods of testing for sensitivities are not like the usual skin tests given by allergists

The skin test is only about 20 percent accurate in diagnosing food allergies—a fact you can verify by consulting any allergist or any textbook on allergy.

Even if the skin does react abnormally to a substance, this does not necessarily mean that the central nervous system will react in the same way. For example, the skin on your hands may be hypersensitive to a brand of soap and break out in a rash. But that doesn't mean you will necessarily also become depressed as a reaction to the soap.

My colleagues and I introduce the food (or other substances that we suspect of being allergenic) directly into the body itself. Then we observe the reaction of the whole system; we don't merely look for a local reaction such as a rash. Specifically we look for a reaction of the central nervous system—unusual behavior, or thinking, or mood.

We have found two tests particularly effective.

1. For the first and simpler one, we drop a diluted solution of the suspect substance beneath the tongue, where it is quickly absorbed into the bloodstream and distributed throughout the body. This method of introducing foreign substances into the system has long been recognized as a rapid and efficient one. You probably know that a patient with heart pain from constricted coronary arteries (angina pectoris) places a nitroglycerin tablet beneath the tongue, because this route puts the medication directly into the bloodstream so it can be quickly carried to the heart. (That's what's going on in those television shows where the overwrought executive suddenly slumps over, gasping, "Ahhh . . . pills . . . left pocket . . . put under tongue . . .")

2. The second testing method is more complicated. First, we remove all possibly allergenic compounds from the patient's environment,

including substances like toothpaste, deodorants, perfumes, tobacco, alcohol, pesticides, automobile exhaust fumes, gas-operated appliances, or any other chemical compounds that could cause symptoms.

Then we put the patient on a water fast, which means that he may eat absolutely nothing, and drink nothing except untreated spring water. The fast itself is not dangerous, although sometimes withdrawal symptoms may be uncomfortable. After four to twelve days (usually four to five days) the patient is free of allergic symptoms and is ready for the tests to begin. We then feed him one food at a time, three times a day. The fast temporarily renders the patient much more susceptible to foods to which he is allergic. If he happens to be allergic to, say, wheat, he will usually show a strong reaction to wheat very shortly after he has eaten it.

We run through the suspected foods one at a time, over about a two-week period. Each tested food may be eaten in fairly large amounts—three potatoes, for instance, or a pound of steak. After the food-testing period is over, we add environmental chemicals one at a time: toothpaste, deodorants, hair spray, perfume, and all the rest.

Obviously the procedure is rather cumbersome and time-consuming, and requires the patient's complete cooperation. But it provides a bonus: The fast itself tends to be therapeutic, since the patient's general level of sensitivity is often lower for a period after the whole procedure is completed.

Also, the fast itself tells us a great deal about the patient's allergic condition, and lets us make a good estimate as to whether allergies are playing a strong role in his emotional illness. If allergies *are* important, many or all of the emotional symptoms will become clear during the course of the fast.

A case in point is John, a twenty-six-year-old man who had been clearly schizophrenic for more than five years. His illness had reached such heights that he had been completely unable to work and had been in and out of psychiatric hospitals. When I saw him, he was delusional: He believed Jesus had made him a saint and told him to start a new religion—a combination of Zen Buddhism and Southern Baptist. To prove he had become a sort of assistant to Christ, he wanted to fly over the city (by flapping his arms) and drop pamphlets. His face reddened with rage whenever he saw his mother, because he believed she added paralyzing drugs to his food, and that these prevented him from flying and thereby frustrated his life's mission.

After six days of fasting, John's symptoms cleared completely. He was as logical as a computer programmer. Quite clearly, allergies had played a crucial role in the formation of his illness.

The sad side of this story (the last I heard of John he was sick again—eating everything), and of so many similar ones, is that very sick people often intentionally expose themselves to chemicals or foods that cause their symptoms. When he was feeling better, John realized that he was just one more unimportant human who hadn't been able to make a significant mark in the world. That knowledge was unbearable to him—and he had found a way to avoid it: He needed only to eat wheat or sugar products to become not only the center of his family's and his psychiatrist's attention, but, indeed, an important *world* figure—an assistant to Jesus Christ himself. As is true for many other people, his desire for attention and power overrode his desire for mental health.

Sometimes patients resist their treatment because the foods to which they are allergic are the ones they like best. These foods actually give the patient a lift, or a "rush," a feeling of well-being not experienced with other foods. After some time they slide off the "lift" and plunge into a depression or some other emotional symptom such as nervousness or irritability. The eventual result is the vicious cycle that I shall discuss in the next section: the treadmill of simultaneous allergy *and* addiction.

Can allergies really cause emotional problems for ordinary people —for someone like you?

They certainly can. You will not necessarily become manic or depressive, or succumb to schizophrenia. You may have none of the rashes or have the trouble breathing that we normally associate with allergic people. You may only feel listless or depressed or unable to sleep; or you may get angry for no good reason; or you may have any of a number of other symptoms often labeled "neurotic" for lack of proper identification.

I have observed that the general allergic reactivity level frequently becomes milder or disappears after patients are given a properly balanced diet, placed on adequate vitamins and other nutritional supplements, and are supplied with proper hormones. But the reverse is also often true: Poor nutrition (a diet containing much sugar and bread and low in minerals and vitamins) leads the body to more and more allergic reactions. Poor nutrition can contribute to the serious condition we shall take up in the next section: nutritional allergic addictions.

NUTRITIONAL ADDICTIONS

What's your very favorite food: Ice cream, chocolate, coffee, bread, cheesecake, milk?

Decide which it is, then ask yourself how often you eat it—every day, every second or third day? And now the $64,000 question: What happens when for some reason you must forgo it? Do you crave it more and more violently, think about it constantly, grow nervous, irritable, or depressed?

If the answer is yes, you may suffer from a food addiction, and you may be every bit as truly hooked as any alcoholic or heroin addict. These food addictions have a pernicious relationship with the food allergies we discussed in the last section; indeed, they are a particular type of allergy.

Because the concept of alcoholism is better known to laymen, let me briefly trace the course of that disease for you. The similarities between food and alcohol addictions will quickly become obvious.

Every alcoholic starts out by having no more than an occasional drink. It lifts his spirits, relaxes his tensions, and facilitates communication. As the alcohol spreads through his system, the world takes on a rosy hue.

At first he indulges in this experience infrequently. But each time the same sequence of "drink = happy glow" is repeated and insistently imprinted on his subconscious. Soon the pleasant association springs to his mind—perhaps no more than half-formed—whenever a business deal sours, his wife has a headache at bedtime, or Junior has flawlessly aimed a baseball dead-center through the neighbor's new picture window. He mixes a drink. After a few minutes life begins to look up.

At first he is likely to restrict his drinking to weekends. After all, he must be up to par during the work week—he mustn't fall behind in the rat race. Yet, come to think of it, what's wrong with a drink after office hours? The boss doesn't own him, does he?

So he institutes the pleasant and "gracious" custom of having a leisurely drink before dinner. Then, if he's a commuter, the thought occurs to him how foolish it is to waste all that empty train time. Soon he's having his first pre-dinner drink on the train (or at the corner bar, if he's a city dweller), a second one when he gets home, and perhaps a last one just before retiring.

Now, gradually, he begins to look forward more and more to his late afternoon drink. He finds himself thinking about it several times during the day, earlier and earlier, wishing it were 5:30 so he could settle down into the glowing haze which the genie of alcohol brings out so easily. He's just a hard-working guy, a good husband and father, a conscientious provider for his family, so what's wrong with trying to relax a bit after a hectic day at the office? If anyone were to tell him at this point that he is rapidly becoming addicted to alcohol, he'd either roar with laughter or sputter in honest outrage.

But now it won't be long before the hallmark of addiction begins to manifest itself. In order to maintain his high mood he needs more and more alcohol, and he needs it at more and more frequent intervals. Whenever he is without his crutch—i.e., sober—he now experiences a growing sense of letdown and discomfort, both mental and physical. What he is suffering from are the pangs heralding the justly dreaded withdrawal syndrome; but this he doesn't know, and wouldn't let himself believe even if somewhere deep down in his mind he had any such inkling.

What he does know is a surefire way to treat those unpleasant symptoms—a quick drink or two, and all is well.

And so the noose tightens around his neck. Every drink gives him a temporary lift (each one shorter than the last), followed by a period of depression and remorse (each one worse than the last). A number of additional physiological symptoms now gang up on him as well, including shakiness, slight confusion, and mental dullness—all with a tendency to worsen rapidly. This syndrome soon begins to afflict him the moment he wakes up, and is not dispelled until the first drink is down his gullet. Needless to say, he doesn't waste any time putting it there.

At 10 A.M. he furtively takes a couple of gulps from the bottle in his desk drawer, to keep "the awfuls" at bay. Two martinis at lunch again stave off the threatening symptoms, and so he manages to keep himself together during the day by having alcohol every three or four hours, until he has his large dose at bedtime, after which he passes out. Inevitably, he must drink more and more just to maintain even such minimal functioning; and soon he can no longer maintain it, no matter how high his alcohol intake. At this point even he may admit (at least to himself) that something is very, very wrong, that he is an alcoholic.

Now his only recourse, if he doesn't want to end up as a derelict, is to abstain from alcohol at once, completely. He is up against the physiology of addiction.

After this cram course in the making of an alcoholic, let me tell you about a patient of mine whom we'll call Betty. A social worker with a long history of unsatisfactory love relationships, she had been in continual psychoanalytical therapy for nine years. Her current analyst, whom she had been seeing for five years, sent her to me because she was not making progress, and he wondered whether I had anything to offer her. (For an "orthodox" psychoanalyst to consider the possibility of contributory physical factors was once an unusual feat of openmindedness, but gradually a few analysts are recognizing that biochemistry can strongly influence emotional illnesses.)

Betty, a bright, intelligent woman with a Master's degree in her field, was quite attractive despite her obesity. Like many intellectuals, she was familiar with the tenets of Freudian psychotherapy, and she was certain that it was the answer to her problems. Accordingly, she looked upon emotional problems as totally separate from body chemistry. This inappropriate dichotomy of mind and body is a concept many people find very difficult to set aside; for some reason they make it a keystone of their personal philosophy and approach to life.

Chemical analysis revealed that Betty's system was low in estrogen and iron. These deficiencies were corrected but this brought no change in her basic complaints, which included intractable obesity, inability to form meaningful relationships with men, a great deal of suppressed anger, and chronic depression. What I am describing, in other words, is a lonely, withdrawn woman, trying to keep the lid on the seething cauldron of her rage over being unable to get the things she felt she deserved from life.

And all the time, every waking hour of every day, she waged an unceasing battle to control her voracious hunger . . .

On Saturday nights, for example, she would be determined to stick with her diet, have a modest dinner, and sip tea while watching TV. But by eleven or twelve she found herself growing almost uncontrollably restless and irritable. Her refrigerator was always empty, since she intentionally kept everything out of her house that could make her gain weight. Eventually, after a vain struggle with herself, frustration would get the best of her. She'd grab up her dog in her arms, rush out of the house, and try to make it to the neighborhood delicatessen before it closed. As often as not, she got there too late. She would then take a cab and set off across the city, feverishly trying to locate two or three chocolate cakes. Sometimes she was desperate enough to drive from one restaurant to another, buying whole chocolate cakes but having to pay for them by the slice.

On the way home she began eating and often she had finished a cake and a half by the time she reached her apartment. Once there, she poured herself a glass of wine and polished off the rest. During this process her restlessness gradually subsided, until, some $30 lighter and fifteen thousand calories heavier, she was once more the kindly social worker whom everyone admired at the psychiatric clinic where she worked. After watching a late TV movie, she would go to bed and practically pass out in a coma.

When she awakened on Sundays around eleven or twelve she was invariably in what she described as her "black sack of depression." She felt as if her entire apartment were enclosed in a plastic black sack, which no ray of light could penetrate. It was stifling hot, and gave her a sense of utter hopelessness and futility—a feeling that she had been totally abandoned and was no longer a member of the human race. Sensitive and cultivated person that she was, she could only abhor the memory of the cake-gorging tub of lard she had been the night before.

Only half-conscious, she would drag through the day, locate another chocolate cake, eat dinner, and have a second cake afterwards. Slowly the black depression gave way as the familiar state of hazy wellbeing enveloped her once again, enabling her to spend a few peaceful hours watching TV with her dog.

By next morning the depression was of course back in full force, but now it was Monday, and a full working day lay ahead. To get herself together she downed a cup of thick hot chocolate with milk and sugar, and on the way to the clinic wolfed down several chocolate cookies. These gave her enough of a lift to enable her to function until the midmorning break, during which she ate half a package of—you guessed it—chocolate cookies.

Betty is a classic example of food addiction, especially dramatic because in her case the process was so far advanced as to constitute a textbook illustration of all the principles involved in the disease. Food-addiction syndromes are quite common. Betty, in case the parallel has escaped you, would be a full-blown alcoholic if her addiction were to alcohol rather than to specific foods.

The first thing I did when she came to see me was to perform a series of sublingual allergy tests. This is the method whereby several drops of various concentrations of food are placed beneath the tongue and the reactions are observed. In Betty's case they weren't long in coming. She responded violently to milk, sugar, chocolate, wheat, and dog hair.

The test for milk produced a sensation of such intensity as to amount to an hallucination. She felt she had left her body and was floating around the room, bobbing against the ceiling. The test for chocolate gave her an equally marked lift, though different—she began to babble nonstop, spouting nonsense, punctuated by incessant, inappropriate giggling. After about ten minutes she came crashing down into a depression, switched to weeping and, between sobs, bemoaned the desolation of her life.

While being tested for wheat sensitivity, she was leafing through a popular magazine. Moments after the diluted wheat solution was placed under her tongue, she was no longer able to follow the story she had been reading, though it was hardly of a kind to make inordinate demands on an above-average mentality. She felt confused, disoriented, totally unable to think clearly.

The test for dog hair produced detonations of sneezing, and gave her a violent headache.

You might think that these demonstrations would have been enough to convince an educated person, intent on improving her health and the quality of her life, that she was extremely sensitive to some substances and would henceforth have to avoid them like the plague. Unfortunately, neither people nor their lives are that simple, and intellectual convictions have a way of withering when confronted by gut reactions, especially when the gut reactions are reinforced by authority figures. A conventional psychoanalyst would analyze the situation surrounding Betty's orgies and decide they were an outlet for her aggressions, a symbolic representation of her wish to be nurtured by a loving mother, or some such. A pharmacologically oriented therapist, on the other hand, would simply give her antidepressants and tranquilizers, possibly followed by a few electroshock treatments, if her depressions grew bad enough.

My problem with Betty was greatly complicated because I knew the real cause of her symptoms and I had to convince her to accept my unwelcome diagnosis rather than the (to her) far more congenial one of her analyst.

Our first discussion about the test results appeared to be productive. She agreed that she suffered from multiple food allergies, that she craved precisely these foods to the point of addiction, and that she basically had the same problem that she would have if she were an alcoholic or a heroin addict. She also made the same resolutions as do most people who are afflicted with the latter addictions. She would gradually cut down on the foods to which she was allergic, and eventually cut them out entirely. She sounded exactly like the alcoholic who vows to have only a couple of drinks an evening from now on, and after a month would cut down to just one; or the three-pack-a-day smoker who's going to reduce his consumption to two packs, then one, then none.

Those of us engaged in clinical medicine know that this route leads to almost guaranteed disaster.

The alcoholic follows the regime for perhaps a week or two, while the tensions within him build up. Then some little thing goes wrong, and in his overwrought state it turns into the proverbial straw that breaks the camel's back. He says to hell with it, and drinks a whole bottle of whiskey practically in one gulp. The same thing happens to the chainsmoker. We all know him—the guy who gives up smoking forever on the first of every month.

After two weeks Betty returned to tell me her story. She *had* cut down her intake of chocolate cake drastically for one week. Then she had gone home to her parents' for a holiday. Her mother welcomed her with the usual huge chocolate cake, and insisted that her little girl have a nice big helping of her favorite homemade peach ice cream along with it.

The milk in the ice cream alone, with the cake, was enough to put Betty in orbit. After a few agonizingly restless hours with her parents she gave an excuse to leave, jumped into a cab, and began one of her familiar, frantic cake hunts. By the time she got home she had gorged herself until she was nearly out of her head, and she collapsed on her bed in a state of stupor.

A second portent of things to come was the fact that she had not been able to bring herself to get rid of her dog. Any allergy-producing substance, whether it be dog hair, dust, or bedding, makes a patient much more vulnerable to all other things she is allergic to. I explained this to her in great detail, and she entirely agreed with me—BUT she had had the dog for seven years, and it was one of the most important things in her life. How could I ask her to give up the only creature she truly loved and that loved her?

If there is one thing on which I wholeheartedly agree with psychoanalysts it's the existence of patient resistances. They can be formidable. Intelligence seems unable to influence them. Here was a bright, educated person fully aware of her catastrophic addiction problem, yet she would not relinquish her dog even though she knew the animal contributed significantly to her illness. Maybe you find such devotion touching. I find it very frustrating.

When will power failed, we took a new tack. After a few weeks it became clear to me that she would never be able to lick her addiction on her own. Whenever she tried to get along without the addictive foods she became so depressed and restless that eventually she always succumbed to the temptation of eating them to gain temporary relief, despite all self-chastisement for such self-defeating behavior.

One day, after a frank discussion of the problem, she and I decided jointly to attack her addiction by giving her small electrical shocks in line with the behavior-modification techniques that are proving increasingly useful. For her next visit to my office, I asked her to bring a supply of cake and ice cream. The power of her addictions is well illustrated by what happened the first two times she tried to comply. The temptation of the food she was bringing to the office was so great that she stopped at the curb before entering the building and ate the entire cake and the ice cream with her fingers, since she had no spoon.

Eventually, on the third try, she made it into my office with cake and ice cream intact. I asked her to begin eating it slowly, bit by bit. And with every bite she took, I administered a brief electric shock, too slight to cause pain, but strong enough to produce distinct discomfort. The idea underlying this treatment was, of course, to condition her by the repeated association of cake and ice cream with discomfort, until the mere thought of the sweets would at once call forth the associated withdrawal reaction.

I repeated this procedure several times during her next few visits, and began to hope that I had finally hit on the solution. And then she once more ate up her props on the street, on her way to my office. I wondered, not for the first time, why any sane human being would choose psychiatry as his profession, gritted my teeth, and worked out a new procedure.

This time I asked her to read aloud detailed directions for making a chocolate cake, and each time she uttered the word "cake," "chocolate," or "sugar," I administered an electric shock of quite disagreeable intensity. Usually this type of behavioral therapy—although not the treatment of choice for food addictions—is a fairly successful conditioning procedure. Taking all factors into consideration, it seemed the most promising approach for her; but it didn't work. After a few weeks she winced at the very mention of these foods—but that didn't keep her from eating them. Her frantic midnight excursions and lost weekends continued.

Finally, I talked her into trying the method most frequently used to break food addictions—a fast of four to seven days' duration.

Other things being equal, fasts can do a great deal to help break an addiction, but it isn't easy. When a person like Betty, who is physiologically addicted to foods, stops eating, what happens to her is essentially the same thing that happens to a drug addict who stops taking drugs. She goes into withdrawal. The withdrawal syndrome involves profound physiological changes in the cells themselves. Experiments have shown that if you deliberately addict artificially grown tissue to hard narcotics and then cut off the narcotic supply, you can actually see the cells changing under the microscope. The effect of these changes on the total organism—i.e., the person whose cells are in withdrawal—can range from discomfort to real agony.

During fasts, all foreign substances must also be removed. The patient must stop smoking, must not take any medication, or even expose himself to such common chemicals as toothpaste, deodorants, perfumes, gas from kitchen stoves, fumes from frying foods, dust stirred by housecleaning, or anything else capable of producing allergic or toxic reactions. All the chemicals removed from the environment should then be added again, one at a time, after the fast is completed, without any overlapping, so that the source of any allergic reaction may be unequivocally determined.

In view of the hardships involved in fasting, and the strength of her addictions, I wasn't too optimistic about the outcome in Betty's case, but it had to be tried.

As expected, the moment the withdrawal symptoms surfaced Betty became extremely restless and depressed and had a strong sense of impending doom. These symptoms continued almost unabated through the second day of the fast. The third day was not quite so bad, and by the fourth day she felt a great deal better. When I saw her on the fifth day, she was cheerful and pleasant and had regained much of her former energy.

I now began giving her one food at a time during each of her three daily meals as a food-challenge test. In Betty's case, my purpose was not so much to diagnose her allergies as to give her the most vivid proof possible of how much worse she felt when she ate her poison.

Betty tested out as expected, reacting to the same foods as during the sublingual tests, only with much greater intensity. Chocolate turned her almost manic—laughing and chattering as if she had taken a handful of speed tablets. An hour later, a trap door seemed to open and she tumbled into an abyss of despair. She cried hysterically for several hours, had fits of shaking, and required sedatives to put her to sleep.

Because the chocolate-produced symptoms were still present the next day, further tests had to wait. I interposed twenty-four hours of complete fast except for water.

After all her tests were complete, there could be no further question in Betty's mind concerning the virulence of her allergic addictions. Once more I urged her to stay away entirely from foods that were so clearly disastrous for her. She promised, and kept her word at first. But, like so many addicts, after a few weeks she began to experiment with small amounts of the forbidden foods. After a fast, as I have mentioned, many patients' general sensitivity levels seem to be temporarily reduced, so that for a while they may get away with eating some of the addictive foods in small quantities. But eventually such piecemeal return to the addictive substances is almost always disastrous. Inevitably the patient increases the quantity, begins to experience small elevations in mood, and as a result continues to increase the intake of the foods to achieve the euphoric effect.

And that, as you may have guessed, is what happened to Betty. Gradually, the unfortunate woman returned to her former eating habits, and was soon back at her midnight rambles, scoring chocolate cake. And once more she became submerged in the vicious cycle of depression, elation, anxiety, and withdrawal.

Only after a near fatal suicidal attempt did she finally face the facts: either she would have to follow her diet, or die. Happily, when the cards were finally down, she chose to live.

Dorothy was another young woman whose history illustrates the virulence of food addictions. For four and a half years she languished as a psychiatric in-patient in one of the country's best known psychiatric hospitals. She may not literally have sat and stared at her belly button during that entire period, but for all practical purposes it amounted to that.

When I first saw her, she was immobilized by depression, which was part of the malignant schizophrenic process choking off her life. Although only twenty-five years old, she felt she had no future, that life had absolutely nothing to offer her. She didn't bother to bathe, or even to brush her teeth. She was so withdrawn that later, after she had improved enough to communicate, we discovered that she had even forgotten how to use our monetary system and didn't know that a dime was worth more than a nickel.

At the hospital Dorothy had eaten what I consider a very poor and unbalanced diet, featuring an abnormal quantity of sweets. I thought this was a telling symptom and decided to put her on a fast; the fast turned into a battle of wills. She was so determined to eat the wrong foods that I had to hire a nurse's aide to stay with her at all times to keep her from cadging food from other patients.

During the fast she became extremely hostile and had to be restrained from attacking other patients to get their food. Though the staff members who had to control her found this most inconvenient, I was quite pleased with this development. Her hostility and aggressiveness at least showed that she was capable of feelings, which I felt was better than having her slumped in a corner like a sack of beans.

On the fifth day of her fast, abruptly and dramatically, her emotional fog cleared, revealing glimpses of a human personality. She spoke her first complete sentence, showed interest in her surroundings, and wanted to know where she was.

And then she smiled for the first time in years.

The young woman was so accustomed to hopelessness that despite continuing marked progress she kept insisting that her improvement was only temporary, that nothing could help her in the long run. She seemed unable to realize that the fast had lifted much of the veil of psychosis which had so long blocked her from reality.

Once she was allowed to leave the hospital on a pass for a visit with her parents, but after a few hours at home she grew tense and asked to return to the institution. Much later, after she had improved immeasurably, she admitted that she had been afraid to get better, because she had become adjusted to hospital life. The thought of having to make her own way in the outside world was overwhelmingly terrifying. This syndrome of being afraid to grow well and leave the protective cocoon of the hospital environment is well known to psychotherapists, who refer to it as "hospitalitis" or "institutionalism." It isn't difficult to understand. Many patients, forgetting what they have lost, gain at least a certain relief by surrendering to illness. I need hardly tell you that these are among the most difficult patients to treat.

In any case, it was financially impossible to post round-the-clock guard on Dorothy forever. I told her firmly that she must restrict her food intake so we could feed her one food at a time to test for allergies. After these tests were completed she would have to follow a diet free of the foods harmful to her. I pointed out how much she had already improved under this regimen, but she continued to deny that she might ever be completely well. As soon as supervision was relaxed she began trading and stealing food again, until she got all the sweets she craved.

If I had my way, no psychiatric hospital or ward would ever allow its patients any sweets. But many factors militate against such a policy, not the least being economic ones. Calories from sweets and other carbohydrates are cheaper than calories from meat, vegetables, and fruits. At least on paper they appear to be cheaper. In the long run, by perpetuating the patient's illness, such economies are pretty costly to patients' families, insurance companies, and society as a whole.

Although I do not like to use electroconvulsive therapy, I felt that in Dorothy's case it was necessary. Dorothy had twenty-five treatments, enough to bring her out of her psychosis to the point where she could cooperate in following a diet. Soon after leaving the hospital she was well enough to take a job.

Though she has cut down drastically on her intake of wheat and milk products and has just about eliminated sweets, she still had, until quite recently, a tendency to slip now and then.

One afternoon she was feeling rather jaunty and decided to forget all about her diet. She was feeling fine nowadays, she was going to eat what *she* wanted instead of what her ogre of a psychiatrist prescribed. She happened to want a chocolate bar.

That evening I had an emergency call from her parents. When they brought her to my office she was as psychotic as the first time I had seen her. She was engulfed in hopelessness, could not be reasoned with, and kept begging to be taken back to the hospital.

I gave her an intravenous injection of 5 grams of ascorbic acid and adrenal extract,* and told her to come back the next day. We would then make arrangements for her to be hospitalized, if she still wanted to go. The next afternoon she phoned to cancel her appointment. She was so much better that there was no need for her to visit me.

During her next routine visit she sheepishly admitted that she was beginning to be sold on the importance of keeping a diet, and since that day she has been much more cooperative.

---

* Cerebral allergies may often be alleviated by intravenously administered adrenal cortical extract and ascorbic acid. Dr. William H. Philpott told me of two patients' response to such injections. One had been quite psychotic. He gave her a massive injection of adrenal cortical extract and ascorbic acid. Within minutes she talked to him in a rational manner. The other was a beauty parlor operator, whose sensitivity to the products used in her trade produced physical as well as emotional reactions. She too received these injections, and since then has been symptom-free.

Recently I have also become interested in the use of Cytomel, a thyroid hormone product, which is being employed in the treatment of schizophrenics and depressives. Dr. Arthur J. Prange, Jr., professor of psychiatry at the University of North Carolina, reports on such use in the October 1969 issue of the *American Journal of Psychiatry*. Important work in this area is also being done by Dr. Magda Campbell at the New York University Medical Center. Those interested should have their physicians check with one or both of these sources.

I have been talking about patients with severe emotional illnesses to prove a point. But a vast range of lesser emotional symptoms are also caused by allergies. Ninety-five percent of my patients suffer from simple depressions, anxiety, phobias, migraine headaches, etc. Those who are affected by food allergies respond just as dramatically to corrected diet as do the schizophrenics and psychotics. And remember: food allergies are by no means the only danger. You can also be allergic to alcohol, tobacco, drugs, air pollution, plastics, fluorescent lights, and a variety of other environmental factors, with similarly disastrous results.

Since allergies tend to reinforce each other, a great many people subconsciously develop their whole lifestyle around their addictions. Almost anyone who smokes and drinks reports that he smokes *more* when he is drinking; others smoke more when they are drinking coffee. This happens because the rush they get from either one of those toxic substances is greater when they are both taken together.

Some choose to arrange their addictions in sequence. I am reminded of one patient—a well-known TV star—who knows that eating candy will give him a high for approximately two hours. If at the end of that period he eats a wheat product, he not only forestalls the letdown, but adds a boost to his high. Two hours later he must smoke at least three cigarettes to keep the high going. He continues in this way throughout the day, day after day, riding the crest of his allergies.

It was said by those who knew Winston Churchill that he drank a quart of brandy a day, and his addiction to cigars was a hallmark. Obviously he rode his addictions with a certain aplomb, though he often lost his highs and plunged into his occasional black depressions. But the Churchills of the world are few. For most allergic people, there comes a point of no return when they can no longer control their conditions. Even if that point is forestalled forever, it's a toss-up whether they are controlling the allergies or whether the allergies are controlling them.

Suppose you are allergic to milk, or to corn, or apples, or some other food that makes you drowsy. You may choose to eat that food at bedtime when you want to go to sleep. You can make yourself go to sleep by being hit on the head with a baseball bat too, but that doesn't mean it's good for you, at bedtime or otherwise.

The role of food addiction in causing emotional symptoms is so important, and so nearly universally missed by physicians and others treating emotional illnesses, that I feel duty-bound to harp on it.

Let me therefore emphasize again that emotional symptoms caused by food allergies *are very common*. I would guess that between eighty and ninety percent of patients with emotional problems are significantly affected by allergic addictions, and that their emotional symptoms could be partly, largely, or totally eliminated simply by taking the allergic conditions into consideration.

In my opinion any psychiatrist who does not test for food allergies is neglecting his patients and is fighting emotional illness with one and a half hands tied behind his back. When patients complain at the expense of a proper initial work-up from a chemical, mineral, vitamin, and allergy standpoint, I always remind them that it isn't nearly as expensive as going to a psychiatrist several times a week for years on end, with little or no result.

Let me tell you about Mrs. B, a forty-three-year-old woman who recently consulted me. Twice a week, for six years, she had been going to a psychiatrist, seeking help for her debilitating symptoms: prolonged bouts of palpitations. She had also consulted a cardiologist, who agreed that she was prone to attacks of excessively fast heartbeats (which she knew). Both doctors declared that she was "nervous," and prescribed a tranquilizer. The only effect was to make her sleepy and to interfere with her ability to work.

I performed my routine chemical tests and found her vitamin B_{12} level very low, a condition rather frequently seen in people with severe allergies. (Because inability to absorb vitamin B_{12} is also frequently an inherited disorder, I now make it a policy to test blood relatives of any patient with a low serum B_{12} level. All of Mrs. B's children had low serum B_{12} levels—one at 0.)

Sublingual challenge tests revealed Mrs. B to be quite sensitive to hydrocarbons, and a more careful history established that her palpitation attacks were especially troublesome at three locations: when she went into her basement, where the gas-burning furnace was located; when she was in her kitchen, cooking on a gas stove; and when she was in her car, driving in heavy, slow-moving traffic. On all these occasions she was exposed to high levels of hydrocarbons from the gas-burning furnace, from the gas stove in the kitchen as well as the smoke of frying foods, and from automobile exhausts, which are so often heavy in slow, dense traffic.

With a patient such as this, it is sometimes impractical if not impossible to do *everything* necessary to avoid hydorcarbons. But at least the exposure to them can be greatly reduced. An offending gas furnace can be replaced or relocated in the garage. In Mrs. B's case, her symptoms were greatly reduced by simply having her avoid the basement as much as possible, and opening its windows to improve ventilation. Her gas stove was replaced by an electric range, and a hood was installed to ventilate the stove area. She was told to avoid frying foods, and advised to get an air purifier for her car. (I recommend the type made by Air-Conditioning Engineers of Decatur, Ill. The average electrostatically-operated air purifier puts ozone into the air, and should be rigorously avoided.) This regimen (together with injections of vitamin B_{12b} resulted in a ninety percent reduction in Mrs. B's attacks. As a bonus, she also became more energetic, and lost much of her former tension and depression.

A similar case in many ways was twenty-three-year-old Barbara, who told me that she had been tired, depressed, nervous, and unable to function all of her life. She had finished high school only with the help of special tutors. She felt that life was not worth living, and had prolonged crying spells nearly every day.

Her food history revealed that she had had an early dislike for milk, and had been fed buttermilk as an infant. She was found to have mild hypoglycemia, and had, in fact, been on a hypoglycemic diet for the past two years. As an afterthought she mentioned that she also felt a pounding in her head whenever she ate candy, which proved that she didn't follow her diet.

Although she had been taking vitamin supplements, blood tests revealed a deficiency of vitamin B_3. A test of her hair indicated deficiencies in copper, iron, potassium, and sodium. She had consulted dozens of doctors, and showed me a list of the drugs which they had prescribed at various times. The list included about thirty different medications, none of which had relieved her symptoms. She was so ill the day she came to see me that we could complete only three allergy tests. During the test for wheat she became very excited, laughed uncontrollably for a few minutes, then gradually lapsed back into depression.

When she could not return for further testing, and was too ill even to come to the office for a visit, I put her on a diet which I considered most likely to avoid the major foods and chemicals to which she was allergic. She was told to eat only fresh meat, fresh fruit, and fresh vegetables, to avoid all processed foods and all grains other than rice, and to drink no milk.

As I always do, I warned her mother that her daughter's symptoms would get worse before they got better—allergic patients with addictions go through a brief withdrawal period on an allergen-free diet, and they may feel just as rotten as any other addict in withdrawal.

It's a good thing that I had warned the mother, because the young woman did feel a great deal worse. She was dizzy and unable to get out of bed, and couldn't eat for about three days. At the end of that time she began to improve. A couple of days later she came into my office alert and smiling, remarking that she could not remember ever feeling this good before. Her formerly dull eyes, now sparkling, confirmed her statement. She listened with interest to the therapy I outlined, and proved a very cooperative patient, who improved continually and rapidly.

Another patient of mine is thirty-year-old Harold, who for nine months before consulting me had suffered from a fluttering in his chest, lightheadedness, numbness in his left arm, and periods of great anxiety. He wondered whether he was working up to a heart attack. Several physicians had examined him, and four electrocardiograms had turned out negative.

His hair test revealed low levels of calcium, sodium, potassium, magnesium, and copper. From this it was easy to guess that his dietary habits left a good deal to be desired, and in fact it turned out that because he was divorced and didn't like to cook, he lived on canned junk foods and TV dinners.

I had him take a computerized psychological test—the Minnesota Multiple Personality Inventory (MMPI). The printout stated that "this patient appears to be tense, anxious, and critically worried. He may complain of physical symptoms which are closely related to his tension. He attempts to control his anxiety by compulsive orderliness and by overconcern with his physical complaints. Although these complaints are more frequently imagined than real, frequent demands for reassurance and medical care may be anticipated. This personality pattern is likely to remain stable and be quite resistant to change."

Here we have a computer interpreting a patient's symptoms as functional in nature; that is to say, having no real physical basis. The reason the computer makes the same mistakes as the physicians is, of course, that it was programmed by people who know little about hypoglycemia or allergies or deficiency states. This particular computer was programmed by a professor of psychology at the University of Alabama, and is run by the Hoffman–La Roche Pharmacological Company. I don't mean to say that the computer is of no value; it's quite useful in diagnosing psychiatric illnesses, but it simply fails to take certain factors into consideration, just as the doctors do who see these patients.

A six-hour glucose tolerance test revealed a marked hypoglycemia in Harold. At the end of three hours his blood sugar fell to 40 mg. percent (55 mg. percent is normal) and all the symptoms of which he complained began to appear. Allergy tests revealed him to be sensitive to wheat, milk, and corn. I might add that there are contaminants of corn in sugar; people who are sensitive to corn very commonly react with sensitivity to sugar too. This sensitivity may make the blood sugar go down, even if there is nothing wrong with insulin metabolism itself.

Harold was put on vitamins, mineral supplements, and a diet free of the foods to which he was sensitive. When he returned for his next check-up, he too reported a change for the worse during the three or four days following the change in his diet; but now his symptoms were rapidly disappearing, and he was very pleased with his progress.

Hypoglycemia and food allergies almost always go hand in hand, and both these conditions as a rule are accompanied by mineral and vitamin deficiencies.

It is my strong impression that the whole complex of allergies, emotional disorders, and hypoglycemia constitutes a syndrome caused by a defect or breakdown of enzyme systems, which means a failure of the individual's basic cellular chemistry.

Basically, such disorders are hereditary. Harold, for example, reported a strong family history of allergy and diabetes. Hypoglycemia often precedes diabetes. However, the fact that it is an inherited disorder does not mean that nothing can be done for those who suffer from it. Such patients need special diets and vitamin and mineral supplements. Sometimes they also need adrenal cortical extract and other hormones, as indicated by the individual circumstances. With this kind of support they can often lead normal lives, indeed, more than normal lives. Many of these people seem to be unusually intelligent and creative, and have the capacity to contribute a great deal to our world.

TESTING YOURSELF FOR ALLERGIES

Is it possible to test yourself for allergies? The answer is a qualified yes. Qualified, because it would be far better for you to have these tests given by a knowledgeable doctor. Unfortunately, very few doctors are knowledgeable enough about the subject to test you accurately. A standard allergist may offer you a skin test, which, as I have said, is not more than twenty percent accurate. A non-allergist is likely to know even less about the subject, and to be even less disposed to learn.

Let me say once more, it would be best to be tested with the help of a doctor, so you should do what you can to convince your physician to read the literature. Tell him about the studies described in this chapter and where he can find the articles. If he still won't go along with you, at least let him know what you are going to do, so that if an emergency arises he will have some idea how to handle it.

That said, let me also urge you not to be discouraged by your doctor's skepticism. If you want to test yourself, don't let him embarrass you out of it, unless he can give you a sound medical reason why the test may be dangerous in your case. Most physicians hate to have their judgment questioned, especially by lay people; but that doesn't make them right all the time.

The test of choice (the sublingual test) is to have your doctor use different concentrations of the foods to which you may be sensitive. He would then drop a small amount of the liquid under your tongue and wait to see if any reaction occurs. Possible symptoms include drowsiness, depression, sudden change of mood, headache, palpitations, elation, giddiness, and anger. After the symptoms clear, a second food would be tried, and so on.

The second method is more difficult and more complicated. It is the method described earlier in this chapter: you remove all possible allergens (except bottled water) from your environment, fast completely for a period of four to five days (usually five), then begin a series of challenge feedings—one type of food at each meal. Since your system will be entirely free of allergic reactions at the time you begin these feedings, any reaction you experience will be intense, and you will be able to identify clearly the agent that caused it.

Caution: before you begin

Fasts have been used by mankind throughout history and probably before, usually as cleansing rituals or religious rites. Many people find them very uplifting, and undertake them several times a year simply as a disciplinary exercise. Others find them extremely difficult, and to some people they are dangerous. Therefore you *must* consult your doctor before you begin to be sure there is no serious contraindication in your case. The fast and the later food challenges must be done under your physician's supervision. People with diabetes, cirrhosis of the liver, heart disease, and kidney diseases should not fast. On the other hand, if you tend to be overweight your doctor may be delighted even if he thinks the allergy notion is nonsense.

In any case, even if you have your doctor's approval for a fast, you should not rush things. Fasts can produce severe reactions, and someone should be with you in case you need help. Your physician should know about the fast and be readily available. Especially if you are severely allergic and/or addicted to something, you may feel strange or depressed or physically ill for a few days as your system adjusts to being without it.

Remove all possible allergens from your environment

1. If there are gas appliances in your house, such as a furnace or hot water heater, washer, or dryer, stay away from them during the test and keep the area well ventilated.
2. Eliminate all cosmetics, including toothpaste, hair spray, deodorant, soap, and perfume. You can brush your teeth with baking soda. Don't use sprays of any kind—no air freshener, disinfectant, mouthwash, or cleaners.
3. Stop all medication. This includes even aspirin and birth control pills. You should also avoid contraceptive creams and foams. Unlubricated condoms can tide you over.
4. Avoid air pollution as much as humanly possible. Don't drive in

congested traffic, keep the windows closed, and don't use the air conditioner or air purifier, unless it is the sort that releases no ozone.

5. And of course you must use no alcohol or tobacco, and no one else should smoke in your space during the test.

It goes without saying that to follow all these measures strictly is to disrupt your life considerably. For those with a mild or acute addiction to tobacco or alcohol, giving up the habit can be as hard as the rest of the test combined. On the other hand, remember that this is only a few days out of your life, and what you will learn about yourself will be a revelation.

Most of us have room in our lives for a genuine revelation. And keep in mind that many of my patients have managed to follow this regimen, rigorous as it is. No doubt they are highly motivated by the desire to find a way out of their emotional pain. The point is, you can do it if you really want to and I guarantee you it will be interesting. And it might change your life.

The fast

The fast itself is simple enough. You ingest absolutely nothing except pure untreated spring water. Be sure to drink one or two quarts a day; otherwise you will become dehydrated.

Keeping your environment perfectly free of allergens, as described, maintain the fast for at least four days. The length of time is determined by how long it takes your body to rid itself of allergic reactions. As you have seen earlier in this book, many patients go through two or three days of withdrawal, during which they feel worse than before they started fasting. Then the symptoms disappear and they feel considerably better than before the fast. *That is the sign you are waiting for.* After you have been free of symptoms for a full day, you are ready to begin challenge feedings. This usually happens on the fourth or fifth day.

The challenge feedings

Begin the day with a meal of one food, in the simplest possible form, and don't break the fast in any other way. The foods most people are

allergic to are wheat, corn, sugar, eggs, milk, and chocolate. But don't
begin a challenge feeding of wheat by eating bread, for that may contain
milk, eggs, sugar and even preservatives. Instead, try a bowl of mush
made with wheat germ and hot water. It will taste terrible. If you can
stand the fast you can certainly stand plain wheat germ; there's more to
life than having all foods taste good all the time.

If you are going to have a reaction, it will usually surface any time
from five minutes to two hours after you have eaten. I recommend that
you keep a written record of what you eat at each meal and how you feel
afterward. I also recommend very strongly that there be someone with
you, if at all possible, to observe your reactions. This will provide a
reality check against your impressions, since it is entirely possible that an
allergic reaction could distort your perceptions.

For your next meal choose a source of protein; a piece of broiled
meat, chicken, or fish, or eggs or cheese. Then for the third meal, go back
to a carbohydrate, perhaps fruit, or corn, or some other grain. Don't take
several protein meals in a row.

If you get a severe reaction from one meal, and the symptoms
continue until time for the next feeding, eat nothing and drink only
water. Keep this up until you are free of symptoms again, then continue
the test.

If you get no reaction to something you have good reason to suspect
you are allergic to, eat one feeding of it a day *for several days*. This can
provoke a response when more widely-spaced feedings do not. You will
have to be very honest with yourself about this. You may get no response
the first time you have coffee or chocolate or ice cream, and you may be
delighted because you favor that particular food and want to believe you
are not allergic to it.

Try to vary the kinds of food you are testing. Don't test two kinds of
fish two days in succession, or two kinds of fruit the same day. When you
have tested all the foods that you eat most regularly, test those you eat
occasionally.

Then, at the rate of one per day, return the environmental allergens
to your environment. You can start with toothpaste, then add deodorant
the next day, and so on. During this time eat nothing that caused a
reaction during the challenge feedings and continue to keep a daily
record of what you're eating and using and doing, and how you feel.

This record will be of use to you for years, for you may feel a mild reaction to something now and later develop fullblown acute symptoms from it. It happens all the time. People suddenly develop sensitivities they never noticed before, just as people sometimes "outgrow" even the most acute allergies.

We don't know all the reasons for these changes, but with the record you keep through these days, you will have a good idea where to find any new culprit that may turn up in the future.

When you are finished testing you will reap a number of rewards. First, you will probably be thinner, a boon to most of us. Second you will know how to avoid foods that affect your emotional wellbeing. Third, your general state of "allergicness" will probably be considerably lowered for a period following the fast. That means that things in your environment to which you are sensitive but which you can't well avoid (like pollen or air pollution) will bother you much less than they usually do. Just be careful so you won't trick yourself and decide that you are also less allergic to foods which you know are bad for you; it's true you can probably tolerate small doses for a while following the fast, but in the end you will wind up as hooked as ever. Then the only way to break the cycle will be to go through the fast—and withdrawal—all over again!

A BREAKTHROUGH IN ALLERGY TREATMENT

I want to tell you about a fascinating approach to food allergies that is still in the experimental stage.

While visiting Los Angeles some years ago, I heard of Dr. Carl L. Eckhardt of Riverside, California, who was using a unique desensitization method for allergies, based on a 1947 article on urine therapy by Professor Johan Plesch.[1] Plesch wrote of it as of a new discovery, though I later turned up some 130 references to auto-urine therapy (treatment by injections of the patient's own urine) when I searched the literature. As a matter of fact, I traced its use all the way back to 1863, when it was mentioned in *The Physiological Memoirs of Surgeon-General Hammond, U.S. Army.*

Wishing to learn more about Professor Plesch and his therapy, I wrote to his last known address, the Palace Hotel in Montreux,

Switzerland, but the management there could provide no news of him. The British Medical Directory last lists him in 1957, so it must be presumed that he died shortly thereafter.

Dr. Plesch was evidently a man of parts. He had received his first M.D. in 1900 from the University of Budapest, and a second one in Germany in 1909. In addition to a number of scientific papers he wrote his autobiography, *Janos: The Story of A Doctor*, published in three editions and translated into Spanish, German, and Italian. He also wrote a book called *Rembrandts within Rembrandts*, which was published in Spanish, German, and English in 1953.

Plesch had been a professor of medicine at the University of Berlin, but had left Germany after the Nazi takeover and settled in London, where he developed a very fashionable Mayfair practice. Even reading his work I had been struck by the man's charm and grace, and I could well understand that he appealed to the Beautiful People of his day.

Around 1950, a member of Dr. Eckhardt's family consulted Eckhardt for chronic eczema, a skin rash often associated with allergies, which had tortured her for years. Eckhardt remembered Plesch's paper, and decided to try urine therapy on the woman, since a string of dermatologists and allergists had not been able to help her. He administered the auto-urine injections at weekly intervals. The eczema soon disappeared, and has not returned to this day. Since that time Dr. Eckhardt has administered some fifty thousand auto-urine injections to allergic patients, all of whom had previously been to numerous allergists without obtaining relief. The auto-urine injections produced very significant improvement in eighty percent of cases.

Another California physician, Norman H. Mellor, also reports a high success rate with this treatment. Neither he nor Dr. Eckhardt test patients for allergies beforehand, because most of the people who consult them are only too aware of their allergies already. Those suffering from a food allergy are instructed to eat that food two hours prior to passing the urine to be injected. Those sensitive to a substance like pollen are instructed to expose themselves to massive amounts of it several hours before the injection.

Please don't think that I embarked on this unusual therapeutic approach lightly. Before trying auto-urine therapy on patients, I not only talked with physicians who used the technique and reviewed the extensive world literature on the subject, but I also administered the injections to myself in order to gain firsthand experience concerning their efficacy and possible side effects. I already knew that two or three abscesses per thousand injections had occurred among Dr. Eckhardt's patients, despite the most rigorous precautions to insure sterile conditions. I improved on Eckhardt's technique by using a bacterial filter through which I injected the urine. No bacteria can pass through this filter; thus it eliminates the danger of infection and abscesses.

I gave myself my first injection on a Saturday afternoon, so that I would have the weekend to recover from whatever lay in store for me.

I must have been quite a sight. Picture me standing in the middle of my consultation room with my pants down, twisting my torso to locate the correct spot on my rump to stick in the needle. Behind me lay the twinkling early evening skyline of New York, as seen from the vantage point of my nineteenth-floor office. I wondered whether anyone was observing me from windows which dotted the panorama. All over New York people were giving themselves their Saturday evening fixes, but it seemed a reasonably safe bet that I was the only one in town shooting urine.

About half an hour after the injection a feeling of profound lassitude seeped through my body, all the way down to my hands and feet. The obligatory couch, a relic of my establishment days, suddenly looked more inviting than it had in years. Maybe the old man had a point after all, I thought wryly, and I stretched out for a few minutes' rest.

Three hours later I woke up, not feeling any livelier. With a minimum of enthusiasm I got up, dressed, and ambled home to my apartment, where I went straight to bed without dinner.

I felt none of the emotional depression that some people experience after the injections, but I did suffer a definite flare-up of the allergic rhinitis which has plagued me all my life. Usually I can breathe through one nostril. That afternoon and evening I could breathe through neither.

By next morning the extreme weakness and lassitude had disappeared, but I still felt rather passive, and I left the apartment only for my weekly movie. Monday morning some of my strength returned, and by Tuesday I was my normal energetic self once more. The nasal obstruction had vanished, together with the weakness.

Altogether, I gave myself a total of twelve injections at weekly intervals. My reaction followed the typical pattern described by Dr. Eckhardt. After each of the first four or five shots I felt the same lassitude, but each time it was less severe. Each time, also, my nasal allergy flared up, but this, too, diminished progressively. Toward the end of the injection series I was no longer experiencing any reaction at all, except for a temporary soreness at the injection site.

To me, one of the most interesting side-effects was the abrupt and fairly long-lasting change in my eating pattern. Long after all other side-effects had evaporated I still could not eat nearly as much as before starting the injections. Could it be, I wondered, that I had a mild addiction to several foods which had been counteracted by the injections? Whatever the reason—when I sat down to my meals I simply did not feel like eating my usual portions. With few exceptions, this held true for my patients who were overweight while undergoing auto-urine therapy. Three-fourths lost weight, unless they were taking one of the major tranquilizers.*

My next guinea pig was my secretary, who had been feeling rather depressed, and who went through periods of withdrawal and general malaise. Sublingual tests revealed that she was quite sensitive to milk: During the test she perspired profusely, and felt depressed and confused for about an hour.

I had her drink milk several hours before giving her the injection. Her reaction was more protracted than mine. She felt that her "head wasn't screwed on right" for five or six days, found it difficult to concentrate, and often felt confused. Similar but less severe symptoms followed the next two or three injections. After that, the adverse reactions gradually faded. She, too, lost weight—ten pounds to my twenty—and felt a great upsurge in energy and well-being. A few months after the completion of the injection series she was again tested for milk and found to be no longer allergic. She now drinks a small quantity of milk as part of her regular diet, without experiencing any adverse reactions.

Next on my list was my technician, who lost eighteen pounds during the therapy, though emotional improvement in her case was less clear-cut.

* Thorazine and other major tranquilizers affect the hunger centers of the brain and frequently cause a patient to gain weight.

Having gathered sufficient experience to satisfy myself, I now decided to try auto-urine therapy on various patients.

About three-fourths of my patients with food allergies have been definitely helped by auto-urine injections.

I regret that I have not had time to pursue this promising field of research with the single-mindedness it deserves, but I hope that as more physicians become aware of the importance of food allergies, more will begin to investigate auto-urine therapy. If you are interested in trying it, you should ask your physician to read Professor Plesch's paper on the subject.

NOTES

1. Johan Plesch. "Urine Therapy," *The Medical Press* (London, England), 1947.

HYPOGLYCEMIA:
THE GREAT IMPERSONATOR

CHAPTER NINE

Even though public awareness of hypoglycemia has increased greatly in the last couple of years, this condition is still one of the most frequently undiagnosed diseases in the civilized world. An estimated 20 to 40 million Americans have it.

Most people who have heard of hypoglycemia assume it to be the opposite of diabetes—i.e., diabetes means high blood sugar, and hypoglycemia means low blood sugar. But the opposite of diabetes is normal. Hypoglycemia is the opposite end of the spectrum in the same disease as diabetes. Both represent an inability of the body to metabolize carbohydrates normally. It is possible to have both hypoglycemia and diabetes, and hypoglycemia is often one stage on the way to diabetes.

Medical students are taught almost nothing about hypoglycemia. They *are* taught that when a patient has a tumor in the insulin-producing glands in the pancreas, his blood insulin levels increase and drive down the blood sugar level, producing hypoglycemia. The patient is hungry all the time, eats a lot, and gets fat even though he may be dying from a malignant tumor. But such tumors are exceedingly rare. Students are also taught that hypoglycemia may occur when a damaged liver is unable to store sugar properly, a condition that occurs more frequently than pancreatic tumors. Medical students hear only a fleeting mention of functional hypoglycemia, a diagnosis which applies to more than ninety-nine percent of people suffering from the disease. (In medical jargon, "functional" means that the cause is unknown. Actually, I think the cause is not far to seek, but more of that later.)

Nine out of ten schizophrenics have acute hypoglycemia. The majority of obese people have hypoglycemia. In addition, millions of people suffer occasional hypoglycemic attacks brought on by alcohol, allergies, diets, hormone changes, stress or anxiety.

Because the cells of the central nervous system mainly use glucose (sugar) in their metabolism, any malfunction in the blood sugar level will almost surely produce a malfunction in the nervous system. Low blood sugar produces emotional symptoms ranging from temporary depression or anxiety to acute insanity. It can also produce any physical symptoms.

As a critical connector between nutrition and the state of your nerves, the importance of hypoglycemia cannot be overstated. Since everybody's personality and biochemical make-up is different, the ways in which individual brains may react to hypoglycemia are so numerous that they can hardly be described; symptoms include just about every complaint imaginable, and hardly a month goes by that I do not see a hypoglycemic patient with a new one. That's why I call hypoglycemia the great impersonator; a partial list of possible symptoms includes depression, fatigue, anxiety, thoughts of suicide, all kinds of allergies, headaches, drug abuse, fainting spells, nightmares, insomnia, forgetfulness, confusion, anger, palpitations, some forms of arthritis, and alcoholism, not to mention such physical symptoms as post-nasal drip, asthma, hay fever, eczema, dizziness, and sweating. In effect, what I am saying is that if you feel bad in any way for more than a few days, hypoglycemia is at least a possibility.

Recently I was consulted by a prominent psychologist who had begun to have such severe symptoms of weakness and depression, that she was forced to stop working. First she had herself examined at Columbia–Presbyterian Hospital where they were unable to establish a definite diagnosis. They told her that she might have an unusual type of liver disease. Next she went to Yale (New Haven) Hospital where, to their great credit and my great surprise, they diagnosed hydrocarbon sensitivity. That is to say, they told her that she was allergic to such substances as automobile exhaust fumes and gas from the kitchen stove.

I retested her and confirmed the diagnosis, but removing these substances from her environment only provided a little relief. She continued to work, but she was still so anxious and depressed that she eventually became addicted to illegal drugs. After a valiant effort to hold herself together enough to practice her profession, she finally had herself admitted to a clinic in New Jersey.

The doctors there performed a *three*-hour glucose tolerance test, apparently because they suspected diabetes. The patient had a long-standing craving for sweets, as well as a strong family history of diabetes. Her glucose tolerance test showed a fasting blood sugar of 100 mg. percent. One half hour after being fed the usual test dose of sugar, her blood sugar had risen to 236 mg. percent, and at one hour it stood at 300 mg. percent; in two hours it had fallen to 210 mg. percent, and in three hours to 79 mg. percent.

These are quite abnormal figures. Most doctors confronted with them would say that the blood sugar went too high and stayed high too long. They would conclude that the patient was predisposed toward diabetes, which was, in fact, the interpretation made at the clinic. The patient was told to cut down on sweets. That was good advice and she soon improved enough to return to work—with the added aid of antidepressant drugs and tranquilizers.

Her condition was better, but far from good. Because she felt very depressed in the mornings, she would stay in bed until 11 or 12 o'clock. She saw patients in the afternoon, went home to sit in front of the TV until 10:30, and then took her bedtime medication and retreated into sleep.

When she consulted me I ordered a number of additional tests. I discovered two interesting abnormalities which were missed at the three institutions where she had been hospitalized. The first was a low level of sex hormones—not too surprising in a forty-five-year-old woman. (Male sex hormones tend to stay at a higher level longer.) The second, far more important, finding which had been missed was her serum B_{12} level, which was reported as 59 pg/m by one laboratory and as 104 pg/m by another. By any standard, both these levels are abnormally low. I don't think any physician would take the stand that an abnormally low serum B_{12} level is a desirable condition; but most physicians associate it only with pernicious anemia, and don't realize that emotional problems caused by such a deficiency may precede pernicious anemia by many years. Low serum B_{12} levels are extremely dangerous and can result in damage to the central nervous system. They are also very often associated with hypoglycemia.

It is unfortunate that the clinic did not perform a five- or six-hour glucose tolerance test on the patient. (To properly diagnose hypoglycemia, I prefer a six-hour test though a number of physicians experienced in the field are satisfied with a five-hour one.) The three-hour test done on my patient is useful for diagnosing borderline or potential diabetes, but it may or may not show hypoglycemia.

It so happens that her tolerance test *did* clearly indicate hypoglycemia, but such a diagnosis was not made by the clinic staff. This is not unusual. I would guess that only one physician in five thousand can properly interpret a glucose tolerance test. Most of them think in terms of absolute blood sugar levels, instead of looking at the curve, or pattern of blood levels taken throughout the test.

Since your doctor is not likely to know how to interpret your glucose tolerance curve, I advise you to have him give you the figures so that you can review them yourself and draw your own conclusions in accordance with the guidelines I'm about to give you. Those of us interested in hypoglycemia (and most of us became interested in it because we have it ourselves) follow these criteria for diagnosing it:

Hypoglycemia is indicated:
1. when the blood sugar, in the course of a six-hour glucose tolerance test, fails to rise more than fifty percent above the fasting level;
2. by a glucose curve which falls during a six-hour test to 20 mg. percent below the fasting level;
3. by a glucose tolerance test in which blood sugar falls 50 mg. percent or more during any one hour of the test;
4. by a glucose tolerance test in which the absolute blood sugar level falls in the range of 50 mg. percent or lower (anything below 65 mg. percent is suspicious);
5. by clinical symptoms such as dizziness, headache, confusion, palpitations, depression, etc., appearing during the course of a

glucose tolerance test—regardless of what the blood sugar readings may be.

The last criterion is important, because glucose levels may fluctuate quickly in the course of a tolerance test. The low point may occur *between* the blood sugar levels measured at one-hour intervals. You should, therefore, take into account any symptoms you exhibit during the test. Ideally, if any clinical symptoms make their appearance, extra blood should be drawn at once, to find out what the sugar level is at that point.

The clinic doctors failed to make the diagnosis because they fell into the common error of looking at the glucose tolerance curve in terms of absolute values. The blood sugar level did not fall below 79 mg. percent. If you ask the average physician whether 79 mg. percent represents hypoglycemia, he will reply that it does not. However, if you examine this patient's test figures again, you will note that the blood sugar level fell from 300 mg. percent to 210 mg. percent between the first and second hour—a drop of 90 mg. percent. Between the second and third hour it dropped from 210 mg. percent to 79 mg. percent—a drop of 121 mg. percent in one hour. This fall is much more than the 50 mg. percent which is considered abnormal by physicians experienced with hypoglycemia. In addition, the patient had severe emotional symptoms—depression, restlessness, and a sense of impending doom during the course of the test.

As noted, brain cells rely heavily on glucose for their metabolism. Also, brain cells, unlike others, are not able to store glucose. This makes blood sugar levels all the more important to the functioning of the nervous system. If the cell metabolism becomes conditioned, over a period of time, to functioning with a blood sugar supply between 80 and 120 mg. percent, the cell will accommodate itself to this sugar level. However, if the blood sugar level changes radically, the whole chemistry of the nerve cell is thrown off balance, resulting in marked emotional symptoms.

Once a patient consulted me because of a depression. I did a glucose tolerance test, and between the third and fourth hour she became paranoid and suspicious of the laboratory technicians, believing that they were going to harm her. Checking back, we found that during this period there had been a rapid fall in her blood sugar level. This was the first and only time this woman had ever had paranoid symptoms.

Strange as it may seem, a startling number of physicians still don't know that sugar is the last thing a person with hypoglycemia should eat. Like a lay person, many physicians falsely conclude that if the blood sugar is low, sugar should make it go up. They base their conclusions on their experience with diabetics who have taken an overdose of insulin which makes their blood sugar levels dive down to dangerously low levels. In such cases of insulin reaction the proper treatment *is* to eat sugar.

Not so in functional hypoglycemia. Such a patient's blood sugar also rises after eating sugar. But the relief will be quite temporary, and soon the patient is in real trouble. Whenever sugar enters the bloodstream, the insulin-producing glands are activated. The insulin in the bloodstream causes the sugar to be stored in the liver. This lowers the level of sugar in the blood, making less sugar available to the central nervous system. This process takes place in all so-called normal people. But people with functional hypoglycemia overreact to stimulation by sugar: they produce too much insulin and their blood sugar is driven down too far and too fast.

Other factors besides excessive insulin may be involved in hypoglycemia

In describing how to interpret your glucose tolerance curve, I mentioned a "flat" curve, which sounds like a contradiction in terms. This refers to a line on a graph recording the rise of sugar in the blood. If the line fails to rise 50 mg. percent above the fasting level, the line forms a very shallow, or flat curve. This may indicate excessive and very rapid insulin production. Or it may indicate that the person cannot absorb sugar. Or it may indicate low thyroid levels, and the thyroid should certainly be tested at once. If thyroid gland tests are normal, many patients with flat glucose tolerance tests do better when given thyroid tablets (60 –120 mg. daily).

Many hypoglycemics are allergic to sugar

Hypoglycemics do not, ordinarily, have hives, asthma, or other classical allergy symptoms. Their allergic response may take the form of a lowering of blood sugar, with all the myriad symptoms this syndrome can produce.

Allergic reaction to foods other than sugar may also cause blood sugar to drop. In fact, it is even possible that allergies *other* than food allergies may also drive blood sugar levels down. In turn, a low blood sugar level tends to aggravate allergic reactions—so you can see how quickly the patient can be enmeshed in a vicious cycle.

In my opinion, no patient with hypoglycemia can be properly treated without an allergy workup as outlined in this book. Almost all people with hypoglycemia also have food allergies.

I urge my patients to treat sugar as if it were arsenic

When I first became interested in hypoglycemia, I ran glucose tolerance tests on all my new patients. After a while, I grew so dismayed at the prevalence of hypoglycemia that I did glucose tolerance tests less often because I'd begun to believe that absolutely *no one* should eat sugar. As I've mentioned before, our enzyme systems have simply not evolved a capacity for handling it. Sugar has been widely available to the mass of mankind only during the past one hundred years—far too short a time for Mother Nature to adapt our systems to adjust to using it properly.

In addition, sugar contains no minerals, vitamins, or proteins. To metabolize it, one must receive nutrients from other sources, and the "average American diet" simply does not include enough excess nutrients to handle the job. And as if this were not enough, Dr. John Yudkin, professor emeritus of nutrition at London University,[1] convincingly explains how sugar increases hardening of the arteries, contributes to heart attacks and strokes, destroys teeth and joints, and may even be a contributing factor in the development of cancer.

Is raw sugar better than refined sugar?

Not really. Raw sugar, or turbinado, is white table sugar before being stripped of all nutrients. It does contain a few vitamins and minerals, and therefore does not drain your system of nutrients as much as white sugar does, but it still hits your bloodstream as sucrose, and it still triggers the same insulin overreaction or allergic response as white sugar. Light- and dark-brown sugar such as you buy at the supermarket (raw or turbinado sugar is more likely to be found in a health food store) is the sugar equivalent of "enriched" bread. It's sugar that has been stripped or "refined" and then treated with molasses to make it look dark again. True, molasses has some nutrients that white sugar does not; but it is still sucrose.

Honey is perhaps the least damaging. It contains some nutrients and it consists of fructose or fruit sugar, and glucose, which is the kind of sugar found in the bloodstream. Neither of these sugars have to be converted into a useable molecule the way sucrose does; they can be absorbed through the stomach wall directly into the bloodstream. Since this is a simpler chemical process than metabolizing pure sucrose, honey is perhaps less likely to cause a severe allergic reaction, though it will still cause obesity, tooth decay, heart disease, and the rest. As far as I'm concerned the difference among these sweeteners is insignificant, and I repeat: DON'T EAT SUGAR OR HONEY.

Hypoglycemics should also avoid alcohol

Some of the great alcoholics of our age have been hypoglycemics; F. Scott Fitzgerald especially comes to mind. It's been said that a hypoglycemic starts seven drinks ahead of the rest of the world.

I know of one Texas physician who came home from the office one afternoon, had a cocktail, and spent the next hour mowing the grass. Then he showered and went to a cocktail party, where he had one more drink and passed out. At the hospital emergency room they tested his blood sugar level, found it to be very low, administered some intravenous glucose, and within an hour he was back at the party. That's one way to discover hypoglycemia.

One of my patients, a business executive, had two drinks before lunch at a conference. After leaving he got into an argument with a man on the street, then took a taxi home at the insistence of his associates. When he arrived at his apartment building he was confused, went to the wrong door, which his key would not open. He began banging on the door, and eventually succeeded in breaking it down. Police officers arrived. He mauled two of them so badly that five more were called to help subdue him.

Some hours later he woke up in the hospital, surprised to find himself in a somewhat battered condition. He had no memory whatever of anything that happened after he left the meeting. As a consequence of this experience he came to see me. I ordered a six-hour glucose tolerance test, during which he nearly passed out. As I expected, the test showed him to be severely hypoglycemic.

ALCOHOL, ALLERGY, AND HYPOGLYCEMIA —THE TRIPLE WHAMMY

When a person with hypoglycemia has a drink and then eats something he's allergic to, he can more easily develop emotional symptoms including confusion, depression, fatigue, restlessness, irritability, or even outright psychosis.

You get an allergic reaction from food when tiny particles of the toxic substance move from the intestinal tract into the bloodstream. You get a blood sugar drop from alcohol because, like sugar, it is a pure, empty carbohydrate and is metabolized very fast—too fast for your body. When you drink *and* eat something you're allergic to, the alcohol carries much greater than usual amounts of the toxic food into your bloodstream, and it does so with great rapidity. Result: The alcohol drives down the blood sugar, and the allergic reaction drives it down still faster and further.

I once had lunch with a girl friend at the Plaza Hotel in New York. After a martini she began her appetizer of oysters, remarking that she was slightly allergic to them but couldn't resist eating them once or twice a year. Before the main course had arrived she was in such a state of confusion that I had to lead her out of the dining room.

Several months ago I was walking past the Brasserie restaurant in New York when I saw a man struggling in an attempt to lift a limp woman from the sidewalk into a waiting taxi. She was in her mid thirties, rather obese, and practically unconscious.

"She only had two drinks, for God's sake," the man kept saying over and over, while I helped him as best I could with his limp burden.

"What did she have to eat?" I asked.

"Smoked halibut," he replied. "She loves it, but she hardly ever has a chance to eat it."

I suggested that he take her to a hospital emergency room nearby, and to tell the doctors there that she was probably having an allergic reaction from the smoked halibut. She would probably respond best to intravenously administered sodium bicarbonate.

TENSION AND HYPOGLYCEMIA
—A VICIOUS CIRCLE

Hypoglycemics are often tense, depressed people. Tension and depression can make hypoglycemia worse, and hypoglycemia can make tension and anger worse. It's a chicken-and-egg problem.

Adolf Hitler was a candy bar freak and undoubtedly suffered from hypoglycemia and sugar allergy. When blood sugar is low, the brain becomes irritable and hyperactive. This irritability can stimulate a rush of adrenalin which will in turn very likely exaggerate your excited or furious feeling. At the same time the brain stimulates insulin production as a reaction to the blood sugar elevation produced by the adrenalin. The insulin causes a sizable amount of blood sugar to be stored in the liver, leaving you with lower blood sugar than ever—and feeling more tense and depressed than ever.

Hypoglycemics should avoid tense situations as much as possible, just as they should avoid fatigue and the foods that radically alter their blood levels in the first place. In addition, some should be supplied with a sedative, a nerve-blocking medicine to cut down stimulation of the vagus nerve by the brain proper. Once a hypoglycemic has learned to recognize this syndrome in himself he can use the drug to help break the cycle when tension arises. I sometimes recommend the prescription drug Bellergal for this.

If you suspect hypoglycemia, what should you do about it?

One obvious answer is simply to assume you have it, and put yourself on the diet I am about to describe. For many reasons, I feel it is the healthful, well-balanced diet that most humans should eat anyway. But if you want proof, there are several things you can do.

A home glucose test

I have already described how to interpret the curve of a clinical glucose tolerance test. But you may not be sure it's necessary for you to sit somewhere for six hours having blood samples taken. Measuring the level of sugar in the blood is the only way to *prove* you have low blood sugar, but you may be able to get a pretty strong indication of your own reaction to sugar by deliberately inviting a drastic blood sugar drop and then waiting to see if you have any physical or emotional symptoms. These don't always show up, by any means; if they do, it doesn't prove anything in the scientific sense. But it can be an important indicator.

1. The first and simplest test may seem a little primitive, but the results may surprise you. Have nothing to eat after 10 P.M. The next morning, at about 8 o'clock, eat two candy bars. Have no water, coffee, alcohol, or cigarettes for the next six hours. Someone should stay with you during this time. You may be very sleepy, depressed, restless, or angry, or you may have any other symptoms known to mankind. Write down how you feel and have your friend also make notes. Hopefully your doctor will be interested in your symptoms.

2. If you like, you can check yourself for possible diabetes at the same time as you test for low blood sugar. (As you know, you can have both.) At the drugstore, ask for some strips to test for sugar in the urine.

So you have hypoglycemia. Here's good news and bad news

First the bad news. It would be nicer not to have it. Now the good news. It is one disease you can often control yourself with proper diet. Some people also need sedatives to avoid tension. Some others must have hormone levels corrected, especially as they get older. (Hormones can affect blood sugar levels. Thyroid and the adrenal cortical hormones are the most obvious examples, but others can be involved as well.) But a great many people can improve their mental and physical well-being tremendously simply by changing the way they eat.

Most people with hypoglycemia require extra vitamins and minerals also.

EAT PROTEIN AND FATS
FOR HYPOGLYCEMIA AND LIMIT
CARBOHYDRATES

Different foods are absorbed by the body at different rates and affect blood sugar in different ways. For example, sugar is absorbed directly and quickly. The blood sugar rises rapidly and then falls rapidly, and the person is soon hungry again. In the case of a hypoglycemic, the system overreacts to the rapid flood of sugar into the system. It reproduces too much insulin, and the blood sugar level is knocked way down, often to below where it was in the first place, causing the symptoms with which you are now familiar.

Sugar, as you know, is a carbohydrate. More complex carbohydrates, like potatoes and grains, are also converted by the body into sugar. This gets into the bloodstream more slowly than when you eat sugar itself, but it still happens very quickly, and fades quickly, leaving you hungry or worse. Nutritionist Adelle Davis once wrote that when you sit down to a bowl of cereal in the morning, you should imagine that you are about to eat a bowl of pure sugar because that is how it will affect your blood sugar levels.

Proteins and fats, by contrast, are digested much more slowly than carbohydrates. The blood sugar rises slowly and steadily, remains sustained for a longer period of time, and falls slowly. To avoid low blood sugar attacks, simply avoid large amounts of carbohydrates, eat more protein and fat instead, and your body will do the rest.

How much protein and fat should you eat?

To answer the first question first—eat as much as you need to to avoid hunger and other symptoms. Most hypoglycemics do much better on six or more small meals ("feedings" if you like to think of yourself as a snacker), than on two or more large ones, because in the long wait between meals your blood sugar may fall to dangerous levels, no matter what you have eaten. Small, frequent doses of protein and fat can keep the blood sugar level much more stable.

If you are overweight, as so many hypoglycemics are, don't worry about total calories on this diet. People with deranged carbohydrate metabolisms grow fat because their appetite control is knocked out of kilter by the wildly fluctuating blood sugar levels. Half the time they don't know whether they're hungry or not, so they eat constantly just to cover all bases. When you change over to a high-protein diet, you may still eat constantly at first, just out of habit, but eventually your appetite control will regain its equilibrium and you will probably lose weight without consciously trying to. Most weight problems, whether obesity or thinness, correct themselves when you begin to eat a diet that actually nourishes your particular body adequately.

What kind of protein and fat should you eat?

Beef, lamb, and pork satisfy best. Glandular meats such as liver, kidney, and brains are very nourishing, though lean. You will find yourself feeling less hungry less often if you deliberately eat fat as well as lean, no matter how you have been conditioned against it. Fish and poultry are excellent sources of protein, though again, they are mostly too lean to sustain you as a steady diet. By all means eat fatty hamburger instead of leaner (more expensive) ground round. When you do eat lean meat or fish, cook it in safflower oil (providing, of course, that you are not allergic to it). Eggs are also a good source of protein, if you are not allergic to them. Mayonnaise is good, but be sure it is *real* mayonnaise and not imitation "salad dressing" full of sugar and chemicals.

You can also eat nuts except for cashews (which are high in carbohydrates). But you should buy them in the shell or at a health food store, because commercially packed nuts have usually been sprayed with various carbohydrates and monosodium glutamate (MSG).

Breakfast is the most important meal

If you eat a high carbohydrate breakfast, including cereal or toast, and fruit juice, let alone, donuts, sweet rolls or pancakes or waffles your blood sugar will rise and then swoop downward so that two or three hours later you are feeling dragged out, let down, and in need of another lift. This syndrome is so common among devotees of the normal American diet that its corollary, the mid-morning coffee break, has become an American institution. The mid-morning low-blood sugar attack is part of the American way of life. Coffee, tea, sweet rolls, and cigarettes, all of which temporarily elevate blood sugar levels, are used every morning around 10:30 by millions of Americans to correct the effect of their high-sugar breakfasts, just as diabetics use insulin at regular intervals to correct *their* blood sugar levels.

I know of one coffee-addicted executive who considers non-stop coffee consumption so normal that he regularly orders coffee for himself and any visitor without even asking if his visitor wants any. He thought it passing strange when a health-conscious insurance salesman declined coffee at eleven one morning, saying, "No, thank you, I've finished my breakfast."

Tests have shown that if you eat a significant amount of carbohydrate at breakfast, *or* if you eat no breakfast at all, that your blood sugar levels will remain erratic for the rest of the day, no matter what you eat at lunch and dinner. And you tend to feel hungry even when you have consumed more than your share of calories, because hunger is felt when the blood sugar drops below a certain level (about 70 mg. percent), *not* when the stomach is empty.

If you've ever tried to diet by keeping yourself bloated with celery, lettuce, water, and diet soft drinks, you know that you feel as grouchy and hungry as ever even while you're stuffed like a sausage. Now you know why.

Eat meat, fat, and a little carbohydrate for breakfast

A proper breakfast might include eggs and bacon and a piece of fresh fruit, or lamb chops, pork chops, or hamburgers with a small amount of potatoes cooked any way you like. The sucrose in the fruit will be quickly absorbed for the morning lift you want; similarly, the starchy potato will be quickly converted to glucose; the meat and fat are digested much more slowly, releasing a steady supply of sugar into the blood so that your blood sugar stays elevated until lunch time, and falls much more slowly than usual because you have not triggered insulin overkill by filling your empty stomach with carbohydrates.

You should eat the fruit after protein or fat, by the way. Fruit contains fructose, or fruit sugar, a sort of sugar to which your inherited enzyme systems have been accustomed over millions of years. Insulin is not needed in the metabolism of fructose, so there is less risk of producing a hypoglycemic reaction.

Fruit juice contains too concentrated a source of fructose, so I do not recommend it, particularly not at breakfast. Eating the whole fruit will give you roughage, which is important for many reasons which we will discuss later.

(For a complete rundown of what I usually eat, meal by meal, see page 107.)

What to eat for the rest of the day

As with breakfast, each meal should consist mainly of protein and fat. You should include some brown rice or potatoes and some fresh fruit. Feel free to eat plenty of salad and leafy green vegetables. These provide essential roughage, and are mainly water and minerals, with very few carbohydrates. Plenty of dressing is fine, as long as it contains no sugar. Have safflower oil and vinegar, or oil and lemon juice. If you are not allergic to the ingredients, use mayonnaise. Avoid ketchup and other prepared condiments. Most of them contain sugar, or are loaded with artificial preservatives to which many people are allergic. (And remember: a hypoglycemic is allergy prone.)

If you are overweight, you should cut down on carbohydrates. Eat all the leafy vegetables you desire and include such low calorie vegetables as celery and radishes. Avoid all nuts and grains. Limit fruit to one cup three or four times a day. Drink only water. Eat all the fresh meat (with the fat) and eggs you desire. If you never make any exceptions to this diet, your weight loss should be slow but steady. Vitamin supplements and often mineral supplements should be taken, as I will outline later. Your cholesterol level can be kept down easily by the use of niacin, brewers' yeast, vitamin C, lecithin, and safflower oil, as will be detailed later in the book.

In my experience, reducing diets that allow patients to eat only fats and proteins (no carbohydrates) make a large percentage of people feel sick.

You should buy a carbohydrate gram-counter—a list of the

carbohydrate content of foods—they're available in paperback booklets at most bookstores and many drugstores.

At first, limit your daily carbohydrates to about 120 grams. If you tolerate this well, gradually work down to about 60 grams a day. Above all, you should keep in mind which foods are the most likely to cause allergic reactions. Once more, they are: eggs, milk, wheat, sugar, corn, and chocolate. Also beware of peanuts and lettuce. In the chapter on food allergies you will learn how to test foods for allergic reactions.

Bedtime snacks

As I've said before, many small meals throughout the day may suit you better than two or three large ones. You should make sure that each snack consists mainly of protein and fat. The bedtime snack is particularly important for people who tend to awaken during the night or early in the morning—often because their blood sugar has gone down. The same is true of people who awaken in the middle of the night with attacks of allergic asthma. If their blood sugar can be kept up during the night, their condition often improves. Eat a piece of meat, or eggs if you can tolerate them, and perhaps a piece of fruit—*with* protein, not alone. Don't eat a bowl of cereal, or cookies and milk as the commercials urge you to do! Milk is a taboo with me anyway (see page 102).

Avoid coffee, tea, and tobacco

Coffee, tea, and tobacco are stimulants—the square American's legal "speed." They give you a lift by stimulating your adrenalin production which raises your blood sugar. This triggers an insulin reaction, knocking your blood sugar down again, and soon you're in a familiar spiral. Whether you call this an allergic reaction, an addiction, or a chronic low blood sugar syndrome makes little difference. The effect is that you're hooked, and the only way to break the cycle is to avoid it in the first place. If you have the habit of sipping hot coffee or tea half the day, switch to herb teas. They are fragrant, hot and delicious.

Avoid all *candies, soft drinks, and baked goods*

And while we're on the subject, it is not a good idea to use artificial sweeteners either. Some people become so conditioned to the release of insulin as a response to the intake of anything sweet that the body reacts to artificial sweeteners as if they were real sugar, and releases excessive amounts of insulin just as if it *were* real sugar.

Also, if you use artificial sweeteners you tend to keep on desiring sweets, because the flavor constitutes a perpetual reminder of the forbidden taste, and becomes a constant temptation.

Altogether, in my view, food should be nourishing and adequate, but preferably not particularly appetizing. This may not be very popular advice—but believe me, it is good advice, and can add years to your life.

When food becomes too important an element of pleasure in life we tend to indulge in too much of it, become overweight, and from that we go on to all the complications of heart attacks, strokes, diabetes, and even cancer.

Since I have advised you against sweets, tobacco, alcohol, coffee, tea, and milk, you might well ask what pleasures are left to you. I'm happy to report that sexual activity does not bring on hypoglycemic attacks unless it is associated with a great deal of anxiety. An interesting sex life may make up for a boring diet. In fact, any kind of physical activity in moderate amounts is very good for the hypoglycemia sufferer. I strongly advise people with this disorder to get outdoors and walk vigorously every day for several miles, unless some medical contraindication exists.

SOME TESTS TO ASK YOUR DOCTOR FOR

When a doctor works up a patient to check for hypoglycemia it is always a good idea to get a thyroid profile. This should include at least a serum cholesterol, a T3 (thyroid), and a T4 (thyroid) test. The PBI (Protein Bound Iodine), the most commonly used thyroid test in recent years, is now being abandoned by more sophisticated physicians because its result is influenced by many medications and cannot be considered accurate. If your physician is not yet aware of this, try to inform him as tactfully as possible by telling him that your aunt or someone had a positive T3 or T4 test when the PBI was normal. If any irregularity of thyroid function is found, it should be corrected under medical supervision.

Sex hormones play an important role in the control of hypoglycemia

Proper sex hormone levels tend to have a stabilizing effect on the nervous system, which is one of the reasons why they are so important. I have often found that my male patients with hypoglycemia have low testosterone levels. Many women with hypoglycemia have low estrogen, or become worse at time when their estrogen level drops during their periods or at menopause.

Men should have their testosterone level checked either by a blood test, or by having a twenty-four-hour collection of urine tested for urinary testosterone output. The latter method is somewhat more accurate, although it is more cumbersome from the patient's point of view. Women can have their estrogen level estimated while getting a Pap smear. A quick, painless vaginal smear is taken on a sterile swab and analyzed for a maturation index to estimate the estrogen level. Also a twenty-four-hour urinary excretion test for estrogen is often in order.

Any deficiency in the sex hormones should always be corrected. This is a very important point and one that many doctors overlook.

Replace sweets with fresh vegetables and fruit

People with hypoglycemia often have an abnormal desire for sweets. They eat a lot of "empty calorie" foods that not only supply no nutrients, but actually drain the body of vitamins and minerals. As we have seen, an inadequate diet of this kind can, over a period of time, result in chronic vitamin deficiencies. Correcting the diet, removing sweets, and lowering carbohydrates stops the damage from going further. Adding vitamin and mineral supplements begins to correct the damage that has already been done.

Assuming that you have eliminated sweets and baked goods from your diet, your main source of carbohydrates will be fresh fruit and vegetables. Rely heavily on vegetables that are low in carbohydrates; eat least of potatoes and rice. Many patients with hypoglycemia are found to have low mineral levels, largely because they do not eat enough vegetables. And vegetables are very important in your diet for another reason. They provide roughage, which is essential for regular elimination.

A great point has been made lately of the fact that Americans eat a high percentage of low roughage foods and thus suffer from constipation. A low roughage diet has also been tagged as a contributing factor in the development of bowel cancer.

You may feel that the diet I have outlined is too expensive since it contains so much meat and so little of the cheaper carbohydrates. You will save some money by not using processed foods, but this diet *will* take a bigger slice out of your budget. Yet consider the compensations: the improvement in health that comes from proper diet usually results in greater well-being, greater energy, and greater efficiency at work. This should lead to your earning more money. Even if it does not, preventive medicine pays for itself many times over. You will lose depression, fatigue, nervousness, insomnia—surely that is worth something. And by decreasing your susceptibility to colds, emotional illnesses, and serious diseases, including heart ailments and cancers, you cut down on doctor bills and expensive drugs.

By following this diet and generally improving your nutrition you may increase your life span by many years, and living long is more productive than dying young. But before you dismiss this diet as not worth the money, try it for a month. A fair trial will probably add less to your normal expenses than one visit to your doctor for a flu shot. I'm sure you've gambled more before, with less promise of reward.

WARNING: People frequently feel less well the first week on a new diet. This happens because they may be experiencing withdrawal symptoms by getting away from foods to which they had an allergic addiction. Also, the bacterial make-up of the gut will gradually change.

WHAT IF YOU CHEAT?

Since people are not machines, I realize that you will probably not follow all the directions I have given you, at least not all the time. My patients don't. Even I don't. The lure of our addictions is strong, and sometimes life's pleasures seem too few and far between to allow our missing any. The "consume now, pay later" attitude is an American way of life. So, being a realist, I am going to give you some tips on how to cheat in ways that will cause the least havoc.

Please don't assume that I advise cheating; you will be much better off if you follow my diet to the letter. But I doubt that you will, at least at first.

For example, if you can't, or won't, give up smoking I suggest that you smoke only after eating; this will cause less disturbance in your carbohydrate metabolism. Also, you might buy—and use—one of the cigarette holders now on the market that can be twisted to gradually reduce the amount of smoke you take in. These are very useful, and so are the cigarette holders with filters that reduce the amount of tar you inhale.

If you must use alcohol, stay off beer, cordials, and sweet wines. Have an occasional glass of dry wine or champagne. Whiskies, if not to be recommended, are at least preferable to sweetened drinks and beer as long as you drink them straight or mix them with water or club soda. All other sodas are prohibited. Also, have your drink with or after a meal, especially a fat-protein-rich meal. Drinking on an empty stomach is particularly bad for you.

If you are going to cheat by eating sweets, you would again be well advised to eat them only after a meal generous in fats and proteins. Then the sugar will cause fewer fluctuations in your blood sugar level because your blood sugar will be sustained by the fat and protein.

Abram Hoffer, M.D., Ph.D., advocates a very clever method of cheating. He says that if you must cheat on your diet, you should select one day of the week to do all your cheating. That way you will receive a dramatic illustration of how rotten you feel when you go off your diet, and eventually this may cause you to give up your forbidden drinks, smokes, and foods. I have found this an effective method.

VITAMINS NEEDED FOR HYPOGLYCEMIA

As part of my initial work-up on a patient with hypoglycemia, I usually do laboratory tests to estimate vitamin deficiencies. The tests most often used are those for serum B_1, B_6, vitamin A, vitamin C, vitamin E, vitamin B_{12} and folic acid levels. The last two are especially important since deficiencies in these two vitamins are very widespread in our society, often pass unnoticed, and are not alleviated by the tiny amounts contained in the popular multiple vitamin tablets. To get adequate amounts of vitamin B_{12} and folic acid you need a prescription.

Yet most physicians do not test for these deficiencies. As a result, many people suffer immense hardships, because such deficiencies can cause brain damage.

Today in my office I saw a twenty-three-year-old man for the second time. He has suffered from dyslexia (the inability to read and write properly) all his life. He had been seen by a psychologist and by a neurologist. It was clear to me simply from talking with him that he was suffering from brain damage. I discovered he had very low serum B_{12} and folic acid levels. His brain damage is probably due to these vitamin deficiencies. The inability to properly absorb vitamin B_{12} and folic acid may be an inherited biochemical defect.

CHOLESTEROL ON A HYPOGLYCEMIC DIET

You may be wondering what the high animal fat content of my diet would do to your cholesterol level. There are two reasons why you needn't worry about this. First, Professor Yudkin of London University has demonstrated that the amount of sugar you eat is probably much more important in hardening your arteries than the amount of fat you eat. You will be protected from this danger by eliminating sugar from your diet. The second reason is that adequate intake of niacin (vitamin B_3) lowers the serum cholesterol and serum triglyceride levels. (It is the fat in your blood, not in your diet, that causes the danger, and cholesterol and triglycerides both are types of fat.)

My own case provides a good example. Before I started taking niacin, my serum cholesterol was 312. After taking 3000 mg. of niacin a day for several weeks, it fell to 213, which is a very respectable figure, especially since I was following a high fat, high protein diet. Niacin will do the same for you, except under some special circumstances—if you have high blood pressure, gout, or diabetes, you should hesitate about taking niacin.

With hypertension (high blood pressure) you may not feel as well with niacin as without it, in which case you should discontinue it. If you do take it, your blood pressure should be monitored closely to make certain that it does not go up. If you feel good on niacin and your blood pressure does not go up, then it is my personal opinion that you should continue taking niacin in megadoses, especially since it provides a further bonus for the hypoglycemia sufferer. It tends to raise the blood sugar level.

This is an obvious advantage for hypoglycemics, but it may cause difficulties for diabetics. I personally would not be deterred by this. If I had diabetes, I would take niacin and increase my insulin accordingly. People with diabetes are very subject to hardening of the arteries: niacin provides insurance against that.

Niacin may exacerbate gout by raising the uric acid in the blood, which is one of the symptoms of that disease. If I had gout and an elevated serum uric acid level, I think I would take niacin anyway and use one of the drugs that lower serum uric acid level. I have given niacin to patients who suffered from gout, but I have not seen any exacerbation of their symptoms because of it.

OTHER USEFUL FOOD SUPPLEMENTS

Because the use of large doses of niacin may cause a relative deficiency in other B vitamins, I would suggest that 60 mg. of riboflavin be taken daily, 100 to 200 mg. of pyridoxine (vitamin B_6) one to three times daily, and at least 100 mg. daily of thiamine (vitamin B_1). It would also be a good idea to take calcium pantothenate—about 200 mg. at bedtime. Calcium pantothenate often calms the nerves, which helps you sleep. Calcium pantothenate is also important in the metabolism of the adrenal cortex, which can have a significant effect on hypoglycemia, as we shall see later.

A crude, natural source of B vitamins is also essential. One heaping tablespoon of Torula yeast in water after breakfast and the same amount of brewers' yeast after the evening meal is very desirable. This usually lowers the blood cholesterol. Start with one-half teaspoon and gradually work up to the full dose. You'll get accustomed to the taste after a week or two.

Ascorbic acid (vitamin C) also lowers the blood cholesterol level. For this reason, and because people with low blood sugar generally feel much better on liberal amounts of ascorbic acid, I recommend that patients with hypoglycemia take at least 1000 mg. of vitamin C four times a day. When I added ascorbic acid to my vitamins my cholesterol level fell from 213 to 190. When I added two heaping tablespoons of lecithin two times a day plus one tablespoon of safflower oil two times a day, my cholesterol level went on down to a beautiful 165. And this was on a high fat diet—high in animal (saturated) fats.

In my view, cholesterol levels should be controlled with the use of these dietary supplements—not with a low-fat diet. Unfortunately, the average physician is as ignorant about lowering cholesterol with dietary supplements as he is about nutrition in general.

THE ADRENAL CORTEX

Among physicians accustomed to treating large numbers of hypoglycemia patients, adrenal cortical extract (adrenal cortex injection) is frequently used as a part of the treatment program. There is some controversy over the use of adrenal cortical extract. In a book published by the American Medical Association, entitled *AMA Drug Evaluations 1971*, it is dismissed as an obsolete preparation and is not recommended. In the front of this book, there is a list of physicians who acted as consultants in compiling this volume. In reviewing this list I failed to find any physicians with wide clinical experience in the use of adrenal cortical extract in hypoglycemia. Apparently the authors of the AMA book drew their conclusion on a theoretical basis, rather than from their own personal knowledge of the subject.

In general, endocrinologists do not appreciate the more subtle aspects of hormone preparations. They know that a massively excessive amount of thyroid hormone, for example, will produce a tense, excited, insomniac patient. But they usually do not know much about the use of thyroid preparations in conjunction with antidepressant drugs to relieve depressions quickly and effectively.

These same academicians are also very knowledgeable about certain adrenal cortical hormones such as hydrocortisone and cortisone, which are widely used in clinical medicine. But the adrenal cortex puts out more than thirty different hormones. Our knowledge of six to twelve of these hormones is extensive; our knowledge about many of the others is very meager. For anyone to assume that he knows all about adrenal cortical hormones is sheer folly, though so-called authorities frequently pretend to have such knowledge.

I know of one woman who has been treated for arthritis with

adrenal cortical hormones for many years, and has suffered most of the usual side effects. She has developed a moon face. Also, because the hormone has caused a loss of calcium from her bones, she has had bones fracture spontaneously—that is to say, without any injury. These have required repeated surgery. In sum, she has been turned into an invalid by the very medications administered in an attempt to prevent invalidism from arthritis. Her physicians have made no attempt to treat her arthritis by evaluating and eliminating food allergies, by administering large doses of ascorbic acid, or by giving her large doses of niacin.

I mention this to reassure you by contrasting these artificial hormones with the older product known as adrenal cortical extract, adrenal cortical injection, or simply as ACE. ACE is a water extraction of the whole adrenal cortex. This is a natural hormone production and contains all of the adrenal cortical hormones in their natural balance, not just one, such as cortisone. *Because it contains all of the adrenal cortical hormones, adrenal cortical extract does not produce any undesirable side effects like the artificial drugs such as cortisone, which is composed of only one of the many adrenal cortical hormones.*

When only one hormone of the adrenal cortex is administered, the whole adrenal cortex is thrown out of kilter. Your own adrenal gland cuts down production of the single hormone you take, but the other adrenal cortical hormones are secreted. Because the adrenal cortex controls so many different chemical reactions in the body, malfunctions in this gland may have widespread, disastrous results. Excessive salt (sodium chloride) may be retained in the body; or excessive loss of potassium may occur. This may result in profound difficulties such as weakness, high blood pressure, and heart failure.

People on these artificial hormones are also more prone to infections; to an increase of the pressure inside the eyeballs; to acne, excessive hair, mental disorders, weight gain from increased appetite, high blood sugar, headaches, sweating and flushing, inflammation of the pancreas, intestinal perforation, increase in the serum fat, acceleration of hardening of the arteries and heart attacks, to name only a few of the side effects.

This is a formidable array of undesirable side effects, and they are by no means rare. In fact they are almost the rule. ACE, however, has none of these side effects.

WHY NATURAL ACE IS USEFUL

My introduction to natural adrenal cortical extract quickly convinced me of its usefulness. A number of years ago I was treating a physician's wife. Over a two-year period her husband had given her injections of hard narcotics, and her addiction plus a very poor diet had gradually led her into a psychosis so profound that she hardly knew what she was doing. Instead of smoking cigarettes she would sometimes eat them. Her hemoglobin was about half of what it should have been. When I first saw her, she was so depressed that she was almost immobile. Whenever she looked at food, she thought she saw bugs crawling in it and she was close to starving because she could not bring herself to eat anything.

Because there was no time to perform the many laboratory tests that would have been desirable, I assumed that she was hypoglycemic.

I put her on a high-fat, high-protein, low-carbohydrate, sugar-free diet with multiple feedings. She received injections of iron and was given a multiple vitamin capsule that contained vitamins A, D, and six of the B vitamins, in addition to 3000 mg. of vitamin C a day, 100 mg. pyridoxine four times daily and 3000 mg. niacin daily. The niacin was gradually built up to 30,000 mg. daily which meant she was taking sixty capsules a day of niacin alone. Fortunately, she had a cast-iron stomach.

It is the general consensus among orthomolecular psychiatrists that there is no point in pushing niacin beyond 30,000 mg. daily.

("Orthomolecular" refers to straight molecules; in other words, if there are molecular [chemical] defects, then these defects should be corrected. Tradition has it that, if possible, the corrections be made with substances that already exist in the body: vitamins, minerals, etc. The term has been stretched to include all chemicals as well as diet. Orthomolecular psychiatry refers to straightening the molecules that have to do with poor function of the nervous system.) Interestingly, whenever the doctor's wife's niacin was lowered to around 26,000 mg. a day, the "bugs" would return to her food and she was unable to eat. Whenever the niacin was raised back to 30,000 mg., the bugs disappeared. Anyone who doubts the effect of niacin on emotional illness would have been convinced if they had seen how easily her eating could be started and stopped by varying her niacin intake.

After about a month on this regimen she was greatly improved. She had rejoined the human race, could laugh, talk, and carry on a conversation, but she still had periods of marked depression and suffered from insomnia that was not relieved by the usual medications. Because we seemed to have reached a plateau and because I wanted to make certain that we were doing everything possible to help her, I held several telephone consultations with various psychiatrists interested in orthomolecular psychiatry.

Dr. William H. Philpott, M.D., of Dana Point, California, suggested that I try giving her adrenal cortical extract intravenously. This was no easy matter, considering that all except one of her veins had been scarred over by the use of narcotics. But I located a vein and a supply of adrenal cortical extract, and soon began giving it to her in double-strength daily doses. The response was quite impressive, and, to me, unexpected. After the third or fourth injection she experienced a decided lessening of her mood swings, became even more alert and regained enough strength for skiing and other sports. Her night fears began subsiding and her former feeling of self-confidence returned.

Naturally, I began using adrenal cortical extract for selected patients, injecting it intravenously once or twice a week for patients with hypoglycemia. I had a clear impression of greater improvement in this patient group. Meanwhile I had also begun trying the injections on myself. They seemed particularly appropriate because I had recently suffered from influenza which had left me feeling weak and made my hypoglycemia worse. I too began to improve rapidly. My hypoglycemia was under control again, so that I no longer had to eat every two hours. After I began to feel better, I started leaving off the injections to see whether their effect was real or whether I had been experiencing a placebo effect. It did not take me long to become convinced that more than suggestion was at work. I clearly felt better with the injection of adrenal cortical extract.

As the hypoglycemic patient improves with proper diet and nutritional supplements, the adrenal cortex can usually be gradually reduced and, after a while, omitted altogether. This was true in my case too. After about a year and a half I was able to discontinue adrenal cortical injections entirely.

I should point out that there is always a good deal of time involved in the recovery from metabolic disorders, so treatment should not be discontinued prematurely.

Among doctors, the question is often asked whether or not adrenal cortex is effective if given intramuscularly rather than intravenously. I recently saw a patient whose case illuminates this subject. The middle-aged woman had visited many physicians without receiving any help, and it was easy to see why physicians had indirectly rejected her. She had an aggressive, abrasive personality and very little insight into the effect she had on others. She continually complained of discomfort in just about every organ of her body. She was aware that she had multiple allergies and her husband had been taught by one physician to give her adrenal cortical injections intramuscularly every day. She felt she could not exist without these injections, but still they did not give her the feeling of well-being which she sought. Her behavior—especially her high-pitched nasal voice—suggested to me that she might have suffered brain damage, and a blood test revealed a very low serum B_{12} level, which can often *cause* brain damage.

After prescribing corrective doses of vitamins, I also started this patient on intravenous cortical extract. Her improvement was dramatic. Immediately she developed a feeling of well-being that intramuscular injections had never given her. The explanation seems to be that when ACE is given in the vein, the adrenal cortex shuts down hormone production for a few hours and recuperates so that it functions more effectively later.

In summary, if you feel sick for any length of time and your physician can find no explanation, it is very likely that you have hypoglycemia. Have a six-hour glucose tolerance test and have it interpreted according to the criteria I have laid down. If you cannot get a six-hour glucose tolerance test, it would be safe to assume that you have hypoglycemia. If your physician approves, go on the diet I recommend, and take multiple vitamins. Frankly, the hypoglycemic diet is nothing but a well-balanced, nutritious diet which almost everyone would be well advised to follow. Nutritional supplements are almost always indicated as well.

NOTES

1. John Yudkin. *Sweet and Dangerous* (New York: Peter H. Wyden, Inc.), 1972.

THE MEGA-NUTRIENT DIET

CHAPTER TEN

I have news for you: Almost all your fellow travelers through time experience periods of anxiety, insecurity, insomnia, depression, withdrawal, shyness, rage, aggression, suspiciousness, and all the other symptoms we label neurotic or psychotic.

If you find this hard to believe, it's because you, like most people, are simply unaware of how much your neighbor suffers. You meet someone in the elevator on your way to work and exchange pleasantries about the weather. You marvel at the other fellow's serenity, wishing your problems were as few and innocuous as his.

But you only see him on stage. You are not present when he gnashes his teeth in rage, sobs in agony, curses the world, and wonders how many sleeping pills it'll take to get him out of it.

The truth is, we're all more or less twisted up, and could well use more tranquility. One reason people are often a bit on guard in the presence of psychiatrists—even in the neutral territory of a cocktail or dinner party—is their suspicion that they, too, harbor a small but dangerous seed of madness. What's more, such suspicion is well founded. Sanity and insanity are not two discrete entities, but two points along the same continuum.

Most people feel secretly ambivalent about emotional illness. They fear and resent any suggestion that they are not straight as sticks themselves, and yet—how often have you heard people say something like, "Let's go out tonight, we'll go crazy and have fun!" Or, "You'll love him—he's a crazy guy." Running amuck, letting go—going crazy—can be an appealing notion.

As Freud pointed out, two conflicting impulses work within all of us: one urging us toward life, the other toward death. And it is this conflict, I believe, that leads so many of us to make self-destructive habits a way of life.

How many times, would you guess, has a smoker, a heavy drinker, or a drug addict said, "I can quit whenever I want to, but I don't want to"? On one hand, such a person is saying that there is nothing wrong with him, that he is not out of control; on the other hand, he is also saying that he is abusing himself on purpose, because he likes to. Is that sane? Probably not. But it *is* normal.

The point is: To protest that you are "sane" is irrelevant, just as it is irrelevant to insist that you can't be suffering from a vitamin C deficiency because you don't have scurvy.

While most of us are functioning adequately, we could feel a great deal better than we do. Still, for many reasons, we resist changing old patterns.

Clinging to the known, the familiar, even when it may be dangerous or even fatal, is an inherited trait in higher primates. In nature, the animal who refuses to venture into unknown territory, avoids confrontation with unfamiliar adversaries and resists the temptation to sample every odd-looking nut or berry he comes across has a better chance of surviving than one who routinely gets lost in the woods, hasn't the sense to avoid snakes and lions, or poisons himself out of curiosity.

Professor Irvin Devore of Harvard conducted an experiment with modern baboons to find out which was stronger—the animals' fear of an enemy they knew to be deadly, or the fear of the unknown. A group of anthropologists, driving jeeps and firing rifles, chased a baboon troop across the veld. The baboons, who had been hunted by man before, ran at breakneck speed until they reached the invisible line that marked the edge of their territory; then they stopped and waited to be shot, rather than cross the line.

People tend to resist the unfamiliar in much the same way. They may stop short of waiting to be shot, but they scorn what they don't know, or make fun of it, trying to defuse it. They pretend to believe that the only people preoccupied with a natural diet are drug-crazed hippies, or old ladies in tennis shoes. They call them "health nuts." That's an interesting concept—to be concerned with health is to be crazy. A person who rejects a diet of pizza and "toastem popups" makes others uncomfortable, like a psychiatrist at a dinner-party, or a teetotaler in a roomful of drinkers. And few of us like to be set apart, or to make others uncomfortable, so we resist changing our eating habits on two counts— it's unfamiliar; and there is peer pressure not to rock the boat.

Besides, most of us really *like* our poisons. We have accumulated a set of crutches—sugar, tobacco, alcohol, and so on—and while it may not be a perfect system, it works in its way. Many of us remember a time when we didn't need two cups of coffee to get our eyes open; when we didn't have a drink every night, let alone four or five; when we could charge through an afternoon so full of energy and appetite for sheer adventure that we hated to have to stop and go home for supper. But those are dim, long lost times.

Do you feel older now, more tired, under much more pressure? Is the memory that is really strong and clear a memory of the lift you got from this morning's coffee or the ease of the first drink at night? Then those crutches are important to you because they are the reality of your life now. To contemplate giving them up, to try to believe that you could feel better without them is frightening. Especially when you count on some of these crutches most heavily to make you feel good.

And last, there is the more subtle problem—some of us don't really want to feel better.

The other day I saw a young girl in my office whom I had earlier diagnosed as extremely sensitive to wheat and sugar. After a stormy period of recovery from an emotional illness, she had begun to feel almost normal again. She had improved to the point where she was ready to re-enter the community by doing some volunteer work. The Sunday before she was to begin, she ate a plateful of macaroni, which she knew contained wheat. She followed this up with two hefty slices of cake. The predictable result was a two-week period of extreme emotional stress.

This girl was terrified of being propelled into health so fast, of losing the attention (and security) of her childlike dependency situation, of having to meet the demands society would place on her as a healthy adult. But she was also angry. Often when you feel anger or resentment at people you love, or upon whom you are dependent, you take out your hostility on yourself. This accounts in part for the furious, self-inflicted wounds a psychiatrist sees so often, the slashes on the wrists of rebellious teenagers, as well as for the self-destructive drinking, smoking, and drug use that so many of us depend on.

THE BACK-TO-NATURE DIET

As you know, I believe that the very high rate of debilitating food allergies and metabolic disorders that I see in my practice are aggravated by a diet that the human body generally is not equipped to handle. For millions of years, man's ancestors lived on a diet of meat, fish, occasional eggs, roots (such as potatoes and carrots), fruits, nuts, and vegetables; he ate what he could kill or gather. About ten thousand years ago, he learned to cultivate such grains as wheat, barley, millet, rice, and legumes (beans and peas). Gradually, his life changed from that of a wandering hunter to that of a farmer. When he began to stay settled in villages instead of roaming from place to place, he learned to domesticate animals. He kept sheep, goats, and chickens. For the first time, he could add milk, cheese, and eggs to his regular diet.

If you think of the evolution of man from his beginning to the present as being one day long, grains and dairy products only enter the picture at about fifteen minutes before midnight. Sugar appears as a dietary staple just as the bell begins to toll.

Man is a tool-using animal, a laughing animal, and a language-making animal. Above all, man is a fast-adapting animal. There are people whose chemistry has already managed to develop an ability to handle grains, sugar, and dairy products, although I contend that many of them would feel considerably better if they avoided these "new" foods. Also many young people, whose enzyme systems have not yet broken down from age and cumulative abuse, can handle the new foods more efficiently than older people. The drastic upsurge of reactive hypoglycemia and diabetes in middle age lends support to such a theory.

How much aging, heart disease, hardening of the arteries, depression, anxiety, insomnia, delinquency, alcoholism, and schizophrenia are caused by taxing less well-adaptive enzyme systems with the new foods, we do not know. More to the point: How much sickness or half-sickness do the new foods bring to your home? To find out, try the Back-to-Nature diet that I am about to describe, the diet I myself follow. You will note that it is not really different from the diet that I have discussed for hypoglycemics (see page 81 ff.), and this is perfectly appropriate because hypoglycemia, food allergies and associated conditions *are all part of the same syndrome.*

The milk controversy

Before I describe in more detail the way to design a Back-to-Nature diet for yourself, I want to discuss the question of milk and dairy products, since so many people labor under the delusion that milk is "a natural," "nature's perfect food," as the milk industry constantly tells us in their commercials.

If you are a white, middle-class American, the chances are you didn't even know a milk controversy exists. Americans have been bombarded with advertisements from the dairy industry stating flatly that "adults need at least three glasses daily" and children need a quart of milk a day or more. Perhaps it will come as a shock to you to learn that the great majority of the earth's adult population cannot digest milk properly. It gives them gas, cramps, indigestion and often causes emotional side effects such as depression and mild confusion.

Most children at about age two experience a gradual reduction of the body supply of lactase which is essential for digesting lactose, or milk sugar. In evolutionary terms this was probably one of nature's survival measures, insuring that older children would stop nursing in time for a new baby to receive all the mother's supply of milk.

In Oriental, African, and American Indian cultures adults drink little milk. Studies at Johns Hopkins University revealed that up to seventy percent of Afro-Americans cannot metabolize milk properly, a fact that gives rise to a good deal of well-justified rancor in the black community, because ethnocentric government agencies continue to waste money on milk for school lunch programs in areas where the children badly need nutritional supplements and are only made sick by being fed milk.

It is currently admitted that inability to metabolize milk and dairy products runs as high as forty percent even among adult Caucasians. I believe that our current tests for milk intolerance are incomplete, so that the actual figure is much higher. In truth, I don't believe anyone over the age of two should drink milk.

I am aware that being against milk is like being against the American flag and motherhood, but I want to emphasize that our feelings about milk have been dangerously manipulated by expensive ad campaigns from those who have most to gain by perpetuating the milk myth, just as we have been tricked by cleverly worded misinformation about "refined" sugar and grain products.

It is true that milk is an excellent and relatively inexpensive source of protein, calcium, and many vitamins for those who can handle it. But I have seen a great deal of emotional damage done to adults who are unable to metabolize milk, or who are allergic to it and who have suffered for years without even dreaming that milk could be causing the trouble.

In addition to the milk-related emotional damage I so often see in my practice, recent studies have linked *homogenized* milk to America's extremely high rate of atherosclerosis. This disease, in which the arteries are clogged or hardened by fatty tissue, leads to stroke, heart attack, and senile dementia. Kurt A. Oster, M.D., chief of cardiology at Park City Hospital, Bridgeport, Connecticut, has discovered that cow's milk (but not human milk) contains an enzyme called xanthine oxidase (or XO). Ordinarily the XO is found in fat globules that are too large to pass through your intestinal wall into your bloodstream. But when milk is homogenized, the fat globules are broken down into much smaller units; they pass easily into the bloodstream and collect in the artery walls, especially around the heart, leading to tissue degeneration and heavy cholesterol deposits. Kurt Essel Bacher, M.D., chairman of the Department of Medicine at Harvard Medical School, agrees with Dr. Oster's findings.

Studies have shown that in countries where people use large amounts of homogenized milk the death rate from heart attack is high, while in countries where little milk is consumed (or where the milk is not homogenized) the heart attack rate is much lower, even if the diet is very high in cholesterol. In one year, for example, the United States' milk intake was 273 pounds per person, and the death rate from heart disease was almost 212 per hundred thousand. In the same year the Swedes consumed 374 pounds of milk per person, but the milk was *not* homogenized; it was preboiled, which kills the enzyme XO. Despite a diet rich in cheese, butter, and eggs, the Swedes had a heart disease death rate of only 75 per hundred thousand.

If it were up to me, I would recommend that babies be given mother's milk up to the age of two, and that after that their milk intake should be eliminated. (If for any reason an infant must be given a formula, it should be made without cane sugar. It is entirely possible that the baby whose formula is laced with sucrose may grow up to be an adult with hypoglycemia or diabetes.)

Having raised my objections to milk as forcefully as possible, I must concede that a great many people will be unwilling to forego milk and dairy products. Indeed, many people probably *can* tolerate dairy products, especially in small amounts. And while I believe that many more are allergic to milk than suspect it, surely some are not.

If you plan to continue using dairy products, I urge you to test yourself for allergic reactions to them, following the procedures in the allergy chapter, and be alert for any symptoms you may experience *whenever* you eat them. Avoid homogenized milk, and consider boiling all your milk to destroy the enzyme XO. And avoid process cheeses, choose yogurt without preservatives, and if you must eat cheese, buy those cheeses that are made naturally, without the additives.

MORE OF THE BACK-TO-NATURE DIET
To start with, you should be careful that whatever you eat is in the most natural condition possible.

That means foods that are fresh, unprocessed, uncanned, unfrozen, uncolored, unflavored, and free of chemical additives. At the very least, processing destroys vital nutrients. More important, additives in processed foods can cause (or contribute to) a range of dangerous physical and mental diseases. Some two thousand of these additives are currently allowed by the FDA. Very few of them have been adequately tested. Of the ones that have, many continue in use because of pressure from wealthy food processors, *even though there is strong evidence that they are dangerous.* Several have been found to cause cancer in laboratory animals; many others speed up the growth of cancers already present. Equally important, they cause emotional disorders in a great many people.

To give one example, Dr. Ben Feingold, director emeritus of the department of allergy, Kaiser-Permanente Medical Center in San Francisco, has been studying hyperkinetic children. Hyperkinesis affects hundreds of thousands of children and adolescents. The symptoms are extreme hyperactivity, aggressive behavior, short attention span, insomnia, a very low frustration threshold, and other forms of behavior so disruptive that many of these children have to be put in special schools.

When it was discovered that, unlike adults, hyperkinetic children calmed down when given amphetamines (or "speed"), a furor developed over the practice in many schools of urging the parents to put their children on permanent doses of speed to make the youngsters easier to handle.

Dr. Feingold took the opposite approach by prescribing a diet that was completely drug-free and contained no preservatives, flavorings, colorings, pesticides, or hormones. Within one week, many of the children in his study were completely symptom-free. But their hyperkinesis could be reactivated in some cases by as little as a single commercially-baked doughnut.

In my own practice, I have found many individuals who develop emotional reactions to pesticides, food colorings, chemical preservatives, and the antibiotics and hormones fed to cattle, chickens, and other livestock.

For these people, a diet of "organic" food is essential, especially during the first phases of therapy, no matter how difficult it may be to obtain it. They should buy all fruits, vegetables, meats, and nuts from a reliable source of organic produce. This is usually, of necessity, the local health food store, although it is cheaper to join or form an organic food cooperative whose members pool time and resources and buy directly from a reliable grower, in bulk.

If it is not possible for you to find or afford pure food, at least see that your fruits and vegetables are clean.

To remove pesticides and chemical fertilizer as much as possible, scrub fruit and vegetables with a vegetable brush, using warm water and Ivory soap (Ivory soap is low in perfumes and has low allergenicity.) Rinse well, first in warm water, then cold. Grapes should be removed from the stems, placed in a bowl of warm water, and washed like other fruit. Some people recommend removing the peels of fruit and vegetables. Since the peel often contains most of the nutrients, I hesitate to suggest that you discard it.

I regret that there are plenty of unscrupulous retailers who will be happy to sell you "organic" produce at greatly inflated prices that is not organic at all. But you can often tell if the food you buy is really organically produced.

Organic vegetables often have much more intense (and better) flavor than those grown with synthetic chemicals. If you have a garden and grow your own vegetables, you already know how much difference it makes to have a tomato ripen naturally on the vine. Organic fruits also *look* different from fruits grown with benefit of pesticide. They are not so large, perfectly shaped, or plastic looking. Nor do they have that glossy wax coat that makes supermarket fruit so appealing—and so likely to make you ill. Organically produced meats, which you can buy frozen at some health food stores, tend to be tough, very lean, and a little gamey tasting—like game, in fact, which is also "organically" grown. This new taste is an interesting adventure. I strongly recommend that you try a completely organic diet at least for a couple of weeks to see if it makes a difference in the way you feel.

If you think that this is unnecessary, if you wonder what could be wrong with a nice, fresh, nationally advertised brand of chicken, consider that a commercially grown chicken goes from egg to butcher block in six weeks—six weeks! What if you fed the same growth hormones to your own children? They would grow up in two years instead of twenty and you'd save a fortune in groceries. Unfortunately, in addition to making chickens grow faster, the chemicals in ordinary commercial chicken can also make cancers grow faster. During butchering, these chickens are often found to have abnormal growths and tumors. It is common practice for cancerous parts to be thrown away (or used in pet food) while the rest is packaged and sold as "cut up chicken parts." Bon appétit!

Always stay away from processed meats such as Spam, bologna, commercial sausage, bacon, and ham. They are often loaded with sodium nitrate, among other chemicals, one of the most dangerous of the common food additives. I know firsthand that sodium nitrate produces many emotional symptoms in adults as well as children.

WHAT I EAT, MEAL BY MEAL

I have already described the many differences in individual nutritional needs. Obviously, then, I am not going to turn about and give you a rigid diet and assure you that it will be just right for you. Even though I champion meats and fats, I have some patients who must totally avoid all animal products. In the chapter on allergy I help you establish your own proper diet.

First, a little introduction. Assume you have hypoglycemia. It's very common, especially among people who think enough about food to buy a book such as this. The same goes for people who have nutrition allergies.

For these reasons, unless proved otherwise your diet should be based mostly on meats and animal fats, laced with roots (such as potatoes), berries and fruits (for desserts), and nuts (if you aren't fighting the weight problem). Multiple small meals are usually better than three large meals. Brown rice is the best grain. Why we handle rice well, I cannot say. But clinical experience has proven to me that rice is usually handled well by the body. To re-emphasize: our ancestors ate the foods I have mentioned for many millions of years, so evolution has equipped us with enzyme systems to handle these foods. We weren't designed to live in a zoo and eat over-engineered food. Some hardy souls thrive on such treatment, but many of us fail to bloom under such adverse conditions.

Now I am going to describe what I eat and why, and what I don't eat and why. From this you will be able to form guidelines for your own diet. You should, as I've said, start with the most natural diet you can manage. In this chapter I will deal with foods, but you should keep in mind that this diet is only part of a nutritional program that includes vitamin and mineral supplements as well. These will be dealt with in subsequent chapters.

MY BREAKFAST

I start the day with a hot cup of weak tea, mainly because my body interprets it as a friendly way to start the day. Then I have the lazy man's food: two heaping tablespoons of granular lecithin mixed with one tablespoon safflower oil, followed by a whole grapefruit and a heaping tablespoon of Torula yeast in water. Sometimes I include a hard-boiled egg, a chop, or a chicken leg. Next, I take my morning vitamins and minerals. After this boost, I enter the day full sail.

A high-protein, high-fat breakfast will help you maintain steady blood sugar levels throughout the day. You might follow my example or have eggs or meat, usually hamburger, chops, or steak. Don't overcook the meat because that drains away the fat, and the fat is important in keeping your blood sugar up.

Many people would rather starve than cook in the morning. But don't use that as an excuse to eat toast and corn flakes! You can cook the meat the night before and eat it cold in the morning, or you can hard-boil some eggs. By way of fruit, you might substitute bananas, apples, oranges, or anything you like instead of grapefruit. For many reasons, it's much better to have the whole fruit rather than the juice.

Most people should have a mid-morning snack. I don't need it.

MY LUNCH

At lunch, I eat a large portion of meat. My lifestyle is such that I must eat many of my meals in restaurants. I might eat differently if I were at home (and if I were a better cook than I am). In a restaurant I consider it safest to order broiled meat—steak or pork or lamb chops or liver. From the standpoint of both allergies and hypoglycemia, plain foods are safest unless you know the cook. I never order anything with a sauce. If I were at home, I could, presumably, make stews and meat loaves.

With my large portion of meat at lunch I eat a salad with safflower oil and lemon dressing, a vegetable, perhaps a small potato or some brown rice, and fresh fruit for dessert. If you, too, are eating in a restaurant, be wary of "fresh fruit cocktail." Insist that it contain *no* canned fruit. Almost all canned fruit contains extra sugar even when it's labeled dietetic. You'll be better off ordering whole fruit. Most restaurants can at least produce an orange or grapefruit; if not, skip dessert and get a piece of fruit at a grocery store.

Three big meals or six small ones?

You may feel that what I've just described is an awful lot to eat for lunch. Perhaps it would be, for you. I find that I look, feel, and perform better on this diet than I ever did before. I don't get hungry between meals, and I experience none of the restless cravings that accompany most diets.

Some people find themselves growing hungry and uncomfortable in the middle of the morning or afternoon, no matter what they had at mealtime. For them, it would be better to eat six small meals a day than three large ones. After all, eating three meals is an arbitrary social convention. An animal in the wild eats when he's hungry and stops when he's satisfied.

The last point is important. Many of us have so abused our natural appetite controls that we scarcely know whether we're hungry or not; or, rather, we seem to want food all the time and therefore develop very unnatural eating habits that have little to do with the messages we get from our bodies.

A conventional diet describes what to eat at breakfast, lunch, and dinner. It forbids you to swallow anything in between even if you're going into a low-blood sugar coma, and makes you feel so irritable and deprived that you eat every scrap on your plate at meals, even if you don't need or want it all. Instead of following a diet on a piece of paper, it is important to get back in touch with your body. Eat slowly, and give your body time to let you know when it's had enough. When it has, *stop eating!* When you're actually hungry again, you can eat again.

Think of all the times when you've arrived at a meal feeling hungry, and very quickly ate everything in sight. What happens? By the time your blood sugar has gone up and your system shouts "stop," you have already eaten much more than you need, and your stomach feels painfully stretched, as if you had swallowed a brick. You've tricked your appetite control mechanism, but the joke is on you.

If you eat at home, you can easily arrange to have small meals when you need them instead of the arbitrary big three. If you work in an office it is harder to explain that you require three lunch periods (although if you dart out quickly several times a day you may get away with it). Or you can have meat sandwiches sent in, and discard the bread; or you can bring what you need from home.

For snacks, the usual raw vegetables are fine. Organically grown or unprocessed nuts are fine (again, watch cashews because they're high in carbohydrates). Roasted soynuts are high in protein. Beef tea or bouillon would be an ideal protein snack, if you can find one that isn't loaded with chemical additives. Fresh fruit should only be eaten with protein for snacks—say an apple with a piece of cold chicken. Try half a banana, sprinkled with lecithin and two tablespoons of safflower oil. The safflower oil can substitute for the protein since, like meat, it will tend to stabilize your blood sugar.

MY DINNER

For dinner I recommend a really large piece of meat, a pound or a pound and a half. When I tell my patients to eat large amounts of meat, they sometimes interpret this as meaning a middling size piece once a day. That may be enough to satisfy the minimum daily protein requirement set forth by the AMA and the FDA, but we have no way of knowing whether this is truly adequate. We do have strong evidence that our ancestors were heavy meat eaters for millions of years. I believe the real "minimum daily requirement" is considerably higher than currently suspected.

The rest of my dinner is the same as lunch. I have a vegetable, a salad with safflower oil dressing, a potato or brown rice, and perhaps some fruit. (Of course if you aren't hungry for all that, don't eat it.) Many people with hypoglycemia can't tolerate nearly as much fruit and starch as that. I have found I do fine on that diet as long as I completely eliminate bakery goods, and as far as I'm concerned, there is every reason to eliminate them. But if you think or know you have hypoglycemia, and the diet I take is not making you feel all that much better, cut out some or all of the fruit, rice and potatoes, and see how that works for you.

Those essential fatty acids

You will have noticed that several times I have mentioned the need for including safflower oil in your diet. Of course this would be anathema on a conventional low-calorie diet, but fats help keep your blood sugar up, as I have said before, and make you feel less hungry. Unsaturated fats also contain important nutrients which, for want of a better term, are called "essential fatty acids." Since they *are* essential they might well be called vitamins, except that you need them in daily amounts of several grams, and convention dictates that a "vitamin" be taken in quantities of milligrams or less. Fatty acids are essential for proper growth and reproduction, for healthy skin and hair, and for resistance to environmental stresses such as X-rays. They are present in corn, peanut, and cottonseed oil, but the best sources are sunflower and safflower oil (olive oil, butter and coconut butter contain little or none).

You should buy safflower or sunflower oil at a health food store (they are not generally available elsewhere). Cold-pressed (this is indicated on the label) oil is preferable; the heat used in normal oil processing destroys some beneficial qualities. Use these oils for cooking and on fruits and raw vegetables, and try to take at least two tablespoons a day. If you don't like oil undisguised, you can buy safflower oil mayonnaise at a health food store. Be certain that the safflower oil and mayonnaise contain no preservatives. Keep them in the refrigerator, along with the lecithin, after opening.

COOKING FOR MAXIMUM NUTRITION

In general, avoid cooking anything (except eggs) in liquid, unless you plan to eat the liquid as well as the solid. If you braise or marinate meat or vegetables, be sure you eat the liquid as sauce or gravy. If you boil or stew or poach meat, fish, fruit, or vegetables, eat the liquid or save it in the freezer and use it in soup stock. Avoid overcooking meat or vegetables; many nutrients are drained away during cooking and others are lost in the steam. If you can smell the food cooking, then you are losing nutrients and flavor.

For vegetables, the method of cooking is especially critical, and in the United States they are routinely cooked in a way that seems calculated to destroy their nutritional value. Soaking and/or boiling is the worst; so many vitamins and minerals leach out into the water that you'd probably be better off throwing out the vegetable and drinking the cooking water.

Steaming vegetables is far better, although in most American restaurants they are badly overcooked so that, again, much of the food value is lost in the steam. The best plan is to steam vegetables only until they are tender and not a moment longer, or to sauté them very quickly in a little hot fresh oil as the Chinese do (vegetables should be warmed through, but still crunchy and barely wilted). But be warned: In American-Chinese restaurants, vegetables are usually deliberately over-cooked because Americans demand vegetables with the consistency of mush. And beware of MSG in Chinese restaurants. Their cooks seem to be addicted to it. When you quiz them about MSG they will smile and give you the polite answer they think you want. Usually they haven't understood your question.

If you are not sensitive to MSG, it often makes food taste better. But it is a chemical to which people are very commonly sensitive, and it can cause any sort of reaction. Some people become confused. Other people get depressed or even schizophrenic. I myself become very sleepy and lethargic. Any emotional symptom that you can name can be produced by MSG. MSG is widely known to bring on a "Chinese food headache."

An insufficient intake of vegetables is one of the major deficiencies in the American diet, even among people who think they eat a lot of vegetables.

WHAT TO DRINK

You will not be surprised that I suggest that milk be omitted. Also, omit soft drinks, since sugar and sugar substitutes both cause problems. A small amount of fruit juice might be needed to disguise the taste of the yeast you take twice a day. But again: fruit juices are not otherwise recommended. Vegetable juices are acceptable. They are high in nutrients and low in carbohydrates. They make a nice change of pace in your diet, and they are handy.

I'm lucky enough to get away with drinking coffee, though for several years after starting my hypoglycemic program coffee would only lift me to an abnormal high and then, an hour later, bang me down as if I had been hit over the head with a two-by-four. Most people should cut down or give up tea and coffee. Decaffinated coffee may be suitable for you. Herb teas are usually well tolerated. Plenty of water is a good idea.

CAUTION: You may be allergic to fluorine and chlorine and other additives and impurities that turn up increasingly in public water supplies. In that case, you should buy bottled spring water, or distill your own. A naturally sparkling mineral water with a twist of lemon will taste great after living in a liquid Sahara.

You should, of course, cut out alcohol. But if you can't, or won't, stick to dry (non-sweet) drinks: Scotch, gin, bourbon, a dry wine, etc. The kind of mix you use is very important, since many contain sugar. A natural mineral water is your best choice. After water, club soda is the second-best mix.

NOTE: Cheap wines and liquors contain fewer impurities (it is the impurities that give wines and liquors their character, not the straight alcohol they contain) so they are recommended over the expensive brands. Hangovers are really severe allergic reactions. I myself have occasionally been so depressed by good wine that I felt like doing myself in, though I can tolerate an occasional glass of inexpensive white wine.

People with hypoglycemia who use alcohol should drink it with meals or after meals. Hypoglycemics may never improve unless they completely eliminate alcohol for the first few years of their treatment. And alcohol can be harmful for people with food allergies.

IS IT WORTH IT?

We are all constantly engaged in assigning values to what we do. If longevity is not among your overriding ambitions, if you don't much care whether you grow senile or spend your most productive years feeling less than your best, by all means follow your own dietary inclinations. If you *are* considering trying my way, the first decision you must make is not whether you want to feel your best—of course you do.

The question is: Do you want it badly enough to make some sacrifice for it—not for a day, a week, or a month, but for good?

Remember—the body goes through a period of adjustment on a new diet. As a result, you may feel worse during the first seven or eight days on a different diet. So a bit of extra patience is valuable.

HOW VITAMINS HELP
CONTROL YOUR NERVES

CHAPTER ELEVEN

Vitamins are organic substances, as opposed to inorganic substances such as a rock or a steel bar. They are needed in minute amounts for us to grow and reproduce. We must have them if we are to live, because vitamins help the chemical changes that take place in our bodies.

Vitamins often have help from minerals (such as iron or calcium) and from proteins. This collection of vitamins, minerals, and proteins makes up an enzyme system. For example, the enzyme called *carboxylase* is made up of *thiamin* (vitamin B_1) and *magnesium* (mineral) and a *protein.*

Enzymes make possible the chemical changes that take place in our bodies. Don't let the word "chemical" throw you. There's nothing difficult about "chemical."

Everything is a chemical—or a collection of chemicals. The gasoline in your car is a chemical. When the gas explodes in the cylinders of your car engine, that is a chemical change. The sparks from the sparkplugs cause the explosion, the chemical change.

Enzymes act like your spark plug. Enzymes, for example, help the

115

cells of your body turn a steak (a collection of chemicals) into energy so you can breathe and walk and shake your fist at a baseball umpire.

Our bodies cannot make vitamins. We must either eat them or have them by injection. We have learned to recreate in the laboratory the vitamins that occur in nature. These are called synthetic vitamins.

NATURAL VS. SYNTHETIC VITAMINS

Most chemists maintain that for biological purposes no difference exists between manufactured vitamins and those occurring in nature. I am not so sure. Some of our foremost scientists, perhaps secure enough to be able to admit ignorance, stress that we have not yet worked out the entire vitamin puzzle.

For example, one evening before dinner I was talking with Albert Szent-Gyorgy, Nobel Prize-winner for artificially making vitamic C. He remarked that vitamin C needs substances to work with it, substances still unknown to us.

"Whatever the unknown substance might be, it's not in those," he remarked as he pointed at a table heavy with French pastries. "It's something in there," and he indicated a salad bowl.

A London aquarium acquired some fish that could only survive in seawater. Since the formula for seawater is known, the chemicals needed to make it were assembled and mixed. But when the fish were placed in it, they died. Several times, with meticulous care, the ingredients were mixed again—each time with the same result. Finally, still another batch was made, and to it was added a small amount of real seawater. And in this mixture the fish thrived. Obviously, the addition of real seawater made the difference; but what this difference consists of, no one yet knows.

Some years ago an article in the *Journal of Nutrition*[1] reported the results of a research project carried out at the Agricultural Research Center in Beltsville, Maryland. It was found that rats' growth rates were greatly impaired while they were on an artificial diet that contained all the known substances needed for rat nutrition. When natural food was added to their diet, proper growth promptly resumed. The inference is that the natural food contained substances not present in the artificial product.

Several studies have established that natural vitamins A and D are much less toxic than the artificially produced variety. It has been reported that synthetic vitamin D in the recommended dosage to prevent rickets has caused toxicity in children, while there have been no such reports about natural vitamins A and D taken in normal dosage.[2]

The Canadian Medical Association[3] reported on fifteen cases of skin disease which were treated by injections of synthetic vitamin B with no improvement. When yeast or liver extract (both rich sources of vitamin B) were given to these patients, the benefits became quickly manifest.

The *Vitamin Research News*[4] of the Soviet Union reported on vitamin C-deficient guinea pigs which recovered much more quickly on doses of natural vitamin C than on the synthetic form.

It was reported in the *American Review of Tuberculosis*[5] that patients suffering from tuberculosis responded much better when given natural vitamins A and D in the form of cod liver oil than when the same substances were administered in synthetic form.

In 1934, William P. Murphy, George R. Minot, and George H. Whipple shared a Nobel Prize for discovering that pernicious anemia could be controlled by injections of liver extract. During the late 1940s, Murphy began to switch from crude liver extracts (which contain a wide spectrum of the B-complex vitamins) to purified vitamin B_{12}, which had been demonstrated to control pernicious anemia as well as the crude liver product. Murphy found that purified B_{12} did indeed prevent and control pernicious anemia. Many of his patients insisted, nonetheless, on going back to the crude extract, because they had lost the sense of well-being it had provided. These patients were receiving benefits from the natural substance that were missing from the synthetic product.

Dr. Murphy, one of the great living heroes of the medical world, is still practicing medicine in Brookline, Massachusetts. In correspondence with me, he said that crude liver probably contains a vitamin or some other similar substance that we have not yet discovered.

My own case provides an interesting example of the desirability of taking natural vitamins, as well as of the variable effects of different forms of administration. Last winter I developed a severe case of allergic dermatitis on my hands. The two dermatologists I consulted recommended cortisone and superficial X-ray therapy. Neither inquired into my dietary habits or vitamin intake. An injection of cortisone did almost completely heal my hands for a week, but when the cortisone wore off the inflammation promptly returned. Other preparations were tried, with similar results.

It became more and more obvious to me that these two specialists were concentrating exclusively on the local disease process while ignoring possibly underlying nutritional and metabolic factors. On my own, I decided to give myself an injection of crude liver extract. Though I was already taking large amounts of all the *known* B-complex vitamins by pill, the effect of the crude liver injection was prompt and dramatic. My hands cleared up completely.

I still require one crude liver extract injection weekly. Whenever I skip it, I invariably develop a lesion near the nail on the fourth finger of my right hand. Equally invariably, it clears up again after the injection. When I take desiccated liver capsules by mouth, or eat another vitamin B-rich compound such as brewers' yeast, the finger dermatitis is not prevented. Hence, I conclude that not only do I need crude B-complex vitamins, but that these must be taken by injection to be effective in my case. Apparently the oral route evidently does not result in sufficient absorption.

The modern environment is murder on our vitamin intake. Not only is the vitamin content of food greatly reduced by the way it is handled before we eat it, but factors such as smog vastly increase our need for several vitamins—notably C and E. We end up with a reduced intake of vitamins and an increased need for them. Remember that smog is not limited to Los Angeles and New York. It is a blight that covers almost all of the country and much of the world. Even in remote mountain regions of Appalachia the natives speak of the deterioration of visibility during their lifetime.

Freezing destroys vitamin K, and vitamin C is destroyed by cooking. What few vegetables we get in our modern diet are overcooked, so that much of the vitamin content is lost.

Drugs are another hazard. Many widely-used ones (such as aspirin, birth control pills, and antibiotics) either destroy vitamins, keep them from being absorbed, or interfere with their utilization. Diuretics are frequently prescribed for women who suffer from so-called idiopathic (cause unknown) edema (fluid accumulation).* These drugs effectively

* Usually there is nothing idiopathic about it: it's often caused by food and environmental allergies, by vitamin B_6 deficiency, or a thyroid deficiency.

eliminate their excess fluid along with vital sodium, potassium, magnesium, and B vitamins. Birth control pills interfere with vitamin B_{12}, folic acid, and vitamin B_6 metabolism.

Recently, Louis F. Wertalik, of the Ohio State University College of Medicine, reported that in a group of healthy young women, birth control pills had greatly reduced serum B_{12} levels, and had also somewhat diminished serum folic acid levels. He was unable to explain the mechanism by which the oral contraceptives produced this effect. Despite the low serum B_{12} levels, he had found the women's tissue levels to be adequate. It may therefore be that the serum levels were simply not reduced for a sufficiently long time to cause a reduction in the tissue levels, and that if oral contraceptives had been continued, the tissue levels would have shown a drop within a year or two.

Mineral oil blocks absorption of the fat-soluble vitamins A, D, and K. Iron, which is frequently prescribed for anemia and forms part of many over-the-counter tonics, interferes with the absorption of vitamin E. The use of tobacco is very destructive to vitamin C. Radiation therapy is destructive to many vitamins.

In recognition of these and many other detrimental circumstances, George M. Owen, M.D., of Ohio State University Children's Hospital, has stated a fact that cannot be sufficiently emphasized: The current nutritional status of the people of the United States is simply *not known.* But we have plenty of alarming clues: The U.S. Department of Agriculture, through Assistant Secretary of Agriculture George L. Mehren, has stated that at least thirty-eight percent of the families in this country live on diets that do not even meet the minimal nutrition requirements set forth by the National Academy of Sciences. As a matter of fact, *even the Food and Nutritional Board of the FDA has admitted that its guidelines concerning allowances for nutritional substances don't necessarily reflect the needs of any one person or group, since these can only be determined by clinical and biochemical examination.*

Nor is sub-standard nutrition confined to "backward" rural areas in the poorer Southern states. A survey of 642 New York City children revealed that seventy-three percent subsisted on diets that did not measure up to the National Research Council's recommendation for daily allowances. According to the Bureau of Nutrition of the New York Department of Health, these children had low blood levels of many of the B vitamins, especially vitamin B_{12}, and niacin, and suffered significant reading disabilities. Dr. George Christakis, director of the survey, urged that these children be given vitamin supplements.

Since excess amounts of the water-soluble vitamins are excreted by the body, it is my firm opinion that large quantities of these vitamins can and should be taken. For the fat-soluble vitamins A, D, and E, on the other hand, the possibility of toxicity does exist under certain circumstances, and much closer attention must therefore be paid to their dosage. The guidelines of the FDA are, however, worse than useless. Most of its recommendations are based on no discernible logic, and some are downright contradictory.

I dislike writing about one vitamin at a time, saying vitamin C helps wound-healing or that vitamin D is needed to absorb calcium, for example. *Each cell in the body needs every vitamin.* Indeed, vitamins do not occur in the food we eat one at a time, isolated from each other.

Space makes it impossible for me to expand on the subject as I would like. This is a practical book in which I hope to teach you what vitamins to take and how to take them.

If you want to know about the separate vitamins intimately, you will find many books by experts without clinical experience who can enlighten you. But not many people who write about vitamins are physicians who sit across the desk from patients day after day, year after year, helping people work out their dietary supplements. This is the unique information I have. This special knowledge is what you bought the book for.

With this preview in mind, let me give you a very brief introduction to vitamins to help you nod hello to them.

YOUR VITAMIN A NEEDS

Numerous studies have established vitamin A as one of the vitamins most frequently missed in the American diet. This deficiency has been noted many times in surveys of children in New York City. Remember, vitamin D and calcium cannot work properly without vitamin A, since vitamin A deficiency affects the skeleton and limits its growth. The central nervous system of growing children can sustain severe mechanical damage because the brain and other parts of the central nervous system continue to grow without a corresponding increase in size of the bony structures. In adults, this deficiency causes a number of symptoms, among them the well-known "night blindness," and the appearance of rough, scaly skin patches, especially on the upper arms. I well remember suffering from the latter condition myself during my teens, and have no doubt that it was brought on by vitamin A deficiency.

The vitamin protects us against colds, pneumonia, and influenza, and a deficiency may result in inadequate protection of the mucous membranes against infection. Bladder stones have also been produced in rats in a vitamin A deficiency state.

The vitamin occurs in large amounts in carrots, liver, and sweet potatoes, and in smaller amounts in many other vegetables. But I do not think it wise to depend upon food intake for an adequate supply. This applies especially to diabetics, who have difficulty in transforming the carotene of yellow vegetables into vitamin A.

Because synthetic forms of vitamins A and D are apparently more toxic than natural ones, I suggest that you confine yourself to supplements made from natural sources of these two vitamins.

Dr. Henry Sherman of Columbia University[6] was able to increase the longevity of rats by giving them added amounts of vitamin A. In his experiments he used the Osborne-Mendel strain of rats, that had been doing quite well on a diet of whole wheat and milk for sixty-seven generations, and whose lifespan was precisely known. If there had been any significant defects in this diet, they would of course have shown up long before sixty-seven generations had come and gone. Nonetheless, by doubling the amount of vitamin A in their standard diet, Dr. Sherman caused the male rats to live five percent longer, and the female ones to live ten percent longer than expected. When he redoubled the amount of vitamin A, the males lived ten percent longer and the females twenty percent longer. A second doubling of the vitamin A dose did not result in any further increase of lifespan. Extrapolating from these figures to human terms might mean that our lifespan could be increased from about 70 to about 110 or 120 years.

No one as yet knows whether these or similar findings are applicable to humans. But since we are betting our health and our lives on our intake of nutrients, I, for one, am going to place one of my bets on supplements of vitamin A.

F. C. H. Ross, M.D., and H. A. H. Campbell, M.D.,[7] reported on an interesting study in which they administered vitamins A and D for ten years to a group of patients. In the treated group, the incidence of coronary heart disease was 5.8 percent; in the untreated group it was 15.8 percent. This may tie in with the well-known fact that the cholesterol level has a tendency to drop when vitamin A is administered.

In laboratory animals many birth defects have occurred in the offspring of mothers deficient in vitamin A. Do you want to take the chance of having malformed children or do you want to take vitamin A?

Medical textbooks state that toxic effects of vitamin A may be noted if more than 50,000 units a day are taken over a long period of time. In my opinion, this is a very conservative figure. Vitamin A intoxication is an extremely rare occurrence, and usually involves the artificially produced vitamin. (One of the signs of toxicity of vitamin A may be emotional instability.)

I take 10,000 units of natural vitamin A daily. Whenever I have any upper respiratory symptoms, I double this amount for a week or so. Ten thousand units is also the minimal dose level I recommend to all my patients, whatever the degree of their emotional symptoms.

YOUR VITAMIN B₁ NEEDS

Thiamin (vitamin B_1) is the granddaddy of the "nerve" vitamins. It is essential for the proper functioning of the central nervous system, and its lack can result in almost any nervous manifestation you can name: depression, difficulty in concentration, fatigue, tension, hyperactivity, confusion, disorientation, hallucinations, numbness in the arms or legs, and many more. Although the brain makes up only two percent of the total body weight, twenty-five percent of total metabolic activity takes place within it. Therefore the brain is extremely sensitive to a lack of vitamins.

Thiamin also acts as a co-enzyme necessary for the oxidation of pyruvic acid, which is a step in the process of carbohydrate metabolism. Since carbohydrates are the central nervous system's prime source of energy, thiamin is particularly important to the proper functioning of that system.

A person who does heavy physical labor needs extra thiamin to compensate for a stepped-up carbohydrate metabolism. For this reason the amounts required for good health vary somewhat, but the FDA (Food and Drug Administration) states that 1.5 mg. of thiamin per day is your recommended daily allowance. Vitamin B_1 is present in many foods but tends to be depleted by the consumption of sugar, alcohol, and tobacco. Vitamin B_1 is lost in storing and preparing food, especially when an alkaline salt like sodium bicarbonate (baking soda) is added to foods during cooking. High temperatures destroy much of the thiamin in meat. When water is used for cooking vegetables, thiamin is leached out.

One of the greatest losses of thiamin is caused by the milling of grains. When the outer husk of the grain is removed, much of the vitamin and mineral content is removed with it. White bread and white rice are, therefore, relatively thiamin-deficient foods. Even though thiamin may be added to enriched bread, it is partially destroyed again by toasting. The symptoms of thiamin deficiency were described by a Chinese physician as early as 2600 B.C., and the problem has not abated since then.

In 1872 a young Japanese navy scientist, Kanehiro Takaki, became appalled at the amount of beri-beri occurring among sailors on long voyages. It seemed logical to suspect a dietetic cause. A crew of 276 left Japan for a trip to New Zealand, South America, Hawaii, and back. Of this crew, 169 developed beri-beri and 25 died of it. Another ship was sent on the same voyage, but with increased rations of meat, fish, and vegetables, and decreased amounts of rice. Wheat and milk were also added to the sailors' diet. On this second voyage no deaths from beri-beri occurred, though fourteen men developed the disease. These fourteen, it developed, had not eaten the full diet as prescribed. Takaki reported his findings in the British medical journal *Lancet*, but the article was ignored by the medical profession, which at the time was convinced that beri-beri was an infectious disease. The struggles proving it to be a nutritional deficiency disease were much like those undergone by James Lind in proving ascorbic acid to be the factor causing scurvy in the British Navy, and the struggles of Joseph Goldberger early in this century to prove pellagra a disease of nutritional rather than infectious origin.

Since thiamin is water soluble, it is rather quickly excreted by the body and cannot build up to toxic levels like vitamins A, D, and E. I therefore have no qualms about taking and prescribing it in substantial amounts. For myself, I buy the 500 mg. sugar-free, starch-free thiamin tablet, and generally take anywhere from a fourth to a half to a whole one after breakfast every morning.

Patients sometimes get such a lift from thiamin that they need a sedative to calm them down. I vividly remember one doubting physician to whom I once gave a 500 mg. tablet. A few hours later he called to tell me that he felt as if he had taken a handful of speed tablets. A sodium amytal capsule was necessary to bring him "down" to working level. This memorable experience convinced him of the tremendous chemical changes which vitamins can evoke. Oddly enough, thiamin in large amounts can have a lifting effect on tired or depressed people and a tranquilizing effect on excited people. To some patients I administer as much as 2000 mg. of thiamin three times a day, and find it to be the decisive nutritional supplement which makes the difference between their feeling ill or well.

Some individuals do much better on thiamin by injection. Occasionally, people need as much as 1000 mg. daily by injection either to raise themselves out of the valley of depression or to pull themselves down from cloud nine. Physicians experienced in the treatment of alcoholics have often found that thiamin in massive doses helps provide relief from the emotional and physical symptoms of alcoholism.

YOUR VITAMIN B₂ NEEDS

The next vitamin on our list is riboflavin, or vitamin B_2. Although widely available in nature, it too is among the most common dietary deficiencies in our society. Cooking does not destroy a great deal of it, unless baking soda is used. Light causes some destruction; but probably the most common cause of riboflavin deficiency is poor dietary habits. The vitamin is available in relatively large amounts in liver and brewers' yeast, and there is a fair amount in many vegetables. But these items do not form a significant part of modern man's diet. Even when you do eat riboflavin, you need proper amounts of hydrochloric acid in the gastric secretions to absorb it efficiently. I am now beginning to test patients with emotional disorders for hydrochloric acid in the stomach, and I frequently find it to be low, especially among the elderly.

 • If you take a relatively large dose of riboflavin it is fairly easy to prove whether or not you are absorbing it properly. If you are absorbing substantial amounts, your urine will turn a rich yellow color.

Riboflavin is active in several enzyme systems, and its lack may cause a wide spectrum of symptoms, including cracks in the corners of the mouth, scaly rashes on nose and forehead, burning and dryness of the eyes, inability to tolerate bright lights, burning of feet, depression, dizziness, and numbness in the arms and legs. Any or all of these deficiency symptoms may coexist, as well as night blindness similar to that caused by lack of vitamin A. Riboflavin is necessary for proper growth, and there is evidence that its lack may increase your susceptibility to infections.

For a number of years I suffered from a mild scaliness of the skin around my nose. I consulted a dermatologist at the University of Chicago clinic, whose only comment was that the condition would probably improve after I passed middle age. He did not check my dietary habits, nor did he perform any vitamin determinations to see whether I was getting the proper amounts of vitamins. In 1961 I consulted a physician at Columbia-Presbyterian Hospital in New York because of numbness in my fingers. Again no history of my dietary habits was taken, and no measurements made to determine my body's vitamin levels. Both symptoms have disappeared now that I take multiple vitamins including riboflavin (and I have not yet passed middle age).

Lack of riboflavin has produced nerve degeneration and malformed offspring in laboratory animals. My usual riboflavin intake is 60 mg. daily. Some authorities believe that riboflavin intake should equal B_6 intake. My clinical experience does not agree with them. Personally, I do quite well on this intake of riboflavin even though I take 400 mg. daily of vitamin B_6.

YOUR VITAMIN B_3 NEEDS

The first vitamin that fascinated me was vitamin B_3, also known as niacin, niacinamide, nicotinic acid, or nicotinamide. Niacin has been one of the vitamins neglected by mankind during the entire course of civilization. Its severe lack has resulted in dermatitis, diarrhea, dementia, pellagra, and even death. But perhaps more germane to our discussion are the innumerable cases of people who have missed out on optimal emotional and physical health because of their less-than-optimal niacin levels.

There is evidence that niacin may prolong life and put off the senility which too frequently mars our final years. Edwin Boyle, M.D., director of research at the Miami Heart Institute, states that when he administers niacin to middle-aged people for the prevention of heart attacks, they almost invariably return to his office with dramatically increased vigor. Their faces are shining. They have an increased feeling of well-being. They are as full of hope and plans as they were twenty years earlier.[8]

The primitive diet I recommend is high in proteins and fats. Such a diet might be open to criticism on the grounds that it could raise the cholesterol level of some people, thus causing increased hardening of the arteries. But niacin has a wonderful ability to reduce cholesterol. Most people probably should take niacin in megadoses, provided they have their physician's approval.

Until I caught infectious hepatitis two years ago I took four 250 mg. capsules of niacin three times a day with meals or 3000 mg. in all. Niacin gives false positive liver tests and it is impossible to know whether one's liver disorder is getting better or worse, if one has hepatitis and takes massive doses of niacin. It did a very good job of keeping my cholesterol down. But now other nutritional supplements do just as well. I will tell more about this later. I might add that many people should take all vitamins and nutritional supplements, except iron, with food to avoid an upset stomach.

For many of my patients I usually prescribe a starting dose of 250 or 500 mg. of niacin three times a day. Because niacin releases the histamine from the basal cells, most people develop a flush when they first begin taking it. This flush is harmless, and usually disappears within an hour, even though it may be severe at first, so severe that you even feel it in your eardrums. It can be reduced by taking two aspirin or an antihistamine an hour before the niacin, or by taking it with food and cold water.

Some people tend to be over-stimulated by niacin during the first month. This can be handled by reducing the dosage or having your physician prescribe a mild tranquilizer to take along with it. Sometimes such restlessness persists in a minor form, consisting mostly of a good deal of drive. Your life may simply take on a more active cast, involving more participation and less standing on the sidelines. Some people engaged in meticulous, sedentary work like bookkeeping or mechanical drawing may find it somewhat difficult to carry on their occupation after going on niacin. But this is far from universal, and can only be tested through trial and error. I have seen many people who have done much *better* at their occupations, including artists who had reached an impasse and inability to create but were able to resume work with new vigor and creativity after being placed on niacin.

Not only does niacin lower serum cholesterol, but it also tends to keep the blood from clotting too easily and increases the oxygen-carrying capacity of red blood cells. Another important property is its tendency to raise blood sugar. A good many depressed or tense people suffer from errors in carbohydrate metabolism resulting in hypoglycemia. For them niacin is particularly useful. If, on the other hand, you have diabetes, ulcers, high blood pressure, or porphyria, niacin must be taken strictly under the supervision of a physician with wide experience in vitamin therapy.

Niacinamide and nicotinamide (so-called, though it has nothing to do with nicotine) have the vitamin effects of niacin but do not cause a flush, and they lack the cholesterol-lowering effects and some of the other beneficial properties of niacin.

Beware: Sometimes the niacinamide form of B_3 causes depression.

FOLIC ACID AND PANTOTHENIC ACID NEEDS

Pantothenic acid was discovered by Roger Williams, the distinguished professor of biochemistry at the University of Texas and, from 1941 to 1963, director of the Clayton Foundation Biochemical Institute, where more vitamins and their variants were discovered than at any other laboratory in the world.

This man, who knows more about pantothenic acid than anyone, believes that if pregnant women were given 50 mg. of this vitamin per day, the incidence of miscarriages and malformed babies would be greatly reduced.[10] He points out that people have taken 250 times this dose without adverse effect—that, indeed, they have been better able to withstand emotional stress with this added vitamin supplement.[11] There is good reason to believe that humans require larger amounts of pantothenic acid than other mammals. Muscle is the most abundant tissue in the body, and our muscles contain about twice as much pantothenic acid as those of other mammals.

Almost every food we eat contains pantothenic acid. As in all other nutritional problems, the question remains: what is the optimal daily amount?

Calcium pantothenate is essential for the formation of steroid hormones, which means that it is particularly important for individuals under stress, since such persons secrete more adrenal cortical hormones than others. But since the vitamin is used in many co-enzyme systems throughout the body, no cell can function properly without its proper supply of pantothenic acid. As yet, we do not know the specific daily requirements of this vitamin. Relatively good sources of it are egg yolk, kidney, yeast, and liver. It is available to some extent in almost all unpurified foods, but fifty-seven percent of it is lost when wheat is turned into white flour, and thirty-three percent is lost during the cooking of meat.[12]

I take 218 mg. of calcium pantothenate at bedtime. Most people, in my opinion, would do well on this, though I may give a tense patient up to 436 mg. of calcium pantothenate four times a day. I often recommend that a patient with insomnia take up to 872 mg. at bedtime to help relaxation.

All of the B vitamins interact with one another. Para-amino-benzoic acid (paba), for instance, helps create a favorable intestinal bacterial flora which enables the organism to utilize folic acid. Dr. William F. Philpott states that sixty percent of his psychiatric patients have low serum folic acid levels.[9] I have begun to incorporate tests for folic acid into my test profile. My findings concur with Dr. Philpott's. Folic acid is necessary to help the body absorb pantothenic acid, which is the vitamin into which the body breaks down calcium pantothenate when taken by mouth. Folic acid is not sold over the counter, except in minute quantities, because if you are deficient in vitamin B_{12}, folic acid may mask that deficiency.

Kurt A. Oster, M.D., chief of cardiology at the Park City Hospital, Bridgeport, Connecticut (whose research proves homogenized milk to be an important cause of hardening of the arteries in man) uses folic acid to combat hardening of the arteries. Indeed, he may use up to 80 mg. a day of folic acid.

I have recently tried up to 80 mg. daily of folic acid in patients with emotional disorders and find that many patients respond well to it. Depending upon the individual, megadoses of folic acid may either stimulate or sedate. Often people simply experience an increased feeling of well-being, which, after all, is the prize we all seek.

After taking large amounts of folic acid for several weeks, we may need to lower the intake. As with many other vitamin supplements, the dosage must be "played with," adjusted upward and downward to find the right level.

I take 10 mg. of folic acid four times daily. Everyone should have his serum folic acid level tested.

YOUR VITAMIN B$_6$ NEEDS

I have a special interest in this vitamin, also called pyridoxin, since I apparently managed to produce a deficiency in myself by neglecting this vitamin while taking large doses of the other B-complex components. My original interest in vitamins centered around niacin and ascorbic acid, and in my ignorance of the subject I emphasized these two at the expense of most others. I developed cheilosis (cracks in the mouth corners) a typical sign of B-vitamin deficiency, usually cured by riboflavin. In my case, riboflavin had little effect on the fissures; by prolonged experimentation with various vitamins, I eventually discovered that pyridoxin made the cheilosis disappear and stay away.

Pyridoxin is involved in many stages of protein metabolism, and thus assumes special importance in my vitamin regimens, because of the high-protein diet I advocate.

In rats, we find that vitamin B$_6$ deficiency causes a puffy swelling of tissues, weakness, anemia, abnormal deposits of iron in the body, restlessness, and convulsions. Many allergic, sniffling children are suffering from pyridoxin deficiency.[13] These children often exhibit stunted growth, high-arched palates, crooked lower teeth, and a pale, puffy complexion.

Dr. Leon Rosenberg,[14] professor and chairman of human genetics, pediatrics and internal medicine at Yale University School of Medicine, has done much work on pyridoxin-dependent children—youngsters who have convulsions and fail to thrive unless given massive doses of vitamin B_6. Roger Williams, too, has drawn attention to the pyridoxin-dependent state.[15] He believes that persons on a high-fat diet need added amounts of vitamin B_6 in order to prevent arteriosclerosis and heart disease, as well as hardening of the cerebral arteries and premature senility.

There is some evidence to indicate that B_6 deficiency is at least a contributory factor in the premenstrual edema of women, and may manifest itself in such diverse symptoms as abdominal upsets or stiffness of the neck.[16]

Vitamin B_6 is also important for the function of the adrenal cortex. I have several times pointed out the high incidence of poor adrenal-cortical function in people with emotional illness.

It would probably be especially important to have large doses of pyridoxin if you are under any kind of stress, whether emotional or physical. The vitamin is also likely to be extremely important for some children who suffer from convulsions, those who do not thrive, and who have allergies and emotional difficulties.

Good sources of pyridoxin are yeast, liver, and—to some extent—eggs and leafy vegetables. I take 100 mg. of pyridoxin three times a day by mouth, again pursuant to my philosophy that everyone should try relatively large doses of the water-soluble vitamins, since they can't hurt and may help.

Let me remind you once more, however, that this is a *general* recommendation. *I can make no specific recommendations for any specific individual without prior examination.* If you take any vitamins, supplements, or follow the diet recommended in this book, it is *your responsibility to check with your physician for any counter-indications that may exist in your case.*

YOUR VITAMIN B_{12} NEEDS

Because of its enormous importance in the treatment of many serious emotional illnesses, this member of the B-complex family will be treated more fully in a later chapter. Let me say here only that I feel very strongly that everyone, whether or not he is suffering from emotional disorders, should have his serum vitamin B_{12} level determined. This is vital because many people can't absorb B_{12} when it is taken orally, so even when they take vitamins in large quantities they may still be deficient in vitamin B_{12}.

The anemia that eventually develops from a vitamin B_{12} deficiency may be corrected by taking 2 to 3 mg. daily of folic acid; however, folic acid will not prevent the nerve damage (brain degeneration, destruction of the nerves in the spinal cord, etc.) which results from a vitamin B_{12} deficiency.

YOUR VITAMIN B_{15} NEEDS

I have in my hand a book put out by the Science Publishing House in Moscow, the title of which is *B_{15} (Pengamic acid): Properties, Functions and Use*. It seems ironic that this vitamin, first discovered, isolated, identified, and synthesized by Dr. E. T. Krebs in the U.S., should find favor in almost every country in the world and be totally neglected by this country. The importance of this vitamin in the Soviet Union could well be summarized by the following statement made by Professor Shprit at a conference of the Institute of Biochemistry of the U.S.S.R. Academy of Sciences: "I believe the time will come when there will be calcium pangamate [vitamin B_{15}] on the table of every family with people past 40."

The chief function so far of vitamin B_{15} seems to be to increase the oxygen intake of tissue and to lower blood cholesterol. People on this vitamin are able to withstand lower oxygen pressures. It has been used extensively for people who have suffered from vascular disorders such as coronary heart disease, but is also valuable in treating cirrhosis of the liver brought about by alcoholism, and it is felt to be a boon to postponing and even helping to relieve signs and symptoms of senility.

This vitamin has been especially valuable in treating withdrawn children who have difficulty learning to speak. Abram Hoffer M.D., Ph.D., of Canada, has reported in a personal communication to me that he has found a number of withdrawn children to be improved with the use of this vitamin. He has come to call it "the speech vitamin."

Pengamic acid is available in many countries around the world. Some of my patients have been able to obtain it from Mexico by way of certain health food stores in the Los Angeles area, and others have picked it up in Germany and Switzerland. The usual doses of the 50 mg. tablets is three times a day. The therapeutic course runs twenty to forty days at which time there is a two- or three-month rest period, after which it is repeated once more.

YOUR VITAMIN C NEEDS (ASCORBIC ACID)

During a recent meeting of the Academy of Orthomolecular Psychiatry I became acquainted with Dr. Albert Szent-Gyorgy, recipient of the 1937 Nobel Prize for working out the chemistry of vitamin C (ascorbic acid).

Even more interesting to me than his address to the assembly were a number of private conversations I had with him, during which he stated, among many other things, his conviction that we are a long way from discovering all the elements required for human nutrition.

For breakfast Dr. Szent-Gyorgy eats a banana sprinkled with two tablespoonfuls of wheat germ. He thinks there is a natural food supplement in wheat germ which is essential to the proper functioning of ascorbic acid, and that this unknown factor is also crucial to vitamin C's role in preventing the common cold. He is also convinced that requirements for vitamin C vary enormously from individual to individual, and that it is tragically naive of the medical profession to think of scurvy as being the only result of a deficiency of vitamin C. Scurvy merely presents the ultimate stage of a disease which manifests itself in many earlier symptoms routinely missed by physicians.

An article by Man-Li S. Yew of the University of Texas, "A Plus for Pauling and Vitamin C," [16] describes that author's studies concerning the effect of vitamin C on growth, wound healing, and resistance to surgical stress in guinea pigs. Dr. Yew found that large amounts of vitamin C are required for optimal functioning within these areas. Small amounts safeguarded the guinea pigs against scurvy, but did not allow them to grow to their ideal size, to heal wounds quickly, or to recover promptly from stressful surgical situations. On the basis of his findings he recommended, among other things, that children should be given approximately 1500 mg. of vitamin C daily.

Last year, I shared a speaker's platform with Irwin Stone, a researcher who has spent much of his life studying vitamin C and introduced its use to Linus Pauling who, in turn, dedicated his book *Vitamin C and the Common Cold* to Stone. Stone addressed his audience as "fellow mutants," meaning that we are each the result of a chance mutation in our genetic code that prevents us from manufacturing vitamin C in our own body like most mammals.

During the last century we have discovered any number of ways to destroy the vitamin C content of food during processing and storage, and our diet has been altered in an extraordinary way, often substituting bare sugar for the vitamin C-rich fruits eaten by our ancestors. This perversion has led to a host of deficiency symptoms, including decreased ability to fight disease and infection, and to emotional illnesses. We know that schizophrenics require as much as one thousand times the vitamin C used by a "normal" person, but we don't know as yet if this is caused by a further chance mutation (causing such people to be born with a wildly exaggerated need for certain vitamins) or whether the enormous stress of being emotionally disturbed creates the need for extra vitamins. Probably both factors are at work.

Vitamin C is a powerful detoxifying agent

It is possible that vitamin C can fight a toxic condition in a schizophrenic because many people with serious emotional problems certainly act as if they were poisoned, even if we cannot identify the toxin. Fred Klenner, M.D., of Reidsville, North Carolina, a leading authority on the use of vitamin C, reports giving ascorbic acid intravenously to a highway patrolman who was overcome and unconscious from carbon monoxide poisoning. Before the needle was removed from the man's arm he was conscious and talking in a rational manner. Tests have also proven that large doses of ascorbic acid will detoxify the venom from snakes (including rattlesnakes) and keep dogs from developing symptoms after having been bitten by these snakes.

I have a number of patients with known hypersensitivities that are greatly reduced or eliminated by ascorbic acid. For example, I have one patient who is so sensitive to tobacco smoke that she can go to a theater where smoking takes place and be so affected that she reels home. Men think that she is intoxicated and try to pick her up on the street. But if she takes about 5 grams of ascorbic acid before going to the theater she can sit through the movie, survive the smoke in the atmosphere, and walk a straight line on the way back to her apartment.

Aside from its connection to emotional illness, vitamin C has been found helpful in combating an impressive array of conditions—from the effects of environmental pollutants like carbon monoxide to the bruises caused by capillary fragility, toxic insect bites, burns, diabetes, high cholesterol, overdoses of barbiturates, colds and other respiratory ailments, and possibly even malignancies like cancer of the bladder. Evidence of more astounding qualities of this vitamin is constantly accumulating.[17]

The optimum daily intake of vitamin C is not yet known, and it is likely that it, too, varies widely not only from person to person but also in the same person at different times and under different conditions. The Food and Nutrition Board of the National Academy of Sciences Research Council suggests an intake of 60 mg. daily for an adult male—and *that,* you may be sure, is *not* the optimum. Linus Pauling takes 6000 mg. of ascorbic acid per day. Dr. Klenner takes 20,000 mg. per day. My own dose is 15,000 mg. a day.

YOUR VITAMIN D NEEDS

Vitamin D is necessary for the formation of a protein in the gut which is active in the absorption of calcium. Calcium is a mineral which exerts a strong effect on the stability of cell membranes, particularly those of the central nervous system. When vitamin D—and therefore calcium—is low, the central nervous system becomes irritable. This irritability can range all the way from simple tension to the ultimate in nervous-system hyperactivity: convulsions.

When I was an infant, vitamin D deficiencies were quite common, and I am certain that I myself suffered from rickets and the hyper-irritability which accompanies lack of calcium. My mother tells me that I cried for most of my first six months of life, and sometimes the only way the family could quiet me was to ride me over bumpy roads in an automobile. Such stimulation would tend to discharge tension in the central nervous system; it would also stimulate the production of adrenal cortical hormone, counteracting any effect of the hypoglycemia and food allergies that had probably been produced in me by the sugar in my formula.

The adult in our society is likely to lack sufficient vitamin D not only because of dietary deficiency but also because he receives very little skin stimulation from sunshine (which produces natural vitamin D). The problem is compounded in the elderly, who lack not only the stimulation produced by adequate light and vitamin D but also live on a diet poor in calcium and magnesium. Older people also produce diminishing amounts of various hormones. Taken together, these factors lead to demineralization of the bones; bone tissue becomes brittle, fractures easily, and heals with difficulty. In addition, depleted calcium reserves can certainly contribute to the emotional problems of old age.

I personally prefer not to depend upon dietary sources of vitamin D such as livers and viscera of fish and animals that feed on fish, and therefore take 400 units of natural vitamin D daily.

Since vitamin D—like vitamin A—is stored in the liver for long periods, it is possible to accumulate toxic amounts of it. The synthetic form of vitamin D is far more toxic than the natural form, but even the former has been used in doses ranging from 50,000 units to 500,000 units daily for relatively long periods, especially for the treatment of myopia (near-sightedness) and for demineralization of bone tissue.

Some people are "vitamin-D fast," and require massive amounts, but I would strongly recommend that no one take this vitamin in large doses without very strict medical supervision.

YOUR VITAMIN K NEEDS

Vitamin K is primarily involved in the clotting mechanism of the blood. It is formed in the intestines of humans, and is of little clinical importance except for persons with specific diseases such as jaundice. For this reason I do not take any vitamin K, and do not generally recommend it.

YOUR VITAMIN E NEEDS

The most important of the fat-soluble vitamins for emotional health is vitamin E. It exerts a powerful influence on the cell membrane and the cell's utilization of oxygen. The brain cells are particularly dependent on a ready supply of oxygen. Also, vitamin E is an aid in hydrogen ion transfers, and thus again affects every cell in the body.

Probably the world's greatest authorities on vitamin E are the Shute brothers in Canada. I have corresponded with Wilfred E. Shute M.D. He informs me that in his opinion most vitamin E preparations in the United States are not reliably labeled, and that one cannot be certain how much vitamin E one is getting unless one uses a reliably labeled product. He recommended the Key-E products put out by the Carlson Laboratories in Chicago.

The Shute brothers are primarily interested in vitamin E for its cardiovascular effect, especially its use to prevent coronary artery disease and ameliorate angina pectoris. Those of us interested in megavitamin therapy for emotional disorders have found it equally useful. It is particularly helpful for patients who are depressed and tired—two very common complaints among persons suffering from emotional illnesses.

Vitamin E has been used extensively for menopausal symptoms, and can often substitute for hormone therapy in women. It probably aids sexual function in the male. All my patients are treated with multiple vitamins, nutritional supplements, and specific dietary recommendations; so when an impotent male becomes potent, it is hard to say which of the elements of his regimen was responsible for his return to the sexual arena. I can only say that, if I had a potency problem, I would certainly include vitamin E in my regimen.

Unfortunately, vitamin E is one vitamin that can cause difficulties. When I first started taking it, I was unable to take more than 150 units daily without raising my blood pressure. Ordinarily, my blood pressure runs around 70 over 110, but whenever I took more than 150 units of vitamin E it quickly rose to 140 over 90, to the accompaniment of a sizeable headache. It took me at least two years to gradually raise my vitamin E intake to its present level of two Key-E capsules of 200 I.U. (international units) at breakfast and lunch.

Although the Shute brothers maintain that the D.-Alpha tocopherol is the only active form of vitamin E, I still take a 400 I.U. E-complex tablet in addition to the Key-E. This E-complex (or mixed tocopherol) tablet contains the D-Alpha as well as the Beta, Delta, and Gamma tocopherols as they occur in nature. I consider this mixture added insurance, just in case we do not yet have the final word on all its active principles. As added insurance I also take 400 I.U. of Alpha-tocopheral acetate at lunch.

It is my feeling that everyone should take vitamin E supplements in amounts of at least 100 or 200 I.U. a day, and possibly much more—for instance, if menopausal symptoms are present, or if there is depression and lack of energy. Some of my patients take as much as 4200 I.U. daily and feel the let-down as soon as they reduce their dose level.

Vitamin E should not be taken more than twice daily, since it interferes with iron absorption. Take vitamin E with breakfast and lunch. This leaves your gut free to absorb iron later in the day. Your family doctor should make certain your blood pressure does not go up too high as you increase your vitamin E. If your blood pressure does increase, it often normalizes if you stay on the same dosage level of vitamin E for several weeks. Your elevated blood pressure will fall quickly if you interrupt your vitamin E intake for a few days and then go back to a reduced level.

WHY USE CRUDE SOURCES OF VITAMINS?

Since it is likely that we have not yet discovered all vitamins and vitamin-like substances, I feel it is desirable to include many sources of crude vitamins. If a Nobel Prize-winning nutritional chemist such as Szent-Gyorgy includes these substances in his diet, I think it wise for you and me to do the same.

Yeast is an excellent crude source of B vitamins, high-grade proteins, and readily assimilated minerals. I take two tablespoons a day mixed in water, one of brewers', or primary, yeast, and one of torula yeast. Each type of yeast has slightly different properties, so I consider it good insurance to take both. I cannot stress too much the importance of yeast. Unless sensitive to it, everyone should take it.

In my list of essentials in life I rank: air, water, food, yeast, ascorbic acid. If need be I would sleep on the streets in a blanket roll if I had to choose between adequate shelter and yeast.

Bakers' yeast. Many nutritionists will tell you that bakers' yeast is not a good source of vitamins because the live yeast in the gastrointestinal tract will itself use up vitamins. If a person has a normal amount of gastric acid, the yeast will be killed. Bakers' yeast supplies cocarboxylase, an important metabolic enzyme to the liver. Many people feel better if they eat a one-half inch cube of bakers' yeast cake three or four times daily. Cake yeast has largely vanished from supermarkets, though some specialty stores still carry it. In any event you can probably talk your neighborhood bakery into selling you a brick. If you get gas from this, it means your gastric acid is not killing the yeast. Take bakers' yeast on an empty stomach. Wait two hours after eating to take bakers' yeast, then do not eat or drink anything for one hour after having the yeast.

Liver. Liver is also an excellent source of crude B vitamins best taken in the form of powder or capsules. Baby liver is preferred because it has not accumulated as many environmental impurities as the liver of a full-grown animal.

Lecithin. While it is not strictly a vitamin, I believe that a regular intake of lecithin is essential to good health.

Lecithin is an emulsifier, but also contains the two B vitamins inositol and choline. It is used in making chocolate and margarine, because it breaks down their gummy consistency and allows them to flow readily through the production process. Similarly, it works like soap in the bloodstream to emulsify fats and reduce cholesterols to a form that can be readily burned, instead of coagulating in your arteries.

Lecithin is abundant in egg yolk, sunflower seeds, melons, safflower oil and seeds and cereal seeds. Lecithin not only helps to dispose of cholesterol, but it also aids in the absorption of the fat-soluble vitamins, and may act to prevent gallstones.

Your body can manufacture lecithin, but to do so it needs three substances: the B vitamins inositol and choline, both of which are present in lecithin itself and also in yeast; and a particular amino acid (a building block of protein) called methionine, which is also present in yeast. But in addition to yeast I feel you should take lecithin itself, particularly if you are on a high-protein and -fat diet. It comes in granules, capsules, and syrup. Granules are best, because it is almost impossible to take enough capsules to do any good. The syrup sticks to the spoon and to the roof of your mouth; also it is not delicious. Take two to four tablespoonfuls a day, sprinkled on fruit, or eat it straight or mixed with safflower oil. Keep the lecithin in the refrigerator after opening the bottle.

Lecithin is an excellent source of two of the less publicized B vitamins: choline and inositol.

Studies of these two vitamins in man are very incomplete. But the evidence is quite clear that laboratory animals require these vitamins.

Choline protects the liver. When this vitamin is low, massive fatty infiltration of the liver occurs. When puppies are fed choline-deficient diets they die within three weeks. Rats show kidney damage after being fed choline-poor diets for only four or five days. Also, cancer, muscular dystrophy, anemia, and heart and vascular disorders have been reported in laboratory animals on a choline-deficient diet.

Personally, I want plenty of choline and I think you do too. Lecithin gives me mine.

Inositol also remains much of a mystery as to exact human requirements, but we do know that it is part of the phosphatide present in large amounts in brain tissue. Beef heart, as well as lecithin, is a good source. Why is it present in such large amounts in this heart tissue? I don't know. But if the heart needs it, I want it.

Mice growth has been proved to be influenced by inositol, as growth is influenced by so many other vitamins, minerals and hormones. And human tissue maintained under artificial conditions grows better with adequate inositol.

Growth of itself may not seem too important, but lack of growth means that the body cells are being blocked from reaching their full potential. If enough cells are stunted in enough places, this means your child may end up as delivering newspapers when he or she might have had a Nobel Prize for literature.

THE VALUE OF UNSATURATED OILS

Both kinds of fats, saturated and unsaturated, are necessary for good health. Saturated fats come mostly from meats. You probably get more than enough saturated fats in your diet; if you did not, your body would manufacture it. Unsaturated fats come from fish and vegetable sources. They too are essential for good health; they help the body to handle saturated fats. A deficiency can lead to dandruff, acne, eczema, dry, lusterless hair, loss of energy, impaired sex drive, and other symptoms.

The active ingredients in unsaturated oils are three fatty acids. They are present in almost all vegetable oils except olive oil, but the best source is safflower oil. You should have at least two tablespoons of safflower oil daily in salad dressing or mayonnaise, or from a spoon if you have to; oil used in cooking should not be counted since heat destroys some of the beneficial properties. For the same reason, you should choose cold-pressed oils rather than the heat-processed variety (the label will tell you). Be sure the oil contains no preservatives, and keep it in the refrigerator after you open it.

Lecithin and essential fatty acids often occur together in nature. Both help to handle saturated fats in the bloodstream, but in addition, lecithin, like vitamin E, is an anti-oxidant: it prevents the oils from oxidizing. Remember, then, we should take safflower oil *and* lecithin.

YOUR BIOTIN AND PABA NEEDS

Biotin is another of the little-publicized B vitamins. Your body manufactures this vitamin, so you don't need to take it by mouth—just be certain you don't destroy your own biotin by eating raw egg whites. Never, never, never eat raw eggs. They will block this vitamin. Humans have become very ill by producing biotin deficiencies in themselves. How would you like to be tired, have numbness and muscle pains in your limbs, suffer from eczema-like skin rashes, have nausea and loss of appetite?

Para-aminobenzoic acid is the scientific tongue twister that designates another little-publicized vitamin, usually referred to as PABA. S. Ansbacher[18] demonstrated that laboratory animals require PABA as an indispensable nutrient but we still don't know the human requirements. At any rate, it is widely believed that PABA is not required in the diet of humans. PABA would be difficult to avoid in diets since it is present in most foods. Yeast is an especially rich source.

PABA has gained some fame as an "anti-gray hair" vitamin (along with calcium pantothenate). Laboratory animals deficient in this vitamin experience graying hair, which clears up after PABA is returned to their diet. Whether this happens in humans remains to be proven. I once appeared on a talk show with nutritionist Carlton Fredericks, Ph.D., and commented upon the lack of grayness in his hair. He attributed it to the 500 mg. of PABA he takes each day.

I have not been able to make up my mind about the anti-graying effect of PABA. As of now, I have no problem with graying of the hair on my head, although my beard is getting quite gray. A few jokesters have commented that I'm getting old from the bottom up, though I can assure any interested women readers that this is not the case.

Several times I have tried taking PABA for a number of weeks, then stopping, then starting it again. I have never been able to decide whether or not the PABA has any effect on the grayness. But I have frequently seen gray hair on my patients' heads turn dark after the patients have been placed on a proper diet with proper nutritional supplements. These supplements do not ordinarily include PABA except as it occurs in brewers' yeast.

Is the prevention of gray hair really important in the overall scheme of your existence? Who can say for certain? We do know that graying of hair represents the failure of enzyme systems, which gradually takes place as we grow older. And more people die with gray hair than with the original color of their hair. A hundred years from now we may have the answer, but that won't do you and me much good. So again we must decide which horse to bet on—but don't forget you are betting your two most valuable assets: your good health and your life. I choose to place my bets on a proper diet and nutritional supplements.

(In the chapter on aging we will discuss other uses of a form of PABA; the Hungarian physician Ana Aslan, M.D., has developed what is called H_3 or gerovital.)

Let me conclude with a few practical points about taking vitamins. First, you should take in as little binder and artificial coloring as possible with your vitamins. Choose straight powder or clear capsules, or sugar-and-starch-free tablets that are clearly labeled as such. Regular tablets often upset the stomach or cause other undesirable side effects. For instance, diarrhea is often caused by ordinary vitamin C tablets. Sweetened chewable tablets are least desirable of all.

You should be aware that you may be allergic to one line (or brand) of vitamins, but you may well be able to tolerate another brand without difficulty.

And remember: you might conceivably feel worse when you take a particular vitamin. Several times I have found a particular vitamin disagrees with a particular patient, even when the patient is not allergic to the vitamin. Your particular enzyme system may function less well with added megadoses of a particular vitamin. This is not common, but it is possible. Only trial and error will answer this question.

NOTES

1. *Journal of Nutrition.* Vol. 70, No. 4, April 1960.
2. *Journal of the American Medical Association*, Vol. 130, No. 1, January–April 1946, pp. 1208–1215.
3. *Journal of the Canadian Medical Association*, Vol. 44, 1941, p. 20.
4. *Vitamin Research News*, Vol. 1, No. 40, 1946.
5. *American Review of Tuberculosis*, Vol. 72, 1955, p. 218.
6. H. C. Sherman *et al.* "Vitamin A in Relation to Aging and to Length of Life," *Proceedings of the National Academy of Science*, Vol. 31, No. 4, April 15, 1945, pp. 107–109; H. C. Sherman and H. Y. Trupp. "Further Experiments with Vitamin A in Relation to Aging and Length of Life," *Proceedings of the National Academy of Science*, Vol. 35, February 1949, pp. 90–92; M. Chieffi and Esben Kirk. "Vitamin Studies in Middle-Aged and Old Individuals," *Journal of Nutrition*, Vol. 37, January–April 1970, pp. 67–79.
7. F. C. Ross and A. H. Campbell, "The Effects of Vitamin A and Vitamin D Capsules upon the Incidence of Coronary Heart Disease and Blood Cholesterol," *Med. Jrnl. of Australia*, Vol. 48, No. 2, August 19, 1961, pp. 307–311.
8. Personal communication, 1972.
9. Personal communication, 1973.
10. J. Roger Williams, *Nutrition Against Disease* (New York: Pitman Publishing Corporation, 1971).
11. E. P. Ralli *et al.* "Physiologic Changes Occurring in Patients with Cirrhosis of the Liver," *Jrnl. of Amer. Med. Women's Assn.*, Vol. 8, September 1958, pp. 293–300.
12. Harold Harper, *Review of Physiological Chemistry* (Los Altos: Lange Medical Publications, 1971), p. 105.
13. Address to Society for Clincial Ecology, Albuquerque, New Mexico, November 1972.
14. Leon E. Rosenberg.
15. J. Roger Williams, *Biochemical Individuality* (New York: Wiley, 1956).
16. Man-Li S. Yew, "A Plus for Pauling and Vitamin C," *Science News*, May 5, 1973.

Table 1 MY USUAL VITAMIN INTAKE

Vitamin	Total Amount	Frequency of Intake
Vitamin A (natural)	10,000 units	Daily (perle)
The B's		
B_1	125–500 mg.	Daily after breakfast (capsule)
B_2	60 mg.	Daily (capsule)
B_3 (niacin form)	3000 mg.	4 capsules of 250 mg. 3 times daily with meals
B_6	300 mg.	100 mg. 3 times daily (capsule)
Calcium pantothenate	436 mg.	218 mg. 2 capsules daily at bedtime
Folic acid	1 mg.	10 tablets 4 times daily
B_{12}	1000 mcg.	Once a week by injection
Yeast (Brewers' or primary powder)	2 heaping tablespoons (in water)	Daily after supper
Yeast (torula)	2 heaping tablespoons (in water)	Daily after breakfast
Yeast (bakers' cake)	$\frac{1}{2}''$ cube	Daily first thing in the morning
Lecithin granules (soy bean origin)	2 heaping tablespoons	2 times daily
Vitamin C (powder)	10,000 mg.	Daily. Divide into 4 doses (in water)
Vitamin D (natural)	400 units	Daily (perle)
Vitamin E (natural)	1. 800 I.U. D-Alpha tocopheral succinate	400 I.U., breakfast and lunch
	2. 800 I.U. D-Alpha tocopheral acetate	400 I.U., breakfast and lunch
	3. 200 I.U. E-complex	Daily, breakfast
Safflower oil	2 tablespoons	Daily

17. Michael Clark, "Vitamin C Is a Miracle Medicine," *Prevention*, July 1973, pp. 44–56.
18. S. Ansbacher, "P-Aminobenzoic Acid, a Vitamin," *Science*, Vol. 93, 1941, p. 164.

HOW TO FIT
MEGA-NUTRIENTS
INTO YOUR DAILY ROUTINE

CHAPTER TWELVE

At this point some of you may feel that if good nutrition is this complicated, you'll just have to go on feeling below par. I realize that when you read about all this for the first time, it may seem that you could find yourself spending hours every day scooping vitamins by the shovel. I can only assure you from my personal experience and the by now very extensive experience of my patients that the complexity of my system wears off quickly with the novelty and you will soon develop a routine that becomes as natural as eating. In fact it should help you to remember that a sound nutritional regimen *is* merely an extension of eating. I've had patients who seemed scarcely able to tie their shoes and still mastered the program handily; I'm sure you can, too. At the end of this chapter I will give you a foolproof method that will reduce all of this to a single, no-effort reach, four times daily. But to begin with, here are some other, more sophisticated ways of getting started.

AT ONE GLANCE:
FIND OUT WHAT TO TAKE AND WHEN

At first, the biggest problem is keeping your schedule straight. In this chapter you will find two blank forms that will help you to keep a simple record. On the first form, titled Daily Intake, you can keep track of each nutrient separately. In the appropriate box, write the number of times a day you take it, and the total daily intake. For example:

Name	Amount	Times Daily	Total
Vitamin C	½ tsp. (2000 mg.)	3	6000 mg.

I recommend that you keep these forms in pencil, so you can change the entries as you fine-tune your program. You will find several blank forms of each type, and when you have used them up, you can easily make your own.

The second table is called the Time Sheet. It contains the same information as that on the Daily Intake table, but arranged according to times of day, so you can keep track of when you take each group of supplements. Again, I recommend that you fill it in in pencil, so you can easily change dosages when necessary. Fill in the name of the supplement, then the amount you take at that time, and the description. (You will soon have these details memorized, but this may be helpful in the beginning.) For example:

Time: Breakfast

Name	Amount	Description
A & D capsule	1	orange pearl
E	2	yellow capsule

and so on. List the capsules and tablets first, then the powders, because you will probably find it most convenient to mix the powders together and take them in one potion. You will find four separate schedules on this table. For most people, these will be filled in Breakfast, Lunch, Dinner, and Bedtime, but I have left the times blank in case you have an unusual schedule.

WHAT IF YOU MAKE A MISTAKE?

If you let yourself feel intimidated by the amount of information there is to be mastered, you may become anxious and might make mistakes. Occasionally, you probably will make mistakes anyway. I do. It's easy to forget your exact dosage now and then, to skip something once in a while or to take one extra. On the whole, you needn't worry too much about it. If you refer to the appendix, Vitamins at a Glance, page 341, you will see how long each vitamin is stored in the body. With vitamins, it takes some time to build up an overdose in your system or to create a deficiency. Remember that you are taking food supplements, not drugs; and it is unlikely that you will do any more damage by making a mistake now and then than the damage you were doing when you took no supplements at all. (I do *not* mean it's all right to be careless or sloppy; when you have developed a truly beneficial program for yourself it is important to follow it carefully. I'm simply pointing out that vitamins are not like insulin or birth control pills, where one slip can mean serious difficulty.)

HOW TO KEEP EVERYTHING SORTED

The next problem that may concern you is the sheer proliferation of bottles and jars. How are you going to keep them all straight? How will you carry your doses with you? Will you have to quit your job and stay home and take pills?

It's really very simple. At a hardware store, buy a small plexiglas tackle box. This is a clear plastic box and is divided into compartments; they come in different sizes for storing fishing tackle, nails, screws, etc. Put each kind of pill or capsule into a separate compartment and label each compartment with the name of the supplement. This enables you to keep all your mega-nutrients in the same place, and it is actually rather handsome. If necessary, buy a second tackle box to keep in your office.

You can also buy a ready-made vitamin chest in some gift shops, containing glass vials for six different vitamins, but the drawback is that you may well need more than six separate containers.

WHAT TO DO WHEN YOU EAT OUT

If you are going out for one meal, and want to carry only what you need for that time of day, you have a number of choices. One is to get an antique pillbox at a flea market. These are ornate little objects made of metal or enamel to keep in your purse or briefcase. If you prefer, you can buy small empty plastic bottles at a notions store; ask for traveling bottles.

If I am going to eat in a restaurant, I sometimes pack a sandwich baggie in the following way. In the bottom, I measure in the powders I need (vitamin C, lecithin, dolomite). I tie this off with a wire tie (they come with the baggies). Then I count out the capsules or tablets I need into the next section of the bag, and tie that off with a second tie.

WHAT TO DO WHEN YOU TRAVEL

When traveling, I generally carry my tackle box in a briefcase or flight bag, and my powders premeasured and mixed in small plastic bottles, one for each day I will be gone. (If you prefer, you can use one large bottle.) This is perfectly light, portable, and convenient, and I rather enjoy the attention I attract when I produce my tackle box after dinner on an airplane. It is, as they say, a great conversation piece.

As you can see, your new nutritional regimen is not going to take over your life, It is going to *change* it, but for the better. You will have to develop a couple of new routines, but there was probably a time in your life when brushing your teeth twice a day seemed an impossible intrusion into your normal activities. With a little ingenuity, you will master the necessary logistics for your particular lifestyle, and you may even be able to turn your new routines to social advantage.

NOW: THE NO-EFFORT WAY

I promised earlier to give you a no-effort way to handle your daily intake of mega-nutrients, and here it is: prepackage it.

Lay out your Daily Intake and Time Sheet forms. Bring out and line up every bottle and every jar of every supplement you take. Take a pile of inexpensive letter envelopes and label them: "Monday Breakfast," "Monday Lunch," "Monday Dinner," "Monday Bedtime," "Tuesday Breakfast," "Tuesday Lunch," "Tuesday Dinner," "Tuesday Bedtime," and so forth. Then place the correct dosage of each supplement into each envelope. Seal it, and have the right envelope within reach at the right time, and that's it.

I do have some patients who, when they start treatment, cannot cope with sorting out, say, fourteen separate elements to be taken after

DAILY INTAKE TABLE

Name	Amount	Times Daily	Total
Vitamin C	½ tsp. (2000 mg.)	3	6000 mg.

TIME SHEET

Time: _____

Name	Amount	Description

arising. For them, a spouse or friend or other helper can prepare enough envelopes sufficiently far in advance so that even quite helpless patients feel secure: their medication is visibly in readiness and mistakes are pretty much impossible.

One further way to guard against errors is for the patient or the helper to add up how many supplements should be in each envelope; to mark the correct number on each envelope when the envelope has been filled; and to make sure that the correct number is taken every time an envelope is opened. But this is really only for the super-conscientious.

A further guard against the possibility of leaving a small pill unconsumed (and then discarded) in an opened envelope is to use transparent envelopes that are used for stamps by philatelists and are available from any stamp dealer.

HOW MINERALS HELP
CONTROL YOUR NERVES

CHAPTER THIRTEEN

About a year ago, the twenty-three-year-old wife of a law student was brought to my office by her husband and her mother, each holding one arm to prevent her from running away.

At first glance, Mary looked like the happiest soul alive. She babbled about amusing people she had just seen on the street, made fun of her mother-in-law's derrière, and skipped blithely from subject to subject. Her body was as active as her mind; she kept pacing back and forth in my office, ignoring me when I invited her to sit down and talk. Her husband leaned against the door, to keep her from bolting.

Her effervescence—like that of all people suffering from mania— was contagious. I found myself smiling at her jokes and listening in fascination to the flow of witty words that leaped forth like pirouetting dancers.

Mary, the family told me, had been trying to finish college for the past six years, but intermittent periods of depression and elation had repeatedly interfered with her studies. She had earned credit for only a year and a half's work. Although she was intelligent and efficient during her normal periods, she was too depressed and slow-moving during her downswings to study effectively. But the worst times were the upswings, like the one she was experiencing at the moment. During these periods her mind often offered only a word salad. She could not even sit still long enough to attend classes, let alone absorb anything from a lecture.

For the past few years, psychiatrists have been using the mineral lithium carbonate with great success in the treatment of such manic states. I don't know why this wasn't tried with Mary. Perhaps her previous doctors had seen her only during her depressive states, and had not realized that she suffered from the dramatic mood swings that characterize the true manic-depressive illness.

I prescribed lithium at once, and saw her again ten days later. On her second visit she was accompanied only by her mother. This time she appeared neither unduly elated nor depressed. She talked about her difficulties in a thoroughly rational manner. She realized that her life passed through up and down cycles. For no obvious reason she would grow more and more restless, take on too many extracurricular activities at school, lose sleep, and finally become so disorganized that she could no longer function. Weeks later she would descend to a comfortable level for a short while and then pass on down into the black caves of depression.

The transformation which a mineral, lithium carbonate, can bring about in manic-depressive illness such as Mary's is one of the most spectacularly satisfying experiences a psychiatrist can have. This simple mineral can literally transform broken lives into useful ones.

Typically, lithium was ignored for a generation after J. F. Cade, M.D., discovered a medical use for it. In 1949, this general practitioner in the Australian hinterlands learned that lithium carbonate could work what seemed like a miracle in the treatment of manic-depressive illnesses. He wrote a convincing scientific paper describing his findings, but the paper was studiously ignored by the medical establishment. Perhaps if Cade had been a professor of medicine at some prestigious university his findings would have been taken more seriously, but in truth, his story is typical of the neglect the medical establishment often heaps upon men who make new discoveries. At least Cade was luckier than Joseph Goldberger, who discovered that pellagra was caused by a vitamin B_3 deficiency, not by germs, as everyone believed. Goldberger died believing his findings had been rejected. Cade lived to see lithium widely used in the United States a mere twenty years after he developed a new use for it.

Body Minerals. When most of us think of minerals we have visions of quaint novelty shops with spears of gleaming quartz or bookends made of petrified wood. Such minerals seem to have little to do with human emotions. Yet the fact is that our bodies could not function without minerals, and that they are especially important to the nervous system.

Physicians are aware that iron, sodium, potassium, and calcium are needed in the proper amounts for good health. However, their knowledge quickly fades away when it comes to copper, manganese, chromium, magnesium, and zinc, among others. Also, most physicians make the mistake of testing the blood for minerals when (except for acute loss) much more useful information comes from testing solid tissue such as muscle or hair. Clearly it is easier to get two tablespoons of hair than two tablespoons of muscle for testing; therefore, we use hair.

Hair tests were originally developed by nutritionists to plan optimal diets for beef and dairy herds. It happens that much of our hard evidence about nutrition comes from intensive studies in animal husbandry. There is money to be made raising healthy cattle as efficiently as possible. Unhappily, the big money in human health care is made in diagnosing and drugging people after they've gotten sick.

You may be aware from detective stories and mystery shows that coroners sometimes test hair samples of possible murder victims for residues of poison in the tissue. Even Napoleon's hair has been analyzed and found to contain excessive amounts of arsenic. Historians speculate that he was slowly poisoned by his last British physician.

Toxic levels of minerals, particularly lead or mercury salts, may cause illness. Recently a patient came to me for treatment of a depression. Hair tests revealed a dangerously high level of lead in her system. She had exposed herself to lead while removing old lead-based paint from the walls of her home.

Public health officials are increasingly aware that many children have poisoned themselves to the point of brain damage by chewing on wood covered with old lead-based paints. Pewter drinking cups may be a source of lead poisoning, as may exhaust fumes from the burning of leaded gasoline. Also, certain lead-based ceramic glazes on bowls and mugs release toxic lead into the hot soup, tea, or coffee you drink from them. There have been cases of whole families lead-poisoned by their pottery. (When you buy handmade ceramics, be sure to ask if the objects were fired at high heat, which burns off the lead; if not, try to make sure there was no lead in the glaze to begin with.)

HOW TO GET A MINERAL TEST DONE

If you are interested in having your mineral levels checked for a deficiency or for abnormally high levels of toxic minerals, you may give your doctor the following information about the hair sample test: Hair should be cut at scalp level from various spots on the back of the head. Use the first two inches of hair that grow from the scalp since the longer hair reflects past, rather than present, mineral levels.

Two heaping tablespoons of hair should be sent by your doctor to Parmae Laboratories, Inc., P.O. Box 35227, Dallas, Texas, 75235, or Hartley Research Labs, 1495 West Street, Provo, Utah, 84601, telephone: (801) 377-5455.

Your hair will be tested for cadmium, chromium, lithium, cobalt, manganese, lead, mercury, copper, iron, magnesium, potassium, zinc, sodium, and calcium. All of the test results are important; but of special interest will be the analysis for lead and mercury which will indicate the presence of any toxicity of these two metals in your body.

HOW TO INTERPRET YOUR MINERAL LEVELS

The figures from the hair test tell us whether or not your mineral level is normal. Still we must use clinical judgment along with the figures in working out your best mineral level.

As with vitamins, there is probably no such thing as a "normal" requirement of this or that mineral. Some people just feel better on what appear—by our present standards—to be abnormal levels of various minerals. Further, an individual's need for a certain mineral may change with age or at times of physical and emotional stress. Before menopause, women need more iron than men; women also need different levels of certain minerals at different times in their menstrual cycle. (Pre-menstrual cramps can often be controlled with massive doses of calcium.) Older people are more likely than younger ones to have mineral deficiencies, because of poor diet or because they absorb food poorly, or both. Pregnant or lactating women need more minerals than they would otherwise.

Not only is the total amount of a mineral in your body important, but mineral levels should be maintained in certain ratios to each other. Sodium and potassium work together. You need both calcium and magnesium, but to function properly you should have about twice as much calcium as magnesium. In times of stress, magnesium and calcium are particularly important.

CAUTION: You can overdose with minerals. Unlike water soluble excess vitamins, excess minerals are not quickly spilled out in the urine. So toxic levels may be reached. With one exception, I don't recommend that you take mineral supplements without the advice of a physician. If you suspect a deficiency in your diet, or recognize symptoms in the following descriptions of minerals and their actions, have a physician order a hair test sample and interpret the results for you. Use the results as a general guideline for starting mineral supplements.

The exception referred to is the natural calcium and magnesium supplement dolomite powder, which is safe and inexpensive and worth a try for anyone. I will discuss it more fully later.

HOW MINERALS AFFECT YOUR NERVES

To illustrate how minerals affect the way you feel, let me explain how two minerals act in nerve stimulation.

Whenever a nerve is stimulated there is an exchange between *sodium* and *potassium* across the nerve membrane. In the resting state most of the sodium remains outside the cell membrane and most of the potassium inside. But when the nerve is stimulated, sodium moves into the cell and potassium moves out of it. This causes an electrical charge in the cell which is passed down the cell body, releasing "catecolamines." These pass through the neural clef* and stimulate the next nerve. In the

* Nerves are not continuous like the copper electrical wiring in your house. A

meantime, the nerve which was stimulated undergoes a redistribution of sodium and potassium. A magnesium-activated enzyme system known as ATP (adenosine triphosphate) pumps the sodium back out of the cell and allows the potassium back inside.

Obviously, if you have a deficiency or a marked excess of the minerals sodium or potassium, your nerves cannot respond normally to stimulations. Also if the nerve membrane cannot allow the sodium and potassium to pass easily in and out, your nerves cannot function properly. If you lack magnesium, the sodium pump will not work properly.

During convulsions, sodium and potassium have a massive interchange through the cell membrane. According to one of the theories about the effect of electroshock therapy, nerve cell membranes are altered by the shock so that sodium and potassium can pass in a more normal manner.

HOW CALCIUM WORKS AS A NERVE RELAXER

Calcium salts are present in the body in the largest amounts of all the minerals. We all know how important calcium is in developing bones and teeth, but there are also sizeable amounts in the body fluids and cells. Furthermore, calcium has a marked effect on the excitability of the nervous system. Many years ago, I witnessed a dramatic demonstration of this.

While I was a resident in internal medicine, a thirty-four-year-old clerk came to the hospital's emergency room one Saturday night. He hated to bother the doctors at that late hour, he said, but he had a severe headache and couldn't find an open drug store. Could he please have a couple of aspirins?

He was given a check-up by the intern on duty who discovered papilledema—a condition in which the nerve endings in back of the eyes bulge out. This is a common finding associated with increased pressure in the skull due to a brain tumor.

The young man was told that he might have a tumor and was urged to admit himself to the hospital for a complete work-up. He wouldn't

---

space exists between one nerve and the next. This space is called the "neural clef."

hear of it, and continued to demand aspirin, which had always helped his headaches before. The intern continued to insist on hospitalization and eventually called the man's family, who pressured him into entering the hospital.

During the next four days, the patient was subjected to extensive neurological tests, including skull X-rays, brain scans, and all the other special tests performed when brain tumor is suspected. Much to everyone's surprise, the tests showed nothing abnormal. The team of doctors was unable to decide on a likely location for a brain tumor, but after a conference they decided to open the patient's skull anyway for an exploratory operation.

During the night before surgery, he began to complain of severe cramps in both legs. At first, the nurses thought he was simply nervous about his surgery, and paid little attention to him. But at the time of midnight rounds, they found him lying rigid, with the muscles of his arms and legs contracted. His throat was so tight that he made a crowing sound with every breath. They called the resident on neurosurgery, who examined the patient and then called me (I was an assistant resident in internal medicine at the time) for a medical consultation. Just before my arrival the patient suffered a convulsion, and was only semiconscious when I saw him.

I suppose it's only natural for surgeons to think in terms of surgical disorders, and internists to give priority to medical problems. I was immediately struck by the similarity between his condition and that of people suffering from an extremely low calcium level, and began to test my hunch by tapping with two fingers along the course of his facial nerve. This brought on a twitching of the muscles of his mouth, nose, and eyelids. I asked for a syringe and an ampule of calcium gluconate. Before we had finished injecting the solution into the patient's vein his body relaxed, the crowing sound which accompanied respiration ceased, and he was shortly conscious and able to talk rationally. This clinched the diagnosis of "hypocalcemia" and saved the man from unnecessary, and possibly dangerous, surgery.

It happened that this patient was suffering from a deficiency of the parathyroid gland, which reduced his calcium to very low levels. Minerals are greatly affected by body hormones, and such a dramatic calcium deficiency rarely occurs unless there is some accompanying defect like lack of vitamin D or low parathyroid hormone. Nonetheless, this case is a good illustration of the inability of the central nervous system to function properly without an adequate supply of a particular mineral: calcium.

Obviously, we don't often see people collapsing in the street, jerking with muscle spasms and making crowing sounds while breathing. But I wonder how many people might be suffering from milder forms of calcium deficiency, and how much emotional suffering they have because of it. A significant number of my psychiatric patients improve with calcium supplementation alone. The same is likely to be true of much of the non-patient population suffering from nervous tension due to stress.

An ordinary diet supplies calcium in fairly generous amounts through milk, cheese, egg yolk, beans, lentils, nuts, figs, cabbage, turnip greens, cauliflower, and asparagus. (I have already discussed in detail on page 102 why milk and milk products, nevertheless, should be avoided by most people.)

Supplementary calcium can be taken in several forms. I usually recommend one teaspoon of dolomite powder three times daily, since this provides much-needed magnesium as well as calcium. Magnesium deficiency is very common in our society—much more so than calcium deficiency. Three teaspoons of dolomite powder provide approximately 1180 mg. of calcium and 700 mg. of magnesium. This should be adequate for most adults, except at special times and during special circumstances such as pregnancy and lactation. At these times I would be inclined to triple the dosage.

How the ecology of the body affects calcium absorption

On a high-protein diet, approximately fifteen percent of the calcium taken in by mouth is absorbed. On a low-protein diet (that is the sugar and wheat diet so common in our society), only five percent of calcium is absorbed. The phytic acid in grains forms an insoluble compound called calcium phytilate. In this form, calcium is bound in such a manner that it can not be absorbed. Oxalates (organic chemicals) in certain foods (especially spinach) also combine with calcium to form calcium oxalate, an insoluble chemical which the body cannot use.

The absorption of both calcium and iron is reduced if hydrochloric acid is not present in normal amounts in the stomach. Lack of this acid is also associated with poor absorption of some of the B vitamins, notably vitamin B_{12}. Reports state that food allergies are more common in persons with low stomach acid because the food is not broken down completely during digestion. Cancer of the stomach has long been linked to low stomach acid.

I test all patients for free hydrochloric acid in the stomach and prescribe acidulin capsules if more acid is needed. Some patients are given a therapeutic trial on acidulin even if tests show normal gastric acidity.

Who would think a physician would advise patients to swallow bacteria, germs? I do. Why? As you may know, the intestinal tract normally harbors a heavy growth of bacteria—as does the mouth and, if you happen to be the type of human with a vagina, you also have bacteria there.

There are bad bacteria, so-so bacteria, and good bacteria. If you get the bad ones, for example, in your mouth, you may develop a strep throat, an invasion and inflammation of the throat by the streptococcus bacteria. If you get a bad one in your gut (like the typhoid bacillus), you may contract typhoid fever.

Most people have so-so bacteria in their intestinal tracts, neither good nor bad. You live. Things go along pretty well.

But it's also possible to have good bacteria that actively contribute to your best health.

That's why I often advise patients to take acidophilus bacteria, known simply as acidophilus. The massive presence of these bacteria helps you absorb certain vitamins and, even if you are a woman and take it by mouth, the acidophilus grows wherever it helps maintain the favorable acid balance. This greatly reduces infection and hence usually eliminates vaginal discharges.

Actually, vaginal discharges almost always disappear on the diet and nutritional supplements I recommend. The acidophilus merely speeds the process and makes it more complete. Unfortunately, few gynecologists are aware of these facts and go blindly along, prescribing local medication, the effect of which is often incomplete and temporary.

Acidophilus comes in liquid, tablet, or capsule form. I recommend two capsules three times a day. Acidophilus is grown in either a milk culture or a soybean culture. If you are allergic to milk or to soybeans you should of course choose accordingly. Capsule acidophilus is freeze-dried, so it won't spoil, as the liquid may.

WHY PHOSPHOROUS IS IMPORTANT

Phosphorous compounds are minerals of utmost importance to human chemistry. A few pages ago I mentioned adenosine triphosphate (ATP), the enzyme system activated by magnesium, which supplies energy for the sodium pump. As the name suggests, phosphorous is part of this enzyme system.

Although phosphorous abounds in every cell, about eighty percent of the phosphorous in your body is combined with calcium to form bones and teeth. Ten percent is used in various chemical compounds at work in the nervous system. Another ten percent is found in compounds involving proteins and fats in muscle tissue and blood.

Since phosphorous occurs in all living tissue, few people are deficient in it. Vegetarians come closest, but even they manage a relatively adequate intake, especially if they eat eggs and nuts.

Calcium, vitamin D, and phosphorous interconnect. You must have vitamin D to metabolize phosphorous. Phosphorous combines with calcium in a ratio of one part phosphorous to two parts calcium. The best natural sources of B vitamins (liver, yeast, and wheat germ) happen all to be high in phosphorous. Meat, fish, fowl, and eggs are good sources. Wheat flour has seventy-one percent of the phosphorous removed when it is refined for white bread and bakery products.

MAGNESIUM: THE NEGLECTED MINERAL

Magnesium salts are the most neglected minerals in the Western world, though they are amply available in nuts, soybeans, seafoods, beans, and peas, and in the supplement dolomite. The human body contains about 21 grams of magnesium. Something like seventy percent is combined with calcium and phosphorous to make bone; the rest is in the body's soft tissues and fluids. As with phosphorous, about one part magnesium for two parts calcium should be absorbed by the body.

Magnesium, like calcium, affects the permeability of the cell membrane. A defect in the cell membrane may result in distortion of perceptions, and alterations of moods, from euphoria to stupor. Studies have shown that alcoholics tend to be quite deficient in magnesium. This deficiency helps lead to the psychosis brought on by alcoholism: the DT's, the infamous "pink elephant" stage of alcoholism.

About 350 mg. a day is the minimum intake of magnesium that I recommend. Most Western people fall short of this figure. If you take relatively large amounts of calcium, and also indulge in alcohol, you should have at least twice the above minimum daily dosage.

The symptoms of magnesium deficiency

Suspect a magnesium deficiency if you have any of the following symptoms: irregular heart beat, excitability, muscle spasms, twitching, tremors, confusion, disorientation, weakness, depression, easily fractured bones, a wish to die.

If you or your physician suspect a magnesium deficiency, you should have a hair test to check. Also your physician might want to give you a trial on dolomite or some other magnesium supplement. For rich dietary sources of magnesium consider kelp, sea salt (a must if you use salt), brewers' yeast, sunflower and pumpkin seeds, raw or lightly steamed leafy vegetables or raw nuts. Milk, eggs and dairy products are low in magnesium. If you take vitamin D or calcium (dairy products or bone meal) your need for magnesium increases. Pregnancy also increases the body's need for magnesium. If you use alcohol, cortisone, the male hormone testosterone or digitalis you should have extra magnesium.

A case of acute magnesium deficiency

In a letter published in the medical journal *Lancet*[1] Dr. Joan Caddle of the George Washington School of Medicine discussed the importance of adding magnesium when thiamin (vitamin B_1) or other B vitamins are administered. In order to use B_1 the body needs a compound called thiamine pyrophosphate, which cannot be formed without magnesium.

In Nigeria, Dr. Caddle observed extremely malnourished children who had been treated with vitamin B-enriched milk with added protein. She discovered that the addition of these B vitamins actually *increased* the children's physical and emotional symptoms. Some children became immobilized and simply sat and stared, while others developed nervous tics of the eyelids, and still others showed tremors of the hands and feet and became unable to walk with a steady gait. A few even developed convulsions, which constitute the ultimate irritability of the central nervous system. Dr. Caddle uncovered a magnesium deficiency in these children. When magnesium was added to their other nutritional supplements, all their symptoms promptly disappeared.

These children represent an extreme case, but magnesium deficiency on a lower level is extremely common among Westerners. Since magnesium is so critically important to your physical and emotional health, you have little to lose and much to gain by adding a magnesium supplement, dolomite powder to your diet.

If you take vitamins and don't get a lift, or if you got a lift from vitamins that later faded, chances are great that you need more magnesium. Dolomite, a teaspoon in water daily two or three times, may do the trick.

WHY SODIUM IS IMPORTANT

We are all familiar with mineral sodium through our use of table salt (sodium chloride). Sodium, too, is used in the ATP energy transfers that take place in every cell, and is therefore essential to life. But our particular interest is sodium's action on the nerve cells, especially those nerve cells that constitute the brain and affect all our emotions.

There can be no question that sodium imbalance produces a profound effect on the nervous system. In Addison's disease, for example, a lowering of adrenal cortical hormones takes place, and these ordinarily help the body retain sodium. When sodium reserves are low, as they are in Addison's disease, the patient grows profoundly weak, tired, and depressed. Fortunately, full-blown Addison's disease is rather rare. The real question is: how many people who are only *somewhat* tired and depressed suffer from a sodium deficiency?

How sodium affects the mentally ill

Most people assume that Americans eat too much salt. I have been doing hair tests for minerals on my psychiatric patients for many years and have collected hundreds of test results. Although I have seen all sorts of patterns of mineral deficiencies and excesses, the most common findings are *sodium* and *potassium deficiencies.*

I strongly suspect that many emotionally ill people have defects in their sodium metabolism, just as they often have defects in their carbohydrate metabolism. I test patients' sodium metabolism with a "salt-dumping" test. First the patient collects all the urine he passes in twenty-four hours. Then he is given a solution of 10 grams of sodium chloride (table salt) to drink over a half-hour period. Then the urine is collected for another twenty-four-hour period. The first and second twenty-four-hour urine collections are tested for total sodium, potassium, and chloride.

Psychiatric patients frequently "dump" sodium. They lose excessive sodium after being given a test dose. Many such patients feel better when they take sodium supplements, and sometimes improve further with potassium supplements.

On the other hand some patients feel worse with added sodium. We humans are very complicated. Here again, a therapeutic trial is the only answer.

Heat exhaustion ("sunstroke") is a sodium deficiency

Profound changes in the central nervous system take place during heat exhaustion, in which the body is depleted of sodium. Patients with such a syndrome often suffer from headache, weakness, confusion, and drowsiness which can lead to coma. You might not think of coma as a manifestation of a central nervous system disorder; but the contrasting states of coma and convulsion do represent the two extremes of reaction in the nervous system.

Coma represents the ultimate of nervous tissue depression. Convulsions represent the height of nervous overactivity. The medical establishment clearly recognizes both these extremes; but the bigger problem is to diagnose the conditions that lie between the extremes: How much of the average person's fatigue, drowsiness, and depression are caused by low sodium levels?

Avoid low sodium

The normal body can excrete what sodium it does not need. The normal kidney excretes sodium without difficulty. But people with a history of high blood pressure should have their sodium intake supervised by a physician. And many people have high blood pressure (hypertension) without knowing it, so have yours checked. Also, patients with certain types of kidney diseases and heart trouble should not take liberal amounts of sodium without consulting their physicians.

I put some patients on a gram of sodium chloride several times daily. Often I advise patients to season their food liberally with sea salt, which contains not only sodium but also many valuable trace minerals and none of the impurities of ordinary table salt.

Many people get into sodium metabolism difficulties because their physicians prescribe diuretics for edema (swelling) of ankles, legs, hands, or face. The common cause of this edema is food allergies. No patient should have a diuretic without first being tested for food allergies. A diuretic is a medication that causes loss of sodium, along with a reduction of total body fluids. Diuretics are also commonly given to promote weight loss. I strongly disagree with the use of diuretics for weight reduction. Many people on diuretics grow depressed and extremely tired from loss of sodium, occasionally to the point of collapse.

POTASSIUM—A SEA STORY

Some years ago an elderly lady came to see me who insisted that she felt well only when she took kelp tablets. She was in her seventies, a stubborn little woman, determined to discover the reason for this oddity.

I was quite unable to shake her conviction that kelp was of great benefit to her. She had read up on the subject and believed that the iodine in kelp made her feel better by helping her thyroid to function more effectively. At the time I was still rather naive about nutrition, and I suspected that she was simply a foolish old woman with a fixed idea. But as I worked with her I gradually realized that her faith in kelp might not be unwarranted.

I began by putting her on kelp one week and taking her off the next, to see what differences there would be in her condition, if any. While taking kelp she was bright-eyed, alert, and energetic. During the weeks without it she dragged into my office depressed, tired, tense, and argumentative.

I then tried giving her a placebo (a bland tablet) one week and kelp the next. I could still see that she was much better with kelp than with the placebo. Next, I gave her a placebo which I said had a very high iodine content—higher than that of kelp—to test again whether her relief of symptoms was a product of self-suggestion. But even on this supposedly high-iodine placebo she did not feel at all well.

I investigated kelp and quickly discovered it had a high potassium as well as a high iodine content. Could the potassium be making her feel better? I performed hair tests and found her potassium level very low. When I substituted another form of potassium for the kelp, she maintained her feeling of well-being, but she disliked the syrup it came in.

At last I admitted that sea kelp was indeed helping her, and that it was the high potassium content that relieved her symptoms. Her self-therapy had been sound.

Too much potassium means trouble

Excessively high blood levels of potassium, amounting to potassium intoxication, usually occur only in patients with kidney failure; those who are in shock; people who are acutely dehydrated; or people suffering from Addison's disease.

The symptoms of elevated potassium are confined mainly to the central nervous system and to the heart. The heart may be slow and emit poor sounds. Ultimately there may be cardiac arrest. Central nervous system symptoms include mental confusion, tingling in the arms and legs, and numbness, sometimes progressing to the point of paralysis.

I have already mentioned that the hair tests of many of my psychiatric patients reveal *low* potassium levels. But interestingly, among the very sickest patients I often see *elevated* hair potassium levels. I have not been able to correlate these findings with medical conditions ordinarily associated with high potassium levels. These patients are often suffering from schizophrenia and are either hospitalized or struggling mightily to keep from being hospitalized. I have not been able to do controlled tests on this group, but many of them have been helped by the addition of sodium chloride to their diets and by intravenous doses of adrenal cortical extract. Of course I also use conventional psychiatric treatments with these patients, including anti-psychotic drugs. As these patients improve, the potassium level in the hair drops.

SULPHUR-PROTEIN EQUATION

Sulphur compounds make up a part of all body cells, since they are used in the formation of protein complexes that make up enzymes, as well as in the actual structure of the cell itself. Sulphur-containing compounds are also active in various bodily detoxification mechanisms. Man's source of sulphur is the protein he eats, where it is present in two amino acids: systeine and methionine. Sulphur in the inorganic or straight mineral form, unbound to a protein, apparently can't be metabolized. So as far as we know, Grandma's sulphur and molasses tonic didn't do much good.

YOUR IRON NEEDS

Although iron is present in the body in much smaller amounts than magnesium, sodium, sulphur, potassium, phosphorous, and calcium, iron salts are known to everyone because of their widely advertised role in preventing anemia.

People's needs for iron change greatly at different times of life. You need extra iron while you are growing, during pregnancy, and breast-feeding, or whenever you have lost blood (from accident, surgery, heavy menstrual flow, etc.). During these stressful periods, iron supplements may be necessary. But in general, only small traces of iron are needed for healthy adult men and for women past menopause. Even young women need only about 18 mg. a day during periods of stress such as child-bearing and lactation. The best food sources of iron are liver, kidney, heart, and spleen; next best are egg yolk, fish, clams, oysters, nuts, figs, dates, asparagus, beans, molasses, and oatmeal.

For the body to use iron properly, some traces of copper must be present. Also, iron is better absorbed when there is hydrochloric acid in the stomach. This means: if you take an iron pill, take it an hour before meals. Vitamin C also helps iron absorption by reducing it to a more soluble ferrous state. Some iron pills have added vitamin C, which makes sense. Phytic acid, which is found in many cereals, and oxalates (such as occur in spinach) interfere with iron absorption. As mentioned, vitamin

E and iron interfere with each other's absorption. Take E in the morning and, if needed, iron at night.

Because anemia tends to cause exhaustion and depression, proper iron levels are certainly important to the adequate functioning of the nervous system. However, iron is one of the nutritional supplements that you can overdo. Excessive amounts cause harmful iron deposits throughout the body. It's therefore a good idea to *consult your doctor before taking an iron supplement.* Most physicians, I am happy to say, are knowledgeable about iron, more so, perhaps, than about any other aspect of nutrition, and certainly more so than about any other phase of mineral metabolism.

YOUR COPPER NEEDS

Copper, essential for cellular metabolism, works in many enzyme systems. Together with iron, it is necessary for the formation of hemoglobin. Copper is also needed to maintain the myelin sheath around the nerves. The sheaths act as insulators, like insulation around wires, so that impulses traveling along them are not passed on inadvertently to other nerves.

Copper deficiency is rare in "normal" human adults, but occasionally my hair test reveals low copper deposits in a patient. The exact clinical significance of this has not yet been determined, because usually a patient low in copper is also deficient in other minerals. In private practice it is impossible to do control studies by administering only one mineral at a time; patients are not expected to lend themselves to experiments. Whatever deficiencies exist must be treated immediately. But definite copper deficiencies are sometimes found in children on a high milk diet, and in some adults who suffer from severe diarrhea and lack of absorption from the gastrointestinal tract. One result can be copper-deficiency anemia.

For copper eat shellfish, other seafood, liver, kidney, lamb and brewers' or primary yeast.

The most significant disorder associated with copper metabolism is Wilson's disease. This involves profound changes in the brain and liver, due to abnormal copper deposits caused by metabolic defects. The disease causes marked tremors, difficulty in speech, drooling, poor coordination and muscle rigidity due to improper nerve stimulation. Accompanying emotional symptoms include changes in behavior and neurotic and psychotic reactions.

It is felt by some that mildly elevated copper levels are often associated with schizophrenia, and attempts have been made to lower the copper levels of patients suffering from schizophrenia by using penicillamine. Most psychiatrists reject this drug because it frequently causes sensitivity and general toxic reaction. Nevertheless, I feel penicillamine therapy should at least be considered for schizophrenics with high copper levels who do not respond to other forms of treatment. And do be wary of copper cooking utensils, copper water pipes, and copper beer cooling coils!

YOUR IODINE NEEDS

A few generations ago iodine received much publicity after the discovery that an iodine deficiency could cause a goiter, a swelling of the thyroid gland. The deficiency was found in areas distant from the oceans, such as Switzerland or America's Midwest; where vegetables were grown in iodine-poor soil; where the soil had not been submerged under an ocean in recent geological history; and where people ate little seafood.

Iodine deficiency can cause hypothyroidism, a low functioning thyroid. But more about this disorder in the chapter on hormones.

The average adult iodine requirement is only 100 to 150 micrograms daily, which you can easily get from iodized salt. Since iodized salt often contains impurities, including sugar, I consider kelp a much more desirable source. The body stores what iodine it needs and discards the rest, so there is virtually no chance of getting too much. A kelp tablet one to four times a day is your best source of iodine.

NOTE: Iodine in kelp or iodized salt rather frequently causes acne-like skin eruptions.

YOUR MANGANESE NEEDS

Manganese is required in amounts of only about 4 mg. a day, and clear deficiencies in man have not been adequately studied. In my hair tests I rather frequently find patients deficient in manganese, but these people usually have multiple deficiencies and cannot be treated for manganese deficiency. It is difficult to know just what symptoms come from a lack of manganese.

The enzymes arginase and phosphotransferases require manganese as a cofactor. In other words, at least these two enzyme systems require the mineral manganese as an activator. Arginase aids in protein metabolism and phosphotransferases aid energy systems.

Copper, iron, and manganese act as catalysts in the formation of hemoglobin.

In tests on male laboratory animals, manganese deficiency has caused a loss of interest in sex and eventual sterility; female test animals refused to suckle their young.

So, what do you need to know about manganese? Eat nuts or leafy vegetables and take brewers' or primary yeast daily!

If your hair test shows a manganese deficiency, your physician might suggest manganese citrate, 50 mg. daily. (This is not available everywhere but you can find it, along with other rare items such as sugar-free, starch-free tablets, vitamins in colorless capsules, and straight ascorbic acid powder at Willner Chemist, 330 Lexington Avenue, New York, N.Y. 10016. I have no financial interest in this or any other nutrition-related concern, although I sometimes wish that I did!)

YOUR COBALT NEEDS

To date there is not much definite information about cobalt deficiencies in adult humans, though some reports indicate that cobalt therapy has helped anemic children. Typically, we know more about the effects of the deficiency on livestock than on humans. It is well known that cattle and sheep grazing on cobalt-deficient land may develop pernicious anemias and severe disorders of the central nervous system, and that their symptoms are relieved by adding cobalt to the diet.

Cobalt is incorporated into the complex B_{12} vitamin structure. I have already mentioned that I believe *everyone* should have a serum B_{12} level test, and that they should try therapeutic doses of vitamin B_{12} at least for a while. While cobalt deficiency per se has not been proven in humans, vitamin B$_{12}$ deficiencies very definitely have.

For more cobalt in your diet, choose seafood.

YOUR ZINC NEEDS

During the past few years some physicians have become interested in zinc, which has been found to help in wound healing. Pediatricians have prescribed it as a popular ingredient of diaper rash ointment.

Some researchers have concluded that persons suffering from schizophrenia also require extra amounts of zinc. There has been no general confirmation of this stand elsewhere, so far as I know. Zinc is used in widespread enzyme systems throughout the body, including one that works with insulin, and the one required for the metabolism of brain cells.

People suffering from alcoholism may have a special problem with zinc. Once they develop cirrhosis of the liver, their average concentration of zinc is only 66 micrograms per 100 ml., about half the amount found in well people. Apparently, persons suffering from alcoholic cirrhosis are unable to store zinc and lose large amounts in their urine. Since zinc is even required in the metabolism of alcohol itself, it might be a good idea for all heavy drinkers to add a zinc supplement to their diet. Brewers' or primary yeasts are good sources. Tablets or capsules of zinc gluconate are available in 50 to 60 mg. sizes in health food stores. One of these tablets daily is the usual dose.

YOUR CHROMIUM NEEDS

Meat, shellfish, and chicken are good sources of chromium for our diet. And again, include brewers' or primary yeast!

Chromium acts in concert with insulin in the metabolism of sugar. In studies on animals maintained on low chromium diets, the animals developed a diminished sugar tolerance, which could be reversed by the addition of chromium. Rats maintained on severely chromium-restricted diets showed impaired growth, and did not live out their usual life span.

Recent research indicates that chromium deficiency in humans is extremely widespread. Chromium is useful in preventing and lowering high blood pressure. It also helps reduce cholesterol and hardening of the arteries. This means chromium probably helps fight the mental changes accompanying senility.

HOW TO ESTABLISH
YOUR OWN VITAMIN
AND MINERAL REGIMEN

CHAPTER FOURTEEN

As I have emphasized, establishing your true nutritional needs can be complicated, and it is an ongoing process. You can't just "set it and forget it." I have been fine-tuning my own nutrition program for years.

It's a physiological reality that from time to time your body chemistry or general health shifts, and this requires that you raise or lower your levels of this or that nutrient. Inevitably, too, you will experience times of unusual physical or mental stress. You may develop allergies or grow out of them. Your hormone levels will change with age, pregnancy, or menopause.

Don't be discouraged at the thought that you will probably never hit on one particular combination of needs that will suit you for the rest of your life. Look at it this way: Almost nothing important in life remains constant; just when you think you've got everything nailed down you change your job or get a promotion; or your children grow up; or your marriage cracks; or the market drops. Your life then must get changed around to accommodate the new situation. Life is indeed a process, and no process is static.

Be sure to get a doctor's advice.

Before I go on, I must say once more that the information I am about to give is valid *in general;* it works for most people, but it is entirely possible that it will not suit you. If sound nutrition affects your body profoundly—and it does—then it follows that altering your nutrition could have a significant and even harmful effect on a person with certain medical problems. So I urge you again to consult your doctor before you begin a megavitamin regimen.

I am aware that this advice raises problems. If every doctor knew what he should about proper nutrition, you wouldn't need this book in the first place. Instead, your doctor may be less well informed on the subject than you are, and he may be discouraging or even scornful of your interest in it. Nevertheless, I recommend that you go over your medical history with him so you can be sure you know if there is any reason for you to anticipate trouble.

Have you ever had rheumatic fever or any other disease that could weaken your heart? Do you have high blood pressure? Do you have diabetes—or high blood sugar? Do you have low blood sugar? Do you have a tendency toward depression? Do you have an ulcer, or any digestive problem that could be aggravated by large doses of vitamins? Are you taking any drugs (such as antidepressents or anticoagulants) that might be affected by your vitamin intake?

As you know, I cannot prescribe specifically for you without having examined you. If you were my patient, I would test you for the above conditions, order a blood sugar test for you that would reveal any tendency toward hypoglycemia or diabetes; I'd have your hair tested for mineral levels; I'd order a blood test to check your serum levels of B_{12} and folic acid and perform a host of other tests. Then I would design a specific vitamin and mineral program for you based on your symptoms and your special chemistry and metabolism. And I would watch you throughout the course of your treatment.

Even if you decide to design your own nutritional program, I still believe you should arrange to have this sort of medical attention, especially in the beginning. If you can persuade your doctor to read up on nutrition and megavitamin therapy, well and good. If not, at least have him check your blood pressure and your heart, and if he tries to talk you out of taking vitamin supplements, make sure he explains his objections in detail, so that you may separate prejudice from sound medical judgment. If he has objections, ask him for specific medical references you may read. Chances are he won't be able to suggest any because he will be passing a negative judgment without proper information.

THE MINIMUM TESTS YOU NEED

It would be interesting, if not absolutely necessary, to have your doctor test you for blood vitamin, protein, and fat levels. But at the very least you should be tested for blood levels of B_{12} and folic acid. As you know, many people who get adequate amounts of B_{12} in their diet (or who take a B_{12} supplement) cannot absorb the vitamin from their intestines; they may therfore have an unsuspected deficiency that can only be traced by B_{12} injections. If this be true in your case, you will need a doctor's cooperation to get the B_{12} shots anyway, so you might as well meet this issue with him head on.

I have found that as many as one-third of my patients have significant B_{12} and folic acid deficiencies. These deficiencies often painfully affect their emotional well-being.

In the case of folic acid, you should know whether you have a deficiency. You will need a doctor's prescription to get a supply of it. Folic acid cannot be sold over the counter, because by taking it you might possibly mask a case of pernicious anemia.

Also, I think it highly advisable to have your mineral levels checked. (In the chapter on minerals you will find the name of a laboratory that will analyze your hair sample for your doctor. You cannot order these tests yourself.) I do not believe that you should take mineral supplements without a hair test, not even the ever-popular iron pills and tonics that are pushed as if they were mother's milk. Remember: minerals can accumulate in your body until they reach toxic levels and that can be at least as dangerous as a mineral deficiency. I've already mentioned the exception to this rule: natural dolomite powder, which supplies calcium and magnesium in ideal proportion to each other.

If your family doctor refuses to cooperate with you in ordering B_{12} and folic acid tests, a mineral test, or in prescribing a therapeutic dose of vitamins, without giving a sound medical reason for his reluctance, then you have two choices. First, you can try some arm twisting. Your doctor, after all, is providing a service. He can give you advice based on his best scientific judgment, but he shouldn't refuse you a treatment that you want if he does so on the grounds of simple prejudice.

If your lawyer refused to handle your divorce case on the grounds that your wife is a wonderful woman and you shouldn't *want* to divorce her, you would be perfectly justified in seeking legal service elsewhere. You can point this out to your doctor, although I'm sure you're aware that it is not likely to improve relations between you. Perhaps the preferable alternative is to locate a second doctor for this treatment alone. When you call for an appointment, make it clear to him or his secretary that you are coming specifically for a B_{12} and folic acid test (plus a mineral test and whatever other special information you want). If, on your arrival, the doctor says he is disinclined to order these tests for you, you can explain that you will be disinclined to pay him for the visit.

I am sorry to have to recommend such behavior, but if that's what you have to do to get adequate medical care, then that's what you should do. If enough patients put enough such pressure on their physicians, the end result may eventually be that medical men will be as interested in preventing illness as they are in treating it.

WHY YOU NEED A NUTRITIONAL BASE

Megavitamins are doses of vitamins that may be hundreds or even thousands of times higher than the quantities that are needed to prevent clinical symptoms of malnutrition. Each vitamin has different properties, and may be of special benefit to one person or another. The amounts that will help you, you can determine for yourself. But before I begin to explain that process, let me say that, like the FDA, I believe that there is a base level of vitamins that should be taken by virtually every adult. But, unlike the FDA, I think that if you live in modern America and eat modern American food, there is almost no chance that you can get adequate levels of vitamins from your diet alone. Therefore, the first thing you should do is bring your nutritional levels up to normal.

START WITH CRUDE VITAMINS

You will remember, from the chapter on vitamins, that there are probably essential nutrients that we haven't discovered yet. Our best information suggests that essential nutrients exist in such crude foods as yeast, and desiccated liver that you cannot get from any manufactured pill. Many apparently healthy, well-balanced people who add these elements to their diet experience an increased feeling of well-being that seems amazing to them, considering that they thought they felt good before.

The first addition to your diet should be yeast: brewers' or primary, and torula. Yeast is a natural source of B vitamins, and it is generally about 50 percent protein, and it contains many essential amino acids. It also contains trace minerals and unidentified nutrients.

Torula yeast is a richer source of B vitamins than the other yeasts. But no more than 50 percent of your yeast should be in this form. My conclusion is based on research findings that show torula yeast may be higher in some vitamins and minerals than brewers' or primary yeast, but lacks certain unknown growth factors present in the other two yeasts. That is to say, laboratory animals fed torula yeast show a spurt of growth when switched to brewers' or primary yeast. You might conclude that this finding is not important for you since you aren't trying to grow. To me it means torula yeast lacks one or more nutrients. How this lack may affect your nutritional status, no one knows. So let's play it safe and include brewers' or primary yeast. I do. Some people claim to prefer the taste of one yeast or the other, but frankly, they all taste less than delightful at first. All I can tell you is you will learn to tolerate it and in remarkably short order. You will even get to like it if you give your body a chance to appreciate it and to expect the lift it gives you. Start with a teaspoon in half a glass of water. I find yeast tastes better when mixed with ascorbic acid. You might find yeast more acceptable at first mixed with tomato juice. Some of my patients buy blank gelatin capsules and pack them with the powdered yeast. (Yeast tablets are not the answer because you would have to take too many. The filler used to make the tablets upsets many people when taken in large amounts.)

The first time you take yeast you may feel slightly ill for a few hours. This is often followed by an upsurge of energy and good feeling, but not always; this will depend in part upon how badly you need B vitamins.

I have heard people describe their reaction during their first day on a teaspoonful of yeast as something akin to a drug rush, beginning with minor queasiness, and then, as the body adjusts to the new chemical state, a period of such marked good feelings, that it amounts to an altered state of being. Other people must take yeast a number of months to begin feeling its benefit.

I recommend that you gradually increase your daily yeast intake until you are up to one heaping tablespoon twice daily. If you can tolerate them well, I think it wise to take torula yeast in the morning and either brewers' or primary yeast in the evening.

It's only fair to warn you that yeast may give you gas at first. In time your intestinal tract will usually adjust to the yeast. You may also find that one type will give you less gas than another, so try switching. But if the situation doesn't improve at all, you can change to six desiccated liver capsules three times a day. Again, start light and build up the dosage.

ADD BASIC VITAMINS ONE AT A TIME

After two or three days on yeast, start to add the other vitamins—one at a time so that you can watch for possible reactions.

Natural Vitamin A: 1 capsule, 10,000 units.

Natural Vitamin D: 1 capsule, 400 units.

Alpha-tocopherol succinate (Vitamin E): 1 capsule, 200 units.

Ascorbic acid powder: one-quarter teaspoon dissolved in water (1000 mg.) 4 times daily (total of 4000 mg.).

Then add lecithin granules, two heaping tablespoons (eaten straight or on fruit) daily, and one-half teaspoon dolomite powder in water with meals or two teaspoons at bedtime. Dolomite makes some people sleepy. If you are edgy or excitable you may prefer it at breakfast.

I do not advise experimenting with the dosages of vitamin A or D. I have not found that higher doses yield any appreciable benefit, and there is always the chance that if you were to take a great deal of either one for a long period (say, three months) you could accumulate a toxic amount. Let me emphasize that the dosage I have recommended is absolutely safe. You would probably need to take five or ten times these amounts for several months before you *might* reach toxic levels.

NOW STEP UP TO MEGAVITAMIN LEVELS

When you have lived with this base level of vitamins for about a month, you can begin experimenting with higher levels of vitamins E, C, and the B's until you determine whether the megavitamin program is best for you. If you suffer from schizophrenia you would probably be best off to continue megavitamins for several years before deciding whether or not they will help you. As you did in the beginning, you should increase only one vitamin at a time, so that if and when you experience a reaction (beneficial or not) you will know to what to attribute it.

One more tip before you begin. The most common difficulty people experience with megavitamins is indigestion, or a burning feeling in the stomach. As you know, I feel that this is far more likely to happen when you take tablets containing starch, sugar, or artificial dyes. If this happens discontinue the vitamin added last. Then after several days, start taking it again at a lower dosage.

If you find that even low doses of a particular vitamin give you stomach pain, you may have to conclude that you are allergic to the vitamin itself, and eliminate it.

HOW TO ESTABLISH YOUR VITAMIN E LEVEL

As you learned in the chapter on vitamins, E is one of the most important vitamins for treating emotional symptoms. If you are tired, listless, or depressed, if you are experiencing menopausal symptoms, if you are under emotional stress or stress from a polluted environment, increased doses of vitamin E may help you. Research indicates that vitamin E may well prolong your life and many men swear it increases their sexual vigor.

The Drs. Shute in Canada have spent their lives studying vitamin E.

They have thrown the vitamin E advocates into somewhat of a turmoil since one of these two physicians now believes that Alpha-tocopherol *acetate* is the important source of vitamin E, and the other brother believes that Alpha-tocopherol *succinate* is the important source of vitamin E. As a result, many of us are suggesting that patients take each type of vitamin E to make certain they are covered. I think it might be a good idea also to throw in a capsule of natural mixed tocopherols (E complex), about 200 units daily.

It is particularly important that anyone with heart disease receive close supervision while taking vitamin E. I am one of the very many physicians who believe that the use of vitamin E is essential for the proper treatment of many kinds of heart diseases. But the proper dosage differs for different kinds of heart trouble.

Also, some people's blood pressure rises if more than 200 units of vitamin E is taken per day. The blood pressure promptly drops to normal after the dose is reduced. Almost every one of these patients can take high levels of vitamin E if the dose is increased very slowly.

For almost two years I couldn't go above 350 units daily. Then, gradually, I could step this up without having my blood pressure rise. Now I seem to be able to take almost any amount without difficulty.

Since vitamin E may be stimulating, I advise that it be taken early in the day. Because it interferes with the absorption of iron, it should never be spread out over three or four doses a day. The gut should be left to absorb iron at night. The E should be taken at breakfast and lunch.

I suggest that people start on about 100 to 200 units of mixed Alpha-tocopherol acetate and Alpha-tocopherol succinate daily. Almost anyone can take that amount without worrying about increased blood pressure. Then, if you want to increase your level of vitamin E, add 100 to 200 units to your daily dose every week. About half of the vitamin E should be in the form of Alpha-tocopherol *acetate* and half in Alpha-tocopherol *succinate*.

Note as you go along whether or not you experience a feeling of increased well-being.

HOW TO ESTABLISH YOUR VITAMIN C LEVEL

I am convinced that there are large variations in the amount of vitamin C that people need for ideal functioning. Linus Pauling says that about 4000 mg. a day is the minimum amount of vitamin C most people require, and, from my clinical experience, I am inclined to go along with him on this figure. I have observed, however, that many people feel better on much higher doses of vitamin C. Here again, the only way to discover at what level of vitamin C you feel best is to increase it gradually to much larger doses.

You can start with your base dose of one-quarter teaspoon four times a day (4000 mg.), then build up by adding about 2000 mg. every four days. Remember to take it well diluted in room temperature or cold water. It flavors hot tea as if it were lemon, but unfortunately heat destroys the vitamin.

If you have an ulcer or have a tendency toward ulcers, your stomach may not be able to tolerate the acidity. This acidity can be eliminated by adding ordinary baking soda (bicarbonate of soda) to ascorbic acid powder. Use the proportion of about three-quarters part of soda to one part of ascorbic acid (by volume). If, for example, you are up to one teaspoon of ascorbic acid, add three-quarters teaspoon of baking soda. Mix the two powders and add water. The fizzing you see occurs when carbon dioxide is released by the chemical reaction that transforms ascorbic acid into sodium ascorbate, a neutral form of vitamin C that has the same vitamin properties as ascorbic acid.

Remember that bicarbonate of soda contains sodium, so you should check with your physician to be certain you have no medical condition (such as high blood pressure) that demands that your sodium intake be restricted.

Remember, too, that the ordinary vitamin C tablet you buy at the corner drugstore is neither sugar- nor starch-free unless it is so labeled. This common ascorbic acid tablet gives many people diarrhea if taken in reasonably large amounts. A better source of vitamin C is the sugar-free, starch-free tablet (so labeled). Better still is the clear capsule containing vitamin C. The straight powder is the best, although even the powder may produce diarrhea when taken in very large amounts. Again, start slow and build up the dosage gradually.

Two warnings!

1. Use the ascorbic acid powder only if it looks like talcum powder. A granular substance (granular like table sugar) is also often labeled "ascorbic acid *powder*." Avoid this granular form. It

frequently causes all sorts of difficulties: diarrhea, upset stomach, rashes, emotional difficulties, etc. How do I know? Not long ago a shortage of ascorbic acid powder developed and many of my patients (along with me) switched to the granular type. Almost all of us had many reactions from it.

2. Some companies started cutting (diluting) their ascorbic acid powder with inert ingredients. This means you get shortchanged and you will be taking the wrong dose. The proper strength: one teaspoon equals about 4000 mg. of ascorbic acid.

These may seem like small points but they are very important because they can make the difference between success and failure in your vitamin program.

As I have already mentioned, ascorbic acid powder, sugar-free/ starch-free tablets and clear capsules are available at: Willner Chemist, 330 Lexington Avenue, New York City. The same (except for the clear capsule) are also available at: Freeda Pharmacy, 110 East 41st Street, New York City.

Authorities disagree about how high to run up your daily intake of vitamin C. Fred Klenner, M.D., of Reidsville, N.C., whose broad clinical experience with the vitamin extends over a lifetime and who probably knows more about the clinical use of ascorbic acid than anyone else in the world, regularly prescribes doses of 20,000 mg. daily for himself and his patients. I find that many of my patients feel better with a minimum of 10,000 mg. of vitamin C, but I have also found that a large group, particularly those with food allergies, feel better on about 15,000 mg. a day. I feel best at 10,000 mg. daily. A few of my patients feel best on 30,000 mg. a day, and I have one patient with an extremely unusual biochemistry who functions well only on the heroic dosage of 40,000 mg. of vitamin C daily.

This very gifted woman has marked food allergies and was for a number of years an alcoholic. When she stopped drinking she became very obese because of a food allergy addiction syndrome that sent her on eating sprees. Tests revealed that my patient, who had tried a great many other forms of treatment without success, was sensitive to almost every food, but especially to meats. Only when we took her off all meats and gradually increased her ascorbic acid to 40,000 mg. daily was she able to control her weight and feel good. By "good" I mean that she lost her chronic depression and tiredness. She was suicidal when I first saw her, but she has now attained significant heights in her profession, takes pride in her slender figure, and finds that life is worthwhile again.

We have repeatedly tried reducing her ascorbic acid intake but she simply does not feel good at lower levels. As a matter of fact, she sometimes needs a 5 gram intravenous injection if she gets slightly depressed. I might add that I also gave her autourine injections, and these significantly reduced her food allergies so that she was able to keep from going on eating sprees.

Based on Dr. Klenner's long experience with vitamin C therapy, on my reading and my own clinical experience, I feel that up to 20,000 mg. of vitamin C daily is a safe dose for most people.

Caution: If you have ever had an ulcer it *could* be reactivated from a large dose of vitamin C. Of course, if you were about to get an ulcer next week, it might develop in a few days. If your uric acid is elevated, it may go higher with more C, though usually it falls. Your cholesterol will drop markedly with large amounts of C. If you are pregnant, inform your pediatrician-to-be about your vitamin intake. We have not had enough long-range experience with people on doses of 30,000 to 40,000 mg. to know for certain whether these are safe. I would never advise such a large dose to anyone who is not under a doctor's care, and I never prescribe it myself except when many other forms of treatment have been tried and exhausted.

There is plenty of controversy about large doses of vitamin C, as there is controversy about every other facet of human endeavor— whether it be how to construct a bridge, how to get the nation out of a depression, or how to attain true happiness.

I believe that the best test of whether a vitamin is helping you is to observe the way you feel.

If you're curious, you can test your own urine for a general idea of how much vitamin C you are excreting. From a drugstore buy a solution of five percent aqueous silver nitrate. With an eyedropper, put ten drops of this solution in a clean cup. Add ten drops of your urine. Wait two minutes. The solution will be white-beige, smoky gray, or charcoal in color. The darker it is, the more vitamin C you are spilling. If you excrete little or no vitamin C, that means your system is using all it can get, and you might consider increasing your dose still further.

Vitamin C can lower your folic acid and vitamin B_{12} levels. If you take more than 500 mg. a day of vitamin C, you should have your serum folic acid and B_{12} levels checked every six months. Better, take folic acid 10 mg. daily by mouth and have a vitamin B_{12}b injection every three months.

HOW TO ESTABLISH YOUR B VITAMIN LEVELS

Finding your own best levels of B vitamins is a two-part process. After you have found your level for C and E, you begin with the B vitamins, one at a time. Take one until you discover what amount lets you feel best, then stop temporarily while you test the next. You should keep a written record of mental and physical reactions to each new nutrient, so that when you are ready to take them in combination you won't forget what you discovered.

When you have tested each one and arrived at a complete schedule of B vitamins for yourself, you may find that taking them in combination produces different effects than each had separately. So you may then want to experiment with the dose levels, to see whether you can decrease any amounts without loss of good feeling, or whether larger doses of one in combination with another will increase the performance of both.

You may well get lost in the process of all this testing. Never mind. Simply refer to the megavitamin schedule I will give you later in the book and follow that. The process of selecting dose levels is difficult and it may be complicated by the fact that you may be one of those persons who must take a particular vitamin for weeks or months before you feel its benefit—or you may only feel its lack months after you have lowered the dosage.

I mention this in particular connection with testing your B vitamin levels because some people are quite sensitive to levels of certain of the individual B vitamins.

Selecting your dosage of vitamin C and vitamin E is a simpler and a more accurate process, as a rule, than finding your correct level for one of the B vitamins.

Since B and C vitamins are water-soluble and easily discarded, there is no danger that extra amounts will accumulate to a harmful level in your body.

You should also keep in mind that the B vitamins are an interlocking *complex*. You need all of them. The yeast you take will provide a good basic level of B vitamins.

Because people's requirements for B_{12} vary greatly, I would have my serum B_{12} level checked occasionally, if I were following a vegetarian diet. Vegetarians are especially trouble-prone when subjected to unusual stress, since any kind of strain uses up vitamin B_{12} in massive amounts. One of the greatest of these strains is pregnancy, since the fetus receives its nourishment from both what the mother eats and what her body stores.

As reported by N. Hakami[1], it is perfectly possible to have normal serum B_{12} levels and at the same time have low tissue levels. That is: the blood level may be normal, but the amount of B_{12} in the nerve and muscle tissue and other tissues of the body may be too low, because the body may lack a specific protein required to transport the vitamin from the blood into the tissues. When this protein is in short supply, massive doses of vitamin B_{12} are required for the tissue levels to reach their normal functioning state.

This chain effect again illustrates the complexity of nutrition, and the multitude of factors that affect our nutrition. Immense gaps still exist in our knowledge. Physicians must still depend to some extent on clinical knowledge, experience, and logic to advise their patients about correct diet and dietary supplements. But again I insist that, rather than waiting another hundred years until all the still unanswered questions are scientifically settled, we must do our best by using what we have.

Take the individual B vitamins in colorless sugar-free, starch-free tablets, or even better, in capsules. Your riboflavin (B_2) will be yellow because the vitamin itself is this color. As you know, you should avoid dyes and binders whenever possible. If you cannot find at a local source vitamins in colorless capsules, I can only suggest that you write to: Willner Chemists, 330 Lexington Avenue, New York City. They will send you a price list and you can then order whatever you need; they mail vitamins all over the country. *Let me assure you once again that I have absolutely no financial or professional connection with this or any other firm mentioned in this book.* In the present state of the study of food allergies, this is simply the only source I know for B vitamins in this form.

HOW TO ESTABLISH YOUR THIAMIN (B₁) LEVEL

Many people, particularly those who are tired or depressed, feel better when they start taking vitamin B_1 in megadoses.

I suggest that you begin with one 500 mg. capsule of thiamin after breakfast on a Saturday morning. I say 500 mg. because less is rarely worthwhile and Saturday because it is possible that you will experience a high and need some time to come down. (Most people find this a welcome sensation, especially if they were tired out from thiamin deficiency in the first place, but if you were to try sitting on a stool all day to balance the books while you felt like climbing a tree or a mountain, it could be annoying.)

When you have adjusted to one capsule a day, move up to three a day, one with each meal. After a week, try going up to two capsules three times a day. That brings you to 3000 mg. a day, which is a pretty hefty dose considering that the government's so-called "daily requirement" is 1.5 mg. If your good feeling continues to soar, you could go as high as 1500 mg. three times a day; I think there is little reason to go higher than that. If your sense of well-being has not increased at this point, you should drop back to a more modest dose. (You may want to try raising the levels again when you are taking megadoses of each of the B vitamins to see whether your reactions change.)

HOW TO ESTABLISH YOUR RIBOFLAVIN (B₂) LEVEL

I'm not sure I have ever seen emotional difficulties improved by a riboflavin supplement alone. Still, vitamin B_2 has a marked effect on certain physical symptoms such as red, burning tongues, painful cracks at the corners of the mouth, and eyes that are sensitive to light. Many people who wear dark glasses all the time because bright light hurts their eyes are suffering from a riboflavin deficiency; this is harmful both in itself and because the natural sunlight you absorb through your eyes is an important source of stimulation to your nervous system, as you will read in my chapter on light. Riboflavin deficiency can also cause myeline (nerve tissue) degeneration, and it has been found to cause atrophy of male sex glands in rats.

I recommend that you try 60 or 100 mg. of riboflavin three times a day for a week. When you have completed this trial and recorded any change in your physical or emotional condition, put riboflavin aside until you have completed testing the other B vitamins.

HOW TO ESTABLISH YOUR NIACIN OR NIACINAMIDE (B₃) LEVEL

Vitamin B_3 is one of the most important new discoveries in the orthomolecular approach to emotional disorders. As you will read in the chapter on schizophrenia, it has proved to be a most useful weapon in the fight against severe emotional disorders, and it can be of great benefit to many other people who are nervous, tired, depressed, or mildly overwrought. As you know, niacin can also have significant physical effects, reducing blood cholesterol and the danger of blood clots, and it tends to raise blood sugar levels, which is a boon to hypoglycemics but a potential difficulty for diabetics.

Because vitamin B_3 can have such important physical effects, I recommend especially that you take this supplement with the advice of your doctor. Get him to read the medical literature on niacin if he hasn't already; if he won't, find a physician who will.

There are two commonly used types of B_3: niacin and niacinamide. I usually find that people who are slowed down and depressed do better on niacin, and that tense, hyperexcitable people do better on niacinamide. *Please note: niacinamide can act as a depressant in some people.*

I generally start my patients on 500 mg. of niacin three times a day. Double the dose every other day until you are taking 1000 mg. three times a day. Vitamin B_3, especially, should be taken in clear capsule form. Willner Chemists produces a capsule of 250 mg. and one at 500 mg., though you must have a prescription for the latter. Niacin may cause flushing, and occasionally, nausea (see the discussion of niacin in the vitamin chapter for the control of side-effects).

Megadoses of niacin most often give a lift and a feeling of buoyancy to older people in general, and to depressed people in particular. After a few days, the flush from your initial dose of niacin should decrease and disappear. Although the standard minimum dose for people with emotional difficulties is generally 1000 mg. three times a day, some schizophrenics must sometimes go as high as 30,000 mg. per day. You should of course select your own dose according to the level that lets you feel best.

Keep in mind that while most people feel better within days of beginning a niacin regimen, some require months to feel the benefits. It is especially important to give this vitamin a lengthy therapeutic trial because its potential benefits are so great. If you find you do better on niacinamide than on niacin, I do not recommend pushing the dosage beyond 4000 to 8000 mg. per day.

When you reach higher levels of niacinamide or, especially, niacin, you might be plagued by nausea. This nausea is often more marked in the morning and may come on *before* you take your after-breakfast dose of the vitamin. For this reason, you may not suspect the vitamin as the cause of your difficulty. Skip your vitamin B_3 for a day. If it's causing your nausea, it should disappear.

Nausea is very common with the garden variety of niacin tablet you pick up at the corner drugstore. It is less common when taking the starch-free, sugar-free tablets and much less common when taking the colorless, sugar-free, starch-free capsule. Again: don't let a druggist tell you a product is sugar-free and starch-free unless it is so labeled by the manufacturer.

People suffering from schizophrenia should generally build up their niacin dosage gradually over a period of several weeks. When they reach the level of experiencing nausea, as most people do at some level, skip the vitamin for twenty-four hours and go back on a slightly lower dosage, say about 1500 mg. per day lower than the level that produced the nausea.

If you don't experience any nausea with higher doses, don't go beyond 30,000 mg. per day. People who do not improve on this level do not improve on levels higher than this.

NOTE: Niacin and niacinamide in mega (large) amounts produce false positive liver function tests. Tell your physician about it. He is not likely to know. I have seen many patients waste hundreds of dollars on complex liver function tests because their physicians were not aware of these false positive tests.

Niacin is frequently needed in high doses by people with severe food allergies; it seems to act as a nonspecific detoxifier. I once had a patient who could scarcely function on less than 30,000 mg. of niacin per day, but when we discovered that she was allergic to meat and eliminated it from her diet, she needed no more niacin at all. Like many other orthomolecular psychiatrists I have also found that using niacin often decreases a patient's need for tranquilizers. Usually your physician can cut your tranquilizer dose in half soon after you start megavitamins.

HOW TO ESTABLISH YOUR PYRIDOXINE (B₆) LEVEL

Pyridoxine (B₆) is one of the most important B vitamins, especially for anyone on a high-protein diet, because it is involved in protein metabolism and can help to keep blood cholesterol levels low. It also plays a part in carbohydrate metabolism, which makes it particularly important for people with hypoglycemia or diabetes. B₆ is essential to prevent certain types of anemia. It reduces tooth decay, and some important studies indicate that it may reduce the incidence of certain types of cancer. Allergic states are often improved by large amounts of pyridoxine.

A deficiency can make you irritable, tired, or restless; an acute deficiency can even lead to convulsions.

When you begin taking pyridoxine, you may find that you have more energy, feel less tense, lose any bloated feeling in your body; that the bags under your eyes disappear; that your arthritis improves. You may find that it relaxes you to the point of sleepiness, and if this is the case, take your dose at bedtime. Begin with 50 mg. once a day, and increase this over the next week to three or four times a day. For the second week, take two tablets, or 100 mg., three or four times a day.

A few people cannot tolerate high doses of pyridoxine. If it makes you nervous, irritable, or slightly nauseous, take it in clear capsule form, with no coloring or binder. If it still bothers you, ask your doctor for a prescription of injectable B₆. Take the liquid out of the bottle with a needle and syringe, squirt it into water, and drink it. Some people can tolerate this form when they can't take any other. (This is rarely true of all vitamins, but happens more often with pyridoxine.)

HOW TO ESTABLISH YOUR VITAMIN B$_{12}$ LEVEL

As you know, a B$_{12}$ deficiency is often a significant contributing factor in cases of emotional illness. Unfortunately, people with B$_{12}$ deficiencies are generally unable to absorb B$_{12}$ orally, so the more severe your need is for B$_{12}$ the more likely it is that tablets will do you no good. Again: I believe *everyone* should have a blood test for serum B$_{12}$ levels, and, whatever the reading, they should also try therapeutic injections of B$_{12}$ to see whether they then feel better.

The preferred form is hydroxocobalamin (B$_{12b}$) rather than the usual cyanocobalamin (B$_{12}$). Ask your doctor for an injection of 500 mcg. of B$_{12}$b, followed in a few days by a 1000 mcg. injection, and a few days later by 2000 mcg. If your blood test was normal, and you feel no emotional improvement whatever, you may conclude that a prolonged use of B$_{12}$ may produce little change. But keep in mind that it may take a year or two of regular B$_{12}$ treatment for the full benefits to be felt. If you and your doctor agree that you should continue the treatment, you should have a member of the family learn to administer the injections.

If you feel better after the B$_{12b}$ injections, you and your physician must find the proper interval for receiving the injections. If you take, say, 1000 mcg. by injection once a week and get a lift from it each time, your intervals are too long. You should find the interval that *fails* to give you a lift. If you take it every three days and get no lift, try every five days. If you get a lift with the five-day interval, try a four-day interval. Then, if you get a lift on five-day intervals but not on four-day intervals, four days is the correct interval for you. If you wait until you get a lift, then you have allowed your B$_{12}$ level to sink too low.

Some patients require as little as 1000 mcg. every three months; others, 2000 or 3000 mcg. every day. I have one nineteen-year-old who is a hellion if she does not get 2000 mcg. every day. If the doubting Thomases of the medical profession could only take her in their homes to live with them a few weeks, they would be absolutely convinced about what I advocate regarding vitamin B$_{12}$ therapy.

Frequently I see patients who have felt "run down" at some time in the past and visited a physician who gave them a "course" of vitamin B$_{12}$ injections. The patient felt much better after the "course" but then gradually settled down into his or her old "run down" rut. For some reason it seldom seems to occur to either the patient or the doctor that the injections must be continued indefinitely.

If your serum vitamin B_{12} level is low, you must be given injections of 1000 mcg. of vitamin B_{12b} at least every three months for the rest of your life. The risk of destruction of brain cells and degeneration of the spinal column, to say nothing of pernicious (called pernicious because it results in death) anemia, is too great to take any chances.

But if your serum levels prove normal, you should still get one or two test injections of vitamin B_{12} to learn if you are one of those numerous persons who must have a higher than normal blood serum level of vitamin B_{12} in order to feel your best.

Along with my usual biochemical, physiological, vitamin, and mineral work-up I always obtain a serum B_{12} level on my patients. The lower limit of "normal" is given as 150 by some textbooks, and as 200 by others. Every textbook will inform you that 226 is a perfectly normal B_{12} level. Yet several years ago I learned from my patients' experiences that a so-called "normal" B_{12} level is not necessarily normal for just any individual. Since then I have made it an invariable policy to give all my patients a therapeutic trial on vitamin B_{12} by injection. I use hydroxocobalamin, or vitamin B_{12b}, because research in England shows that the usual form of vitamin B_{12}, cyanocobalamin, may be toxic for some people. Dr. W. S. Foulds[2] and his associates have found destruction of the eye nerves from cyanocobalamin in patients sensitive to the cyanide radical which it contains.

There is a movement in England to remove cyanocobalamin—the usual form of vitamin B_{12}—from the market altogether. Scientists there feel, and I strongly agree, that hydroxocobalamin (vitamin B_{12b} should be exclusively used instead. Apart from the problem of toxicity, cyanocobalamin must be transformed in the body and turned into hydroxocobalamin to become biologically active. So why not use the biologically active form in the first place? Also, hydroxocobalamin keeps blood levels of the vitamin at high levels approximately three times as long as cyanocobalamin.

Hydroxocobalamin is *not* expensive, and can readily be obtained by your doctor. If the druggist will not bother to order it for him, your physician can order directly from Henry Schein, Inc., a wholesale drug supply company at 39–01 170th Street, Flushing, New York 11358.

HOW TO ESTABLISH YOUR FOLIC ACID LEVEL

As you know, you should have a serum folic acid test when you have the test for vitamin B_{12}. If you have a borderline or deficiency level, you must take folic acid all your life. You will need a prescription for it since only minute amounts may be sold over the counter in the United States. (In Canada one can buy 5 mg. tablets without prescription.)

The textbooks of medicine say that people absorb folic acid if it is given by mouth, unless they have some rare, serious intestinal disorder such as tropical sprue. Much to my surprise I have discovered that some people without demonstrable gastrointestinal disorders do not absorb folic acid properly. I have checked this finding with Kurt A. Oster, M.D., of Bridgeport, Connecticut, who is possibly the world's greatest authority on folic acid. His clinical experience agrees with mine. I give these people folic acid by injection. Since vitamin C causes a loss of folic acid through the urine, it is particularly important that people on ascorbic acid pay attention to their folic acid levels. Injections of vitamin B_{12} help the gut absorb folic acid.

Deficiency in folic acid has been associated so prominently with anemia that physicians seem to pay little attention to other possible symptoms. It is known that guinea pigs have convulsions and become very lazy if they have deficiencies of folic acid. At least one study at Yale University reveals brain damage caused by folic acid deficiency. I believe that many nervous disorders are caused by folic acid deficiency, that its deficiency causes much depression and indeed may, like vitamin B_{12} deficiency, produce almost any emotional disorder you can name. I strongly recommend that patients who are deficient in folic acid take at least 5 mg. four times a day and that they have a repeat blood test after a month to see if they are absorbing it properly. If not, it should be given by injection.

A fair therapeutic trial would be to start with 1 mg. three times a day and work up to perhaps 10 mg. three times a day. After leaving it at this level for several weeks I often find it worthwhile to go up gradually to as much as 20 mg. four times a day. At these levels people often feel a great deal better or a great deal worse. The effect will be obvious in only a day or two. Even if you feel much improved with the very high levels, it may be necessary for you to drop your level by as much as fifty percent after a few days, if you suddenly find yourself feeling less well.

Some patients feel stimulated by large amounts of folic acid and others feel sedated. Still others just feel rotten.

Only trial and error will help you and your physician find your correct level.

Folic acid is a very neglected vitamin. Since it helps niacin accept methyl groups there is much theoretical reason why folic acid might be helpful to persons suffering from schizophrenia. My clinical experience with this vitamin bears out this impression.

A nasty rumor has been circulating that high doses of folic acid might cause convulsions. This rumor is based on a misinterpretation of work done on an epileptic. Both Dr. Oster and I agree that convulsions are not a risk to persons taking folic acid.

If I had a demonstrated folic acid deficiency, I would take folic acid all my life and I would check my blood serum level twice a year to make certain I was absorbing it. Otherwise I would give myself a trial on it to see whether it seemed to be beneficial to me.

HOW TO ESTABLISH YOUR PANTOTHENIC ACID LEVEL

Pantothenic acid is certainly a neglected vitamin. It is important in the production of the adrenal cortical hormones and in carbohydrate metabolism. A deficiency can cause degeneration of nerve tissue, physical weakness, and depression.

The exact amount needed by humans has not been determined, though it is probably in the order of 10 to 15 mg. per day; more, perhaps double this figure may be desirable in situations of stress. Some people feel better when taking up to a hundred times the basic amount. Since many people are relaxed by the use of this vitamin I think it is a good idea to take it at bedtime. If you are tense, hyperactive, and irritable, you might try it during the day. You can start on 200 mg. at bedtime and increase it every night to 600 mg. or you can take 200 to 400 mg. three or four times a day in a trial to see what level is best for you.

HOW TO ESTABLISH YOUR BIOTIN LEVEL

The chances of your being deficient in biotin are rather slim. A deficiency may occur if you eat raw egg whites, since this deactivates the body's biotin, but otherwise it is generally felt that man's intestinal bacteria supplies adequate biotin. Never eat raw egg whites.

As a trial on biotin you might take 250 to 500 mg. three times daily.

HOW TO ESTABLISH YOUR INOSITOL LEVEL

This vitamin does not loom large in my arsenal. We know that rats on small (or reduced) amounts of inositol lose their hair, but we have no direct proof that humans lose their hair for the same reason. Inositol acts along with choline (another "minor" B vitamin) to help the body to manufacture lecithin—which helps mobilize and decrease fatty substances in the body and tends to lower cholesterol. However, I advise people to take the lecithin directly.

When mice are given such large amounts of caffeine that they become paralyzed, inositol will offset this paralysis. Does that mean that if you are a heavy coffee drinker you need more inositol than normal? We don't know for certain, but it is a possibility. Inositol is available in brewers' or primary yeast. A better source is two heaping tablespoons of lecithin granules daily. If you would like to try it separately, try 500 or 600 mg. daily; if you feel a specific effect from it, follow up your discovery. Who knows? Maybe you will win a Nobel prize.

HOW TO ESTABLISH YOUR CHOLINE LEVEL

Choline, like inositol, is an important minor B vitamin. It too is necessary for the manufacture of lecithin. I believe it is amply supplied in the lecithin and the yeast I recommend, but if you want to experiment with supplements it can't do any harm. Two hundred to a thousand mg. daily would be a fair trial. People who had had liver damage (alcohol, hepatitis, etc.) are often helped.

HOW TO ESTABLISH YOUR PABA LEVEL

Para-aminobenzoic acid (PABA) is one of the "minor" vitamins that appears to be more promising than the two I have just mentioned.

During the late 1940s an obscure Romanian physician, Ana Aslan, M.D., practicing in Transylvania, heard that procaine (novocaine), the common local anesthesia injected into your gums by the dentist, broke down in the body and formed the vitamin para-aminobenzoic acid. She also learned of occasional unpleasant reactions to the alkaline form of procaine, which is the one commonly used in local anesthesia. She made a buffered, acidified form of the procaine which she began injecting into patients and which carries the trade name of Gerovital (or H_3).

Dr. Aslan is particularly interested in preventing aging (see page 318), and she claims that she has increased the lifespan of her patients by an average of some thirty percent. A thirty percent increase in lifespan impresses me. If you are going to pass on at age 70, and you can add thirty percent to that, you would be over ninety when you died. Dr. Aslan has also found PABA useful for many psychological complaints such as depression and fatigue. She reports success in Parkinson's disease and claims an eighty percent cure for schizoid patients—meaning persons who are not frankly schizophrenic but who are still severely disturbed emotionally. She has also reported that her injections help greatly in cases of impotence. Incidentally, Dr. Aslan avoids sweets and advises all of her patients to do the same, since she feels sweets accelerate aging.

With its usual hostility toward new ideas, the American Medical Association did not approve procaine injections for use as anything but an anesthetic. Now, a generation later, the medical profession in this country is being forced to have another look at H_3. Recently several United States congressmen visited Dr. Aslan. They were impressed by the good results they saw and inspired several American physicians to begin research on the subject. While the final results are not in, initial findings appear quite favorable.

I have occasionally used plain procaine for patients, particularly those who were depressed or suffering from schizophrenia, and generally felt that it was useful. Recently a drug company in Florida has produced a procaine that is buffered to an acid level like that of Dr. Aslan's formula and has produced another vial of the buffered potassium solution which she uses, so that one can mix the two solutions and produce Dr. Aslan's formula. This I have used for over a year and find it is frequently helpful in treating depression.

PABA is available in tablet form at your local health food stores but it only comes in strengths of about 60 mg., not an effective dose. Your physician can give you a prescription for this vitamin. It is made under the name of Protaba and manufactured by Glenwood Laboratories, 83 North Summit Street, Tenafly, New Jersey 07670. It is supplied in 500 mg. tablets or capsules. If you really want to see whether PABA has anything to offer you, suggest to your physician that he prescribe one 500 mg. tablet one to three times a day. Should you experience any nausea or loss of appetite, the dose level should be reduced.

Should you not get the results you seek from the oral use of Protaba, then I suggest that your physician give you Dr. Aslan's H_3 solution by injection two or three times a week for twelve weeks. By that time you should know whether this vitamin has anything to offer you. The solution is made by Pharmex, Inc., Hollywood, Florida 33070.

DO YOU NEED VITAMINS BY INJECTION?

For some people, injection is the only effective way to receive water-soluble vitamins.

I have already mentioned the need of giving vitamin B_{12b} by intramuscular or subcutaneous injection because its absorption by the oral route is too unreliable to be depended upon.

If repeat blood serum tests show folic acid is not being absorbed, then it should certainly be given by injection.

A number of patients feel better after they get vitamin C by injection. Although it can be given in the muscle, this route is so painful that I seldom use it except in a multiple vitamin mixture and in conjunction with a local anesthetic.

This means that, in order to get really large doses of vitamin C into patients, we must use the intravenous route.

Giving vitamins intravenously is a special field in itself. Only physicians who are versed in the intricacies of intravenous vitamin therapy should use this route since serious and even fatal reactions can occur unless the physician is aware of a number of seemingly small details that must be observed.

For example, the two ml. vials of ascorbic acid must not be used for intravenous administration because they contain a preservative poorly tolerated by the vein. Rather, the larger multiple dose vials must be used and these absolutely must not contain phenol as a preservative. I use the 30 ml. multiple dose vial put out by Henry Schein Inc., 39–01 170th Street, Flushing, New York 11358. This contains 250 mg. of sodium ascorbate per ml. I generally use 20 ml. (5000 mg.) drawn up into a 30 cc. syringe and diluted with 10 ml. of sodium chloride, the 10 ml. size to be used only once since it does not (and this is important!) contain a preservative. This is put out by Invenex, a division of Mogul Corporation, Chagrin Falls, Ohio 44022.

When large amounts of ascorbic acid (30,000 mg. and more) are administered, the vitamin should be mixed in with 1000 ml. of normal saline to which is added 10 ml. of ten percent calcium gluconate, to be given by slow intravenous drip. Such large amounts are usually employed for infections rather than emotional difficulties.

Interestingly, some patients are allergic to all forms of ascorbic acid given by mouth, even the form that is injected intravenously, but they can tolerate without difficulty intravenous injections of the vitamin.

The B vitamins are rather frequently given intramuscularly with novocaine to keep down the pain. Sometimes I also give these by vein; if so, strict precautions must be taken to use the proper forms of vitamins; to have the correct dilution; and to be given at the proper rate.

Unquestionably some people who respond favorably to injected vitamins show little improvement when given the same products by mouth. How do I know? I have tried giving them, stopping them, giving them again, and substituting placebo injections without the patient's knowledge. I am my own most demanding critic and always question everything I do, as well as everything other physicians do. I never believe what I read in scientific papers or what other physicians tell me, until I have demonstrated the facts to myself.

The other day I was talking on the telephone to Kurt Oster, M.D., the folic acid authority. I happened to mention that some patients, contrary to what is written in the medical textbooks, do not absorb folic even though they are free of demonstrable gastrointestinal disorders.

In a surprised voice he asked how I knew that. He thought he was the only one in the world aware of that fact, since he had discovered it with his own patients but had never reported it in the scientific literature.

I told him I knew because I had tested my patients' serum folate levels before and after giving folic acid by mouth.

HOW TO FINE-TUNE YOUR VITAMIN REGIMEN

As I said earlier, finding (and staying on) your best vitamin level is an on-going process. Once you have been through the one-by-one vitamin check I have described, you have an outline to work with. But the process is not finished by any means. You are now taking yeast, vitamins A and D, and your own level of C and E. You are taking whatever additional doses of B vitamins you have found to be helpful to you. At this point, you should begin again to test higher levels of vitamins in combination. For example, vitamin C and vitamin B_6 are interconnected; when B_6 is low, blood levels of C tend to be low and when B_6 goes up so does the vitamin C. Therefore, you may be able to lower your level of vitamin C if you are taking extra B_6, and still maintain a feeling of well-being; on the other hand, you may find that pushing the doses of both vitamins still higher produces even better results.

Similarly, you may find you can reduce your vitamin E. Vitamin E compensates for stress in the body. So do several B vitamins. When you take them together, you may feel best with a higher or lower level of both.

Over a period of time, you should continue to test your reactions to various combinations of vitamins. Go back to the beginning dosages of the B vitamins; take two together; push the doses of each to the top limits; observe the way you feel. When you hit on a combination that works for you, add the rest of the B vitamins, one by one.

As a rule, people feel best with a certain combination of vitamins, although the proportions and combinations change over time. Throughout, continue to take yeast; this will minimize the possibility of creating a deficiency of one B vitamin while experimenting with another.

FINDING A MINERAL SUPPLEMENT

As you know, I am firmly against taking mineral tablets without first getting a proper hair test to determine what your mineral levels really are. But there are a few exceptions to this. I've said it before: Dolomite powder, supplying calcium and magnesium, is considered fairly harmless. You might try a teaspoon in water at bedtime; many people find it helps them sleep. If you are nervous or edgy, you may prefer to take up to three teaspoons during the day for its calming effect. Many people thrive on a potion they affectionately call "sludge": it's made of yeast, dolomite, and vitamin C powder in water or juice and it's taken two or three times a day.

I think a dolomite supplement is always a wise idea because many people are low in magnesium and because people who eliminate dairy products from their diets need an alternative source of calcium.

If you like, you can also try one kelp tablet a day as an additional source of natural minerals, and I recommend the liberal use of sea salt to supply sodium and other minerals, unless you suffer from hypertension or have some other medical reason to keep your sodium intake low.

When hair tests show mineral deficiencies, the specific minerals missing must be given a trial.

NOTES

1. N. Hakami *et al.*, Neonatal Megaloblastic Anemia Due to Inherited Transcobalamin II Deficiency in Two Siblings," *New England Journal of Medicine*, Vol. 285, No. 21, 1971, p. 1163.
2. Foulds *et al.*, "Cyanocobalamin: A Case for Withdrawal," *Lancet*, Vol. 1, Jan. 3, 1970, p. 35.

WHAT TO DO ABOUT
HORMONE DEFICIENCIES

CHAPTER FIFTEEN

Hormones are the products of the endocrine glands and, like vitamins and minerals, they affect the metabolism of every cell. Without proper nutrition the endocrine glands cannot produce hormones in normal quantities. In innumerable cases, an initial work-up of my patients has revealed hormone deficiencies along with vitamin and mineral deficiencies. When these deficiencies were corrected by proper diet and nutritional supplements, the functions of the glands often normalized themselves.

One such patient was a physician in the prime of life. He had not had intercourse for many years. Besides a low serum B_{12} level and low serum testosterone, he also suffered from a defect in his carbohydrate metabolism. His diet was corrected; he was placed on supplementary vitamin B_{12} injections, and given other nutritive supplements. Soon his testosterone level returned to normal, and therewith his interest in sex.

While we're on the subject of sex, let me tell you about a couple who consulted me regarding their marital difficulties. They had been seeing a marriage counselor together for over a year, but their situation hadn't improved. During our first interview, the husband succinctly summarized the problem by stating that since the birth of their last baby his wife had been "a bitch." Strangely enough, his wife agreed. She said that she simply couldn't control her temper, nor her mounting depression. Yet despite long explorations with the marital counselor, she had been unable to decide exactly why she was so angry and depressed.

A careful history revealed that she had started taking contraceptive pills that contain hormones, a year ago, after the birth of the baby. Since some women react to these pills with emotional disturbances, the obvious first step was to change her method of birth control to see what would happen.

When the couple returned four weeks later, the bad vibes that had been so palpable between them had completely disappeared. Their faces were relaxed. They agreed that their marital difficulties had all but vanished. Where once they had fought over every small issue, they now found themselves laughing over their former shouting matches. They had never lost their affection for each other—or they would not have tried so hard to save their marriage; but in spite of their love, they had been at each other's throats many times a day. All that lay behind them now; their marriage was better than ever.

In 1957, the director of the National Academy of Nutrition, J. S. Walters, M.D.,[1] reported on 726 of his patients who had been receiving hormones for various emotional, psychosomatic, and physical disorders. After a careful work-up, including measurement of hormone, vitamin, and mineral levels, he had put these patients on a proper diet and nutritional supplements. As a result of this regimen, the supplemental hormones could be reduced in most cases, and eliminated in many.

Of special interest were the eighty-one vegetarians among the group. Fifty-six of them agreed to add meat to their diet, at least temporarily. Of these, sixty-five percent increased their levels of estrogens (female sexual hormones), testosterone (male hormones) and adrenal cortical hormones (manufactured by the adrenal glands). The remaining twenty-five vegetarians who could not bring themselves to eat meat cut down on cereals and cooked vegetables, and increased their intake of raw nuts, sunflower seeds, and cold-pressed oils. Those who took at least one to four ounces of raw nuts and seeds experienced a rapid and dramatic increase in hormone levels.

It has long been known that hormone levels drop sharply during periods of semi-starvation or extremely poor nourishment. But here, too, the medical profession has fallen into the trap of considering people either "sick" or "well," while the truth far more frequently lies somewhere in between: Most people are neither wholly sick nor wholly well—and most people follow a diet that is neither all good nor all bad. It is this group, comprising perhaps ninety percent of the population, who do not feel their best, partly because of inadequate hormone levels due to inadequate diet.

The body's nervous and hormone systems are closely interrelated

Low hormone levels often bring about tension, depression, or almost any other emotional symptom you can name. On the other hand, increased tension, depression, and emotional upheaval can in turn affect the hormone system, creating an endless vicious cycle of turmoil.

Any stress affects the endocrine glands: the stress of surgery, of burns, of grief—all these traumas cause hormone levels to change. For example, the adrenal cortical hormone pours out in great quantities to meet a stressful situation. Eventually, if the stress lasts long enough, the adrenal cortex becomes exhausted, and, as a result, the level of adrenal cortical hormone is lowered.

THE THYROID HORMONE

The first hormone system I will discuss in some detail is that of the thyroid because its effect on the emotions was recognized earlier than that of the other hormone systems. When I was a medical student, physicians were greatly preoccupied with the relationship between the thyroid gland and emotional disorders. Almost every patient with any symptom suggesting emotional troubles was given a BMR—a test to measure the rate of metabolism, in which the thyroid plays a large part. Patients suffering from fatigue almost routinely received thyroid tablets, even if their laboratory tests were normal. Almost equally commonly, very tense patients had part of their thyroid gland removed to reduce tension.

In those days, when you saw a woman who was complaining of

emotional instability, it was almost routine to see a scar on her throat—mute testimony to the fact that part of her thyroid gland had been removed. I kept wondering why I kept on hearing the same complaints when the supposed root cause had already been removed.

By now the thyroid removal operation has fallen into disrepute; the supervisory "tissue committees" at reputable hospitals no longer allow a thyroid gland to be removed simply because a patient suffers from nervousness—unless the patient is also demonstrably suffering from excessive secretion of the thyroid gland. (Recently a new twist to this situation has developed, of which I will speak later on.)

Hypothyroidism

The thyroid hormone is essential for the proper development of the nervous system. A child born with a very low supply of thyroid will remain severely mentally retarded unless the hormone is supplied promptly and continually. When thyroid deficiency appears in adulthood, the damage is less dramatic, though it may still be extensive. Low thyroid hormone means lowered cellular metabolism. The brain cells no longer work properly. As a result, intellectual functioning is slowed, and mood disturbances make their appearance.

Linus Pauling, the two-time Nobel Prize-winning chemist, has said that all depressions could be eliminated if it were possible to get sufficient oxygen to the brain cells. The depression that accompanies the lowered oxygen utilization in people low in thyroid hormone would seem to be a good illustration of his point.

In the elderly, the depression, poor memory, and confusion that go with low thyroid levels is often mistaken for senility—i.e., the hardening of the arteries of the brain, which produces similar symptoms. Thyroid disorders are particularly difficult to diagnose in the elderly, who often don't exhibit the classic symptoms of over- or under-active thyroids. It is therefore especially important to perform laboratory tests for thyroid function in this group of patients.

I arrange for a series of thyroid tests on all my patients. I feel that this should be standard procedure. Unfortunately, most psychiatrists neglect to do this. While we're on this subject, I venture that fewer than two percent of them order routine chemical, hormone, vitamin, mineral, or even physical examinations for their patients. It may be up to you to demand such tests from your doctor if you feel that perhaps all may not be well with your internal machinery.

Symptoms of reduced thyroid function may cover the full range of emotional illnesses. Some patients become angry, even paranoid; others grow profoundly depressed—to the point of believing that the world is about to come to an end. Strangely, agitated states may also occur as a result of low thyroid function. These may be due to the memory impairment and confusion that frighten the patient and make him restless.

Even more serious disorders may occur in the adult hypothyroid sufferer when he is subjected to some additional stress such as infection, surgery, or depressant drugs. Such a patient may even go into a coma.

We attribute night blindness to lack of vitamin A, but a low thyroid level may also cause this disorder, and should always be considered when people have trouble getting about at night or in semi-darkness. Deafness may occur. Speech may become hoarse and slurred. Body movements may be slow, faltering, and clumsy. Some patients complain of numbness and tingling in the hands and feet.

As you might guess, low thyroid levels are also accompanied by sexual changes. Men tend toward impotence; if they are able to have an erection, it is usually short-lived. Their sex drive and sperm count tend to be low, so that they are less likely to father children even if they are capable of an erection.

Since women have a much more elaborate reproductive system, they naturally experience even more problems when suffering from hypothyroidism. Their sex drive, too, may be lowered; and they do not ovulate. Frequently they have excessive and irregular menstrual bleeding. If the condition persists long enough, menstruation may cease altogether.

Hypothyroidism also has a profound effect on carbohydrate metabolism—a subject more fully discussed in the chapter on hypoglycemia.

Constipation is a frequent complaint, as well as loss of hair, dry skin, and brittle nails. There may be puffiness around the eyes and mucus accumulations in the eyes, causing the eyelids to be stuck together on awakening in the morning. Symptoms akin to those of arthritis may also be present.

The hypothyroid syndrome often develops very slowly, and may go unrecognized by the patient or his family until it has progressed to a marked degree. The first symptoms, such as fatigue, lack of zest, menstrual disorders, and a special sensitivity to cold, may be shrugged off and blamed on the stresses of life.

It is always important that nutrition be maintained at an optimal level, since this undoubtedly contributes to the adequate functioning of all the glands; but for the thyroid gland it is especially important that iodine intake be adequate, since iodine is used by the gland in the production of its hormone. If iodine amounts are insufficient, the pituitary gland will stimulate the thyroid gland until it becomes enlarged in an attempt to produce more hormone. The resulting protuberance is one type of goiter.

If your physician discovers that your thyroid gland is not functioning adequately, don't jump to the conclusion that all you need is proper diet and nutritive supplements. These are, indeed, vital. But if the thyroid deficiency is marked, you will need a thyroid preparation as well, and your physician will have to recheck your condition from time to time to learn whether you can gradually reduce medication and maintain adequate functioning on proper diet alone. Such improvement is a very individual matter. It occurs fairly rapidly in some people; in others, hypothyroidism may be like diabetes—a deficiency that persists through life, necessitating medication on a permanent basis.

Hyperthyroidism

The second major thyroid disease results from the over-supply of thyroid hormone; it is called hyperthyroidism. (In general, "hypo" means too little; "hyper" means too much.) Although much research has been done on the subject, no one yet knows why some people's thyroid suddenly becomes overactive and starts pouring out torrents of hormone, although it has been noted that this frequently happens after some kind of emotional or physical stress. We know that persons on inadequate diets react more adversely to life stresses; and it is therefore possible that diet may help cause excessive thyroid production because the malnourished person cannot handle stress adequately.

A frankly overactive thyroid requires medical intervention, and in addition to medical treatment it is vital that you receive a proper diet and nutritional supplements. Nutritional balance is particularly important in hyperthyroidism, because the thyroid hormone speeds up the body's metabolism and makes the enzyme systems handle a greater volume of work, which requires more than the normal amounts of vitamin and minerals.

Among the symptoms produced by an overactive thyroid, you may be surprised to learn, fatigue is probably the most common complaint. One tends to think of the thyroid hormone as an "upper," because people with low thyroid function are given thyroid extract for more energy. However, if such medication is pushed beyond a certain point, the patient can go into hyperthyroidism and be tired because of *too much* thyroid just as easily as from *too little* thyroid.

Many physicians, even well-trained and experienced ones, are unaware of this, and tend to prescribe more and more thyroid hormone for their hypothyroid patients in order to increase their energy. In reality, after a certain point is reached, they actually contribute to and exacerbate the patient's fatigue. This fatigue, which then constitutes an early symptom of hyperthyroidism, may in part be due to the relative vitamin and mineral deficiency produced by the speeded-up metabolism.

Other symptoms of hyperthyroidism include a feeling of tension, inner tremulousness, sometimes accompanied by a fine tremor of the hands that causes handwriting to deteriorate. Bowel movements may be increased. Women usually experience reduced menstrual flow. People with overactive thyroids also perspire easily and cannot tolerate much heat. Often they have itchy skin, a condition frequently misdiagnosed as due to tension. The skin tends to be warm and moist, with a velvety quality. The hair is fine-textured. Emotional instability shows itself in irregular life patterns, insomnia, and fluctuating moods. Occasionally, patients have epileptiform seizures, and sometimes they develop a toxic delirium, lose touch with reality, and turn frankly psychotic.

To illustrate how easily one can be fooled by the subtle emotional disturbances of beginning hyperthyroidism, let me tell you about a forty-two-year-old, hard-driving businessman who came to see me about his emotional difficulties.

I ordered my standard laboratory work-up, including a thyroid profile to estimate his thyroid gland's level of functioning. It so happened that he had been referred to me by an internist who requested that his own laboratory do the tests. I readily agreed. The thyroid test results were reported to me as normal.

For the next nine months I tried to help this patient, using many different approaches. I placed him on a proper diet and prescribed the indicated nutritional supplements. When he did not improve, I added medication. Then, since he still did not respond as expected, I switched to a different medication. During subsequent months I changed his medications eight times without any benefit.

It often happens that a patient requiring medication (such as a tranquilizer or anti-depressant) will respond to one but not to another. One must discover through trial and error which one is best for that particular person. But with this patient I seemed to make no headway.

I then began spending more time with him in an attempt to discover any psychological stresses in his life of which I was unaware. True, he had a wife who was less than satisfactory by most standards; but he had lived with her for twenty years, so she must have fulfilled some of his needs.

Then, to my distress, the man began losing his touch in business matters. He was in a highly competitive industry in which it is notoriously easy to be a millionaire one day and bankrupt the next. For a long time he had walked this tightrope very successfully. Now it became more and more evident that he no longer had his former acute grasp of business affairs. His judgment had become poor, and he was allowing his emotions to draw him into some very difficult situations.

Since he was not responding to my therapy, I had a neurosurgical consultation to rule out a brain tumor. A work-up in depth failed to reveal any evidence of a tumor or other neurological disease. The man finally decided that I was not the one to help him and, as it turned out, he was quite correct. After leaving me he went to Duke University Medical Center where, much to my embarrassment, he was discovered to have a small thyroid tumor that was putting out excessive thyroid hormone.

As you know by now, I greatly enjoy tripping up the medical establishment by coming up with a diagnosis they miss; this time the establishment had its revenge.

Checking back on the man's medical history, I realized that the laboratory where the referring internist had had the thyroid tests performed had been in error; that, all along, I had been dealing with a patient suffering from an overactive thyroid. His condition had not been sufficiently advanced to show the obvious symptoms of hyperthyroidism; but the very small tumor had nonetheless put out enough excess hormone to make him irritable, to confuse him, and to cause a deterioration of his business judgment.

New and exciting discoveries are constantly being made in this particular area of medicine. Some years ago, I read an article by Arthur J. Prange, Jr., M.D.,[2] professor of psychiatry at the University of North Carolina, in which he reported on his successful combination of the anti-depressant drug Tofranil with a fraction of the thyroid hormone known as cytomel. Shortly thereafter I happened to hear of Magda Campbell, M.D., who was using cytomel in the treatment of schizophrenic children at New York University Medical School. I contacted Dr. Campbell and learned that she was treating both hyperactive and extremely withdrawn children with cytomel, and that her improvement rate was very high—especially considering the fact that, as a rule, little can be done for these youngsters. She also used cytomel on non-schizophrenic children with behavior problems—again with good results. She pointed out that cytomel has a clear anti-psychotic effect, which makes it much more important than the simple anti-depressant effect reported by Prange.

After talking with Dr. Campbell, I began prescribing cytomel for some of my chronically depressed schizophrenic patients. For the most part, these were patients with whom I had worked for a year or two and who had achieved significant improvement, but still remained on a plateau somewhere between health and illness. They were functioning outside of hospitals, but were only working at undemanding, menial jobs. In many of these previously static patients, improvement was prompt and impressive—especially when cytomel was combined with Tofranil. Some patients were made restless by the hormone, and had to be taken off it. Interestingly enough, children can tolerate much higher doses of cytomel than adults. Children receive anywhere from 25 to 75 mcg. daily; adults usually receive only 25 to 50 mcg. a day.

Both cytomel and Tofranil are prescription drugs, and you will have to have your doctor's cooperation to use them. Most psychiatrists are not aware of the importance of this hormone therapy in a wide spectrum of serious conditions, and it would be quite appropriate for you to bring it to your doctor's attention and invite him to consult the professional literature on the subject. Hopefully he will not shrug it off as "unproven," just to spare himself the trouble of learning a new technique.

PHEOCHROMOCYTOMA

Pheochromocytoma is an endocrine-producing tumor frequently missed in patients because psychiatrists don't take a careful history with pheochromocytoma in mind, and do not, as a rule, take the patient's blood pressure. If these two simple steps were observed, and a twenty-four-hour collection of urine were inspected for vanilmandic acid or norepinephrine-meta-epinephrine excretion, something like ninety percent of patients could be definitely diagnosed as either having or not having pheochromocytoma. The remaining ten percent, if strongly suspected of having it, should be seen by an internist for more specialized laboratory tests.

A pheochromocytoma is a tumor occurring in the so-called chromafin cells which are widely distributed throughout the body and produce the nervous system-stimulating substance known as catacholamine. Its symptoms are frequently nervous in nature: patients tend to suffer from a feeling of apprehension, palpitations, a pounding in the head. They frequently break out in sweat and have what appears to be emotionally triggered nausea and vomiting. Often they have attacks of extreme anxiety that may be episodic, because the tumor may put out its catacholamine intermittently rather than regularly. The patient's blood pressure must therefore be measured *during* an anxiety attack because that may be the only time when a tumor is making discernible trouble.

Ninety-five percent of the time, the tumor is located somewhere in the abdomen, but only fifteen percent can be palpated (felt with the fingers), and it often requires extensive X-rays and other diagnostic means to locate it.

HOW THE PITUITARY GLAND AFFECTS YOUR EMOTIONS

The pituitary gland is the central gland in the hormonal system, since it sends out hormones to stimulate all other glands. It lies against the brain; numerous nerve pathways from the brain lead to it. It is therefore greatly influenced by what takes place in the brain, and its secretions, in turn, have a great effect on brain function. The secretions of the pituitary affect the other glands by, in effect, turning them on and off.

For example, it is the pituitary that stimulates the ovary to start putting out female sex hormones such as estrogen; and in the latter part of the menstrual cycle it brings about a change in stimulation, so that progesterone is added to the ovary's hormone outflow. It also stimulates the adrenal cortex, which causes the cortical hormones to flow out in emergency situations.

Because it is directly connected to the hypothalamus (the brain center for primitive emotions), anything that affects emotional tone affects the pituitary, which in turn affects all other glands. Undoubtedly, the pituitary is involved in some of the various states of semi-health in which so many people find themselves.

You are probably aware that emotional strain from whatever cause can bring about menstrual irregularities in women. In most instances these are due to pituitary dysfunction, which throws the female sex hormones off balance. Quite frequently I see seriously disturbed women who fail to menstruate for months or even years, and then suddenly begin having regular cycles again. This is always a favorable sign in the course of a serious mental illness.

THE ADRENAL CORTEX AFFECTS YOUR EMOTIONS

The adrenal cortex produces at least thirty hormones, but we are intimately familiar with only a few. About seventy percent of adrenal cortical underactivity is due to as yet unknown causes. Whenever we are confronted with a disorder of unknown cause, we must always consider diet as a factor, since cells need proper nutrition to fulfill their normal functions. Those adrenal cortical hormones that we know about do have a strong influence on carbohydrate, water, and mineral metabolism.

In both an overactive and underactive adrenal cortex, sodium and potassium may be present in abnormal amounts. Indeed, the fact that so many of my emotionally disturbed patients have abnormal sodium and potassium hair levels makes me wonder whether adrenal cortical disease is not one of the fundamental disorders in a high percentage of emotional diseases.

We know that during periods of stress, the adrenal cortex pours out its hormones as a protective mechanism. This gland may well be overworked in people who are chronically disturbed. It is difficult to evaluate this possibility because proper testing of adrenal cortical function really requires ten days in the hospital. Even if we find the tests to be within so-called normal limits, there is no guarantee that some state between good health and outright illness may not exist.

We do know that when whole adrenal cortical extract is administered to emotionally ill people, many feel better. As mentioned previously, William F. Philpott, M.D., reports giving a combination of intravenous ascorbic acid and adrenal cortex to psychotic patients, which aroused many of them from their psychotic states. I have observed the same phenomenon in my office, and therefore sometimes use adrenal cortical extract. Incidentally, adrenal cortical injections are also very helpful for patients who have emotional symptoms following the eating of some food to which they are allergic.

Some of my views about adrenal cortical hormones cannot be definitely documented at this time. Much more scientific work on this is being done in Europe than here. My clinical experience leads me to believe, however, that eventually clear scientific proof will be forthcoming to the effect that many emotionally ill people can benefit from adrenal cortical extract.

Modern living, with its lack of exercise, probably increases susceptibility to adrenal cortical insufficiency by not providing the stimulation of physical activity. Rather, it tends to give constant overstimulation from the tensions surrounding us, as well as from the "refined" foods which we eat.

HOW ADRENALIN AFFECTS YOUR EMOTIONS

Another part of the adrenal gland is involved in the well-known "fight-or-flight" mechanism which was so vital for our ancestors. Whenever primitive man met an emergency situation such as a dangerous animal he was forced either to fight or to run to escape. The body's immediate reaction to such emergencies was vital for survival, and it was the adrenal gland that insured it. The adrenal gland shoots adrenalin into the blood stream, which makes the blood sugar go up and thus readies the muscle tissue to work more efficiently. At the same time, adrenalin causes a reduction of the blood supply to the abdominal organs, making more blood fuel and oxygen available to the muscles.

For millions of years this mechanism was most appropriate; it certainly helps to account for our survival as a species. But nowadays this vestige from the past is a liability. If, for example, a woman working in a typing pool feels the need to get up and stretch her legs, and at the same time would like to tell her disapproving supervisor to get off her back, she has a feeling of confinement and repressed hostility which causes adrenalin to shoot into her blood, making her ready for fight or flight. Yet if she needs to earn a living, she can neither fight nor flee. The adrenalin in her blood makes her tremble with repressed hostility. Her blood sugar shoots up because of the increased adrenalin secretion; as a result of the elevated blood sugar her insulin-producing glands secrete insulin which knocks the blood sugar down again—often too low and too rapidly. The result: a hypoglycemic attack.

The stress of going through this frustrated fight or flight reaction and its attendant strain on carbohydrate metabolism is one of the ways for hypoglycemia to get started. If the insult to the carbohydrate metabolism is increased by eating highly refined foods, including sugar, the whole mechanism grows more brittle, and the emotional life of the patient tends to break down rather quickly in many instances. It is not for nothing that we refer to modern life as a rat race. The surprising thing is that the rats hold up as well as they do.

HOW SEX HORMONES AFFECT YOUR EMOTIONS

Testosterone, the male sex hormone, accounts for some of the most neglected hormonal difficulties in all of medicine. I routinely test serum testosterone levels of all male patients, and find that a large number—twenty to thirty percent—suffer from deficiency.

In addition to those who suffer from outright emotional illnesses, other men have damaged testicles which do not secrete the normal amount of testosterone. Many men in the male menopause experience a gradual decline of hormonal output. Others have grossly deficient diets or have excessive alcohol or marijuana consumption. Recently it has also been discovered that male homosexuals as a group have significantly lower serum testosterone levels than heterosexual males, which must be a blow to those who contend that male homosexuality is a purely psychological disorder.

Stress can reduce the testicular output in rats. If male rats are placed in a container of water from which they cannot escape and must swim or drown, the stress of the situation lowers their testosterone levels. It is reasonable to suspect that modern living involves sufficient environmental stress to lower the testosterone levels of human males as well.

Men tend to be neglected when it comes to hormone therapy. Women receive much more attention to their hormone levels and almost routinely get proper hormonal therapy if they can afford it.

This discrepancy can be accounted for in several ways. For one thing, most physicians are males, and seem to be rather preoccupied with female genitalia and hormone functions in general. I don't mean this in a derogatory way. It is only natural for a male doctor to be more interested in the female patient, and especially in her sexual functions. This is simple biology, and I don't think such reactions are restricted to physicians. I suspect that the butcher, the baker, and the candlestick maker are likewise more interested in their female clients.

A second explanation is that men are slower to "doctor." They are much more reluctant to consult physicians than are women. Perhaps this is a consequence of the male's need to see himself as aggressive and competent, while many females more readily accept a dependency situation and do not lose status in their own eyes by admitting to some defects and seeking help for them. Physicians in every specialty except urology have more female patients than males.

Among out-patients, this also holds true for psychiatry. The woman with emotional troubles has sense enough to look for help; the male hangs on as long as he can (possibly with the aid of nightly drinking bouts at the corner tavern) until he has a complete breakdown and must be hospitalized.

A third factor is the relative complexity of male hormone therapy. In general, female sex hormones are effective when given orally. Male hormones are not. They may even cause trouble when given by mouth. Hence, the preferred form of male hormone administration is by injection. This is inconvenient because they must be given at intervals ranging from one to four weeks, often for an indefinite period. An alternative is an implantation of male hormone pellets under the skin, but this involves repeated minor surgery and is even less pleasant to contemplate.

Lastly, endocrinologists do not seem to be fully aware of the emotional importance of male hormones. They may have read about the emotional troubles experienced by males without proper hormone levels, but they seem to be so involved with life-and-death problems like Addison's disease that they tend to neglect the importance of the quality of life.

One of my patients, a twenty-four-year-old man, had an endocrine disorder of unknown origin. At the time of puberty, he did not develop the normal pituitary gland required to stimulate the testicles to put out male hormones. Whether this was an inborn defect or due to some damage to the pituitary could not be determined. Since his genital development did not proceed normally, he was taken to an endocrinologist for a work-up. This sophisticated expert declared that the boy lacked testosterone and let the matter drop, without suggesting any attempts to stimulate testicular function, or advocate replacement hormone therapy.

The young man went to college where he lived the life of a recluse, feeling unhappy and isolated, and harboring a strong dislike for women. Nor did life improve after college. Because he was emotionally volatile, with sharp mood swings and a propensity for snapping back at his superiors, he was condemned to menial positions. Even these he could barely handle, because he was physically awkward and inefficient.

His difficulties finally became so acute that he consulted me. A full allergy, vitamin, mineral, chemical, and endocrinological work-up revealed some minor food allergies that needed correction, and confirmed the low serum testosterone which had been diagnosed years before. I started the young man on injections of testosterone enanthate, gradually increasing the weekly dosage. The result of this treatment has been quite gratifying to him and to me. For one thing, his sense of well-being has increased greatly. This simple statement spans a wealth of meaning for people who have spent their lives feeling that they are balancing on the edge of a volcano, in a state of anxiety and pain which makes life hardly worth living. The world will never know how many people exist in such a state of despair; and the tragedy is that in many cases these lives could be salvaged.

This patient gradually grew interested in women, and started dating. His relationships with men changed too. Having lost his marked mood swings and quick temper, he got along much better with his superiors and coworkers—besides growing more efficient at his job. At work and in his private life, he crawled out of the hole in which he had been hibernating for so long, and became a social human being. Clearly, the whole quality of his life had been changed by hormone administration. I could cite many similar examples.

I must admit that I have also had failures with hormone therapy. Some patients with defective sexual hormones don't improve on supplementary hormones, and some patients even grow worse, becoming hostile and aggressive. We therefore always start hormone therapy at low dosages and gradually build up to find the proper clinical level.

No matter how sophisticated our tests, we cannot predict with one hundred percent accuracy how anyone will react to a modification in his chemistry. In the end, it always comes down to a process of clinical trial. Some patients consider this an imposition, and feel that we are experimenting on them. That is not so. We are, in effect, trying to tailor a program specifically to them so it will fit them and them alone. This is not easy, and often involves much time and effort for both doctor and patient. Perhaps all of us are searching for magic—but in the end we must settle for hard work instead.

You may be interested in knowing something about the use of male sex hormones in women. Women normally have some male sex hormones in their bodies, just as men have some female ones. The injection of additional male hormones in women is useful in several conditions. Where there is a lack of appetite and general loss of interest in life and where the physician is unable to find a specific chemical defect, injections of testosterone may help. They are also particularly useful for women who have lost interest in sex.

I recall one such patient who consulted me years ago. This thirty-eight-year-old woman gave a history of feeling depressed and frigid. Her life was extremely drab, since she had neither energy nor inclination to even leave her house. Her husband had lost interest in her because she not only lacked sexual drive but also had no zest for entering into any kind of meaningful interpersonal relationship with him.

I was rather shocked when she told me that a former family doctor had given her testosterone several years before. The results, she told me, had been very satisfactory. But then she had moved to her present location, had lost touch with the doctor, and had been unable to find anyone who used this form of therapy. Like the others she had consulted, I declined to administer testosterone. The treatment sounded rather wild to me. I had heard of its use in women, but had never pursued the subject and knew little about it.

I gave this patient a work-up from a nutritional standpoint, and corrected some nutritional deficiencies. When this did not improve her condition, I put her on anti-depressants. A lengthy stretch of therapy on a number of successive anti-depressants did not lessen her symptoms, and she became no better when tranquilizers were added. One day she asked me point blank why I did not give her one injection of testosterone as a trial, since my methods did not seem to work, while the hormone used by her former physician had worked. It was a difficult argument to refute, so I began to study the subject and to gather a number of opinions. The general concensus was that if one stayed under 300 or 400 mg. of testosterone enanthate a month by injection, there was little danger of any masculinizing effect on the patient. If any masculinizing effects (such as lowering of the voice) were noted, testosterone should be discontinued, or the dosage reduced.

I started the patient on 50 mg. weekly of testosterone enanthate by injection. By the time she came in for her third shot I could see a clear change both in her appearance and in her outlook on life. Her facial expression was animated, she moved with more vigor, and reported that her interest in sex had picked up and that her family life had begun to have some meaning for her again. She was also making plans to expand her meager social contacts. Testosterone had helped this woman, who had failed to respond to many other approaches. As I have stressed and will continue to stress throughout this book, each person is a unique individual, and each case therefore involves a voyage of exploration for the physician, to discover how to help that particular person.

THE CASE FOR ESTROGEN THERAPY

By far the most frequently used hormonal therapy today is the supplying of estrogen and other female sexual hormones to women. We are all aware of women's menopausal symptoms, which include hot flashes, depression, difficulty in making decisions, inability to concentrate, and regrets over past actions and missed opportunities. Today more than ever before, women in the menopausal years (and beyond) receive estrogen therapy, which is often effective in combating the above symptoms. More and more gynecologists feel that administration of estrogen for an indefinite period is the most sensible way of handling menopausal problems.

In addition to its obvious emotional benefits, estrogen therapy yields other benefits for women. They are less likely to develop osteoporosis or to lose bone calcium (and thus much more likely to avoid fractured hips from brittle bones). The skin maintains a firmer, more youthful texture. Women on hormone therapy keep a vigor and youthfulness not found in similar age groups who do not receive hormone therapy. Perhaps most important is the lowered incidence of post-menopausal coronary disease.

Some women object to taking estrogen because they fear that it might cause them to develop cancer. Estrogen in itself does not cause cancer. If cancer is already present, estrogen may, in some instances, cause it to grow more rapidly. Women who take estrogen should therefore have a breast and pelvic examination (including a Pap smear) every six months (every woman should have this done in any case— whether she is on estrogen therapy or not).

It is also particularly important for menopausal women to receive correct nutrition. This will help them through the difficult transition years, keep their estrogen levels at a higher level for a longer period, and also help them to tolerate lower levels of estrogen. Interestingly, vitamin E in large doses seems to act as a substitute for estrogen in many women, making it possible for them to take smaller amounts of estrogen, or to do without it altogether.

In my opinion, estrogen derived from natural sources is particularly useful, and synthetic estrogens should be avoided. The most commonly prescribed estrogen tablet is called Premarin, and comes in various strengths. But note that Premarin contains at least seven elements to which women may be allergic. Ayerst, the pharmaceutical company that makes Premarin, also manufactures a hypoallergenic form of Premarin for women who cannot tolerate the regular tablet. Hypoallergenic Premarin comes in capsule form without binder and coloring, and may be obtained by your physician directly from Ayerst. It is given away free by the company to physicians, but cannot be purchased through drugstores.

Estrogens are generally prescribed in a cyclic fashion: they are taken for twenty-one days, then discontinued for a week. Some women do better on injectable estrogens, which can be given intramuscularly every three or four weeks.

Women past the menopause frequently suffer from itching, burning, and pain in the vagina following intercourse. This is usually caused by a thinning of the mucous membranes, and this, too, can be alleviated by the administration of female sexual hormones. The disappearance of this problem is often important in the emotional life of older women. Sometimes, in addition to injections or tablets, these hormones are applied locally in the form of a cream or suppository.

Menopausal problems are not limited to women in their fifties. Studies I have done on patients to estimate their estrogen levels have shown that even very young girls may be menopausal because of insufficient estrogen. Since estrogen deficiencies can occur at any time of life, a woman with emotional difficulties should insist that her doctor do a maturation index to estimate her estrogen level. The maturation index is performed like a Pap smear, and tests the vaginal cells to see whether they are being properly stimulated by estrogen.

A second satisfactory way of testing for estrogen is to collect a twenty-four-hour urine sample and measure it for total estrogen excretion. These tests are most important; every woman with emotional or psychosomatic symptoms should have them performed. I have these tests performed on all my new women patients and give hormone treatment as indicated.

Many other hormonal systems exist in the body in addition to those I have discussed, but they have less day-to-day direct influence on emotional factors and therefore are less pertinent to the subject of this book.

NOTES

1. J. S. Walters, *Journal of Applied Nutrition*, Vol. 10, No. 3, 1957.
2. Arthur J. Prange, Jr., *et al.*, "Enhancement of Empramine Antidepressant Activity by Thyroid Hormone," *Amer. Jrnl. of Psychiatry*, Vol. 126, October 1969, p. 4.

DIET IN THE
CURE OF ALCOHOLISM

CHAPTER SIXTEEN

Alcoholics are supposed to be difficult people. Almost any physician will tell you that he does not like to treat alcoholic patients because they are just too difficult to be worth his time and trouble. But if you stop and think about it, aren't a lot of people difficult these days?

I suspect the real reason why so many physicians do not care to treat alcoholics is because physicians do not really know what to do for these patients. In fact, unless a physician is steeped in nutritional knowledge, he cannot treat them adequately.

Consider a patient who recently visited me from Buffalo. Tests revealed he was suffering from severe hypoglycemia and that he had a low NAD (Nicotinamide Adenine Dinucleotide). A hair test demonstrated deficiencies in iron, manganese, calcium, magnesium, and copper. He also had multiple food hypersensitivities as revealed by sublingual allergy tests.

A computerized MMPI gave a printout of his psychological state, and the first paragraph said:

THIS PATIENT SHOWS A PERSONALITY PATTERN WHICH FREQUENTLY
OCCURS AMONG PERSONS WHO SEEK PSYCHIATRIC TREATMENT.
FEELINGS OF INADEQUACY, SEXUAL CONFLICT AND RIGIDITY ARE
ACCOMPANIED BY A LOSS OF EFFICIENCY, INITIATIVE AND SELF
CONFIDENCE. INSOMNIA IS LIKELY TO OCCUR ALONG WITH CHRONIC
ANXIETY, FATIGUE, AND TENSION. HE MAY HAVE SUICIDAL THOUGHTS.
IN THE CLINICAL PICTURE, DEPRESSION IS THE DOMINANT FEATURE.
PSYCHIATRIC PATIENTS WITH THIS PATTERN ARE LIKELY TO BE
DIAGNOSED AS DEPRESSIVES OR ANXIETY REACTIONS. THE BASIC
CHARACTERISTICS ARE RESISTANT TO CHANGE AND WILL TEND TO
REMAIN STABLE WITH TIME. AMONG MEDICAL PATIENTS WITH THIS
PATTERN, A LARGE NUMBER ARE SERIOUSLY DEPRESSED, AND OTHERS
SHOW SOME DEPRESSION, ALONG WITH FATIGUE AND EXHAUSTION.
THERE ARE FEW SPONTANEOUS RECOVERIES, ALTHOUGH THE INTENSITY
OF THE SYMPTOMS MAY BE CYCLIC.

To summarize: Here is a thirty-four-year-old man severely depressed, with multiple vitamin and mineral deficiencies, multiple food hypersensitivities, hypoglycemia—and he drinks about a quart of whiskey every twenty-four hours. "Pitiful" would describe him better than "difficult." His marriage was dissolving. Because of his fuzzy thinking, poor concentration, and frequent absenteeism he was about to be discharged from a responsible position. History revealed that his alcoholism went back at least fifteen years, but had gradually become more serious during the last two years. He visited me only because he realized his life was about to rupture.

Here was a patient in many ways typical of people who have problems with alcoholism: He had multiple deficiencies and multiple food allergies.

I put him on a diet free of alcohol, wheat, rye, barley, corn, sugar, sweets, milk, and processed foods. He was instructed to emphasize fresh meat, fresh vegetables, fresh fruits, eggs, and nuts. He was also given dietary supplements including vitamins A and D, primary yeast, ascorbic acid, lecithin, calcium pantothenate, ferrous gluconate, manganese citrate, glutamine, and dolomite. In addition to these supplements to be taken by mouth, he was given injections of multiple B vitamins, including B_{12b} and vitamin C.

When he stopped drinking he passed through a rough period of withdrawal during which he experienced a mild form of delirium tremens with signs of restlessness, confusion, and disorganization. This lasted for three or four days. Because of nausea during this time, he was unable to take his oral supplements properly, so I administered massive amounts of vitamins and ACE as well as a temporary tranquilizer by injection. After the withdrawal period, he was able to take oral supplements again and rapidly improved. Except for a three-day slipup he has remained alcohol free.

Today he is quite cheerful. He feels that he is "with it," and is again succeeding at his work and his marriage. Several times in the past he stopped drinking for a few months but each time returned to alcohol because of a lingering craving for it. His present period of abstinence is unique. For the first time he no longer has any real craving for alcohol. Indeed, he says that the idea of returning to it bores him.

This response is typical of patients who do pay attention to their allergies, who avoid foods that give them trouble, and take nutritional supplements as directed. If a patient cooperates about his nutrition needs, almost every alcoholic recovers. I do have failures, but ninety-nine percent of these occur in people who do not follow the diet and do not take their supplements properly.

Today almost all "drying out" clinics and hospitals that are particularly geared to helping people with alcoholism use massive doses of vitamins. But many clinics neglect the patients' mineral levels and do not test them for food allergies to learn which foods they should avoid. Their rates of recovery would be much higher if the clinics paid more attention to the fine points of nutrition.

I cannot recall ever having seen an alcoholic who did not suffer from some marked food allergies. These patients are notoriously low in minerals, especially magnesium—a most important mineral for regulating the excitability of the central nervous system.

Typically, physicians also neglect the alcoholic patient's nutritional needs. Many practitioners will give a patient a modest oral vitamin supplement without realizing that these patients often require massive doses of vitamins for an indefinite period, and often require them by injection, at least at first. They also neglect the mineral levels of these patients and the food allergy aspects of alcoholism.

The average psychiatrist in private practice neglects nutrition completely and has almost nothing to offer the patient suffering from alcoholism. For such a psychiatrist the alcoholic patient is a very difficult patient because the psychiatrist can't cure him.

Much interesting information from the laboratory gives us fresh insights into the problems of alcoholism. For example, some laboratory mice inherit the trait for becoming alcoholic. Strain A, for example, will drink no alcohol when it is available. Strain B may drink alcohol in modest amounts. Strain C may be quite fond of alcohol and drink it to the point of malnutrition.

We humans rather dislike thinking of ourselves in biological terms. But the fact is that we are biological creatures. We eat, sleep, defecate, and reproduce and undeniably share these biological traits with grasshoppers, goldfish, and gazelles. Yet only now are psychiatrists beginning to accept the studies done a generation ago at Columbia University showing quite clearly that the trait of schizophrenia can be inherited. We seem to be able to accept the fact that high blood pressure may be an inherited trait or that cancer may "run in the family," but it seems difficult for us to realize that psychological problems are fundamentally also biological problems and that the tendency toward them can also be inherited.

INHERITING ALCOHOLISM

It is my feeling, shared by many workers in the field, that alcoholism is a complex trait based on an inherited biological defect. I have previously pointed out how many biological differences we inherit. Unfortunately, we know less about heredity in humans than in the lower animals, since animals lend themselves more readily to experimentation.

We know, for example, that cattle fed on large amounts of wheat develop "wheat disease," a form of paralysis due to low calcium in the diet. When calcium is given, the paralysis disappears. Not *all* cattle develop this disease when fed large amounts of wheat. Some remain healthy. They happen to inherit a metabolism able to withstand the strain of low calcium diets.

Cattle grazed on grass develop "grass disease" caused by a magnesium deficiency. Again, not all cattle develop this disease. The inherited biological differences in cattle allow some cattle to handle the deficiency better than others.

We are quick to speak of individual rights and to recognize that individuals have different needs and desires. It is repugnant to Americans to dictate where a man should work, where he should live, at what age he should marry, and so forth. We recognize that individual needs, preferences, capacities, and talents vary greatly from individual to individual. This recognition of individuality must be extended to individual biochemistry. By now I trust I have convinced you that individuals are different and that you will concede it is quite possible for humans to possess genetic traits that make them more susceptible to alcohol than their neighbors.

It is traditional among psychiatrists to talk about people turning to alcohol in order to escape problems. Admittedly, alcohol is an escape from problems, but why do not even more people use alcohol as a means of escape? Why does one man escape by becoming a Sanskrit scholar while another may escape by homosexual cruising and still another may escape by eating quarts of ice cream?

In any of these cases the act of escape may become the main facet of their lives and be a disintegrating force. But none of these escapes is likely to be as disintegrating as alcoholism, because alcoholic excesses produce malnutrition and, ultimately, damage to the nervous system and a gradual disintegration of the personality.

I will never forget a young man who visited my office many years ago saying that he was coming to see me because he couldn't work out his problems. He said that during a recent period of unhappiness, he had made a conscious effort to become an alcoholic. He had visited bars. He had drunk himself to sleep every night and had a wake-up drink every morning but he had utterly failed at his attempt to become an alcoholic! Ultimately he developed headaches, depression, nausea, but he never managed to go the alcoholic route. As in other endeavors of life, it requires inborn talents to be a really good alcoholic.

HOW NUTRITION CONTROLS THE DESIRE TO DRINK

Professor Roger Williams at the University of Texas discovered that if alcoholic mice are fed vitamin- and mineral-enriched diets, they soon lose their interest in alcohol. The genetic trait that predisposed them toward alcoholism could be modified by the use of massive nutritional supplements.

Does the same principle hold for people? Psychiatrists who are emphasizing nutritional therapy for alcoholics say, "yes." Most alcoholics are able to stop drinking and even lose interest in alcohol if they are given proper nutritional supplements and are maintained on diets that exclude foods to which they are allergic.

Studies show that alcoholic mice gradually become more and more deficient in vitamins and minerals, since alcohol contains neither vitamins nor minerals. The more the mice drink, the less they eat, and as they drift deeper into their deficiency state, they become more and more interested in alcohol.

In another experiment, mice were gradually fed more and more sugar so that they became more and more deficient in vitamins and minerals (since sugar, like alcohol, provides "empty" calories). Like the alcoholic mice, these animals became progressively more interested in sugar and less interested in other food. In other words, they became addicted to empty calories.

Deficiencies cause a change in the metabolism of mice so they crave the very food that harms them. Hence they perpetuate and even exacerbate their illness, producing more and more deficiencies by consuming more and more of the deficient foods.

This is exactly what happens with human alcoholics. All alcoholics start drinking modestly and gradually increase their intake of alcohol, so that more and more of their diet is composed of empty calories. Hence they increase their deficiencies, which in turn makes them more and more interested in alcohol.

In my view, mice become more interested in alcohol and sugar when they are vitamin deficient because they develop an allergic addiction to alcohol and sugar. In my chapter on food allergies you will have noted that allergic addictions produce a temporary mood lift so that the person (or the mouse) wants to return to the substance time and time again to repeat the lift. Allergic addictions are quite common in life. They frequently result in obesity. People gorge on sweets and bakery products. This produces more and more vitamin deficiencies. And this makes them more and more hungry because it increases their allergic state, just as in the vicious cycle of the alcoholic.

People we call allergic or hypersensitive must have an inborn error of metabolism, but we know from experimental evidence with mice and with people that allergic states and hypersensitivities can be reduced by the use of vitamins and minerals.

It is possible to have an allergic addiction to foods that do not necessarily make vitamin and mineral deficiencies worse. These food addictions are not nearly as serious as addictions to alcohol and sugar. For example, I have patients addicted to such foods as apples, lettuce, or even to concentrated protein powders that some nutritionists advocate (but not I).

It is possible to make some mice drink more heavily if you bang bells and make them generally uncomfortable in their cages. You "drive them to drink." Yet other mice in the same environment cannot be made to drink, no matter how uncomfortable you make them.

We people tend greatly to overemphasize our surroundings and our problems and to blame them for troubles that are really biochemical. If you think you have problems, check out your nutritional supplements and your food allergies. Once all of these are in ideal balance, 95 out of 100 of your problems will have disappeared. You will be able to cope with your remaining problems with a little finger, even if it previously required both arms and both shoulders just to keep your problems from crushing you.

Although this is a book on nutrition and emotional disorders, I would like to commend the work of AA and encourage anyone with alcohol problems to seek AA help. In general, AA has been hostile toward psychiatrists, mainly because of the unpleasant experiences AA members had during the '40s and '50s when psychiatrists routinely gave patients barbiturates, changing them from alcoholics to barbiturate addicts. But one of the AA's co-founders, Bill Wilson, was a very strong advocate of nutritional approaches (including megavitamins) as an aid to anyone who wanted to give up alcohol.

THE SPECIAL NUTRITIONAL NEEDS OF ALCOHOLICS

ANYONE SUFFERING FROM ALCOHOLISM MUST GIVE SPECIAL ATTENTION TO HIS NUTRITIONAL NEEDS. That sentence should be written in flashing red neon letters a yard high and placed in every room of the alcoholic's home.

First he should be on the basic nutritional program as detailed elsewhere: Natural vitamins A, 10,000 units daily; D, 400 units daily; E, 200 units breakfast and lunch; ascorbic acid powder, one-quarter teaspoon in water four times daily; brewers' or primary yeast, one heaping tablespoon in water two times daily; lecithin granules, two heaping tablespoons on fruit twice daily; and safflower oil, one tablespoon twice daily (all with his physician's approval).

Most persons with alcoholism would do well to add megavitamins to their nutritional supplements, again with their physician's approval. See the section on megavitamins for details.

It is most important for alcoholics to check out their food allergies also, since almost everyone with this problem suffers from food allergic addictions. If these are not solved, the chances of recovery will fall drastically.

Some aspects of nutrition are especially important in treating alcoholism. Although these will be discussed in the next few pages, I want to remind the reader that *every* aspect of nutrition is important for the alcoholic.

Each person suffering from alcoholism should be given special tests for food allergies (as detailed in the chapter on food allergies). Skin tests are of no help. If tests are not done, then the alcoholic should assume he is allergic to table sugar, to grains (other than brown rice) and to milk products (other than butter), and these should be eliminated from the diet in most cases.

THE DOLOMITE NEEDS OF ALCOHOLICS

Generally, it is particularly important for a person with alcoholism to get extra amounts of magnesium, taken in the form of two or three teaspoons of powdered dolomite at bedtime in water or one teaspoon three or four times a day, depending on which schedule makes him feel best. Magnesium orate is excellent (but expensive) for people who don't easily assimilate the magnesium from dolomite.

THE GLUTAMINE NEEDS OF ALCOHOLICS

Glutamine, an amino acid, constitutes, along with glucose, the bulk of nourishment used by the nervous system. Glutamine can give an enormous lift to people with a malfunction in the metabolism of the central nervous system, especially people who are tired or depressed. Glutamine can be very stimulating—even overstimulating—to some people. When I take a couple of capsules I feel as if I have been pumped full of speed.

Glutamine often offers special relief to the alcoholic—and here is how. An alcoholic, like a sugar addict, gets more and more hooked on his poison as he becomes more and more malnourished and has more vitamin and mineral deficiencies. Once this damaged metabolism extends to the appetite control in the hypothalamus, addiction to malnutrition itself sets in.

A research scientist, William Shive, at the University of Texas, became interested in an unknown substance present in extracts of many plants and animals able to protect living cells from alcohol poisoning. The unknown substance proved to be glutamine, an amino acid present in many protein foods but frequently destroyed, i.e., turned into glutamic acid. In laboratory tests, bacteria were poisoned by adding alcohol to the medium in which they grew; when glutamine was added to the medium, the bacteria could tolerate much higher doses of alcohol without suffering damage.

When glutamine is given to alcoholic rats and hamsters, they lose their desire for alcohol, or greatly diminish their intake. Although long-range experiments on humans have not yet been conducted, some spectacular results have been documented. J. B. Trunell reports one case of an alcoholic who was given glutamine without his knowledge (glutamine is tasteless). Abruptly and for no apparent reason, the man gave up drinking, got a job, and in a follow-up two years later reported that he no longer had any desire to drink.

Although glutamine is not a miracle cure by itself, and does not necessarily help every alcoholic, I strongly recommend that it be given a trial by anyone with a drinking problem. If your druggist doesn't carry it, you can order it from Willner Chemists (see the vitamin chapter for the address). If you want to take it just for a potential lift, begin at one 200-mg. capsule three times a day, for a week, increasing to two capsules three times a day the second week, as part of your experimental nutrition regimen.

If you are trying to control a drinking problem, take five capsules three times a day. If it speeds you up too much, take it at meals and not at bedtime. If necessary, decrease the dose and build back up more slowly.

There have never been any reports of unfavorable side-effects from glutamine, so you can take as much as you feel you need, though I see little point in exceeding 3000 or 4000 mg. three or four times a day. Remember that the deleterious effects of alcohol may be more acute than the effects of simple malnutrition, so be sure you give glutamine time to help you recoup the losses that your nervous system may have suffered already. As with other recommendations in this book you should follow your doctor's advice. Be sure you are taking *glutamine,* not *glutamic acid* which does not protect against alcohol poisoning. Many doctors and druggists confuse the two.

CHOLINE, INOSITOL, AND ALCOHOLISM

Because nearly everyone who has suffered from alcoholism for any period of time has sustained some liver damage, a source of choline and inositol is especially important. The best source is lecithin, two heaping tablespoons twice a day. Twice this amount would give an added margin of safety. Brewers' or primary yeast also helps supply these important vitamins.

THE THIAMIN NEEDS OF ALCOHOLICS

Special attention should be given to thiamin since some patients with alcoholism have long experienced a thiamin deficiency and often require massive amounts over an indefinite period. I recommend 500 to 1000 or perhaps 1500 mg. three times a day. Again, some people find thiamin quite stimulating. It should be taken in doses that are not *over*stimulating and of course thiamin should be taken in conjunction with the other B vitamins since all the B vitamins work together.

For others, thiamin has a marked calming effect.

THE VITAMIN B_{12b} NEEDS OF ALCOHOLICS

The next emphasis should be placed on vitamin B_{12b} (hydroxoco-balamine). Most alcoholics do better with large injections of vitamin B_{12b}. When I was giving a speech in L.A. not long ago a woman came up to me saying she had for many years been an alcoholic. When she gave up alcohol, she became schizophrenic and then happened to be given an injection of vitamin B_{12} by a family doctor. She immediately felt greatly improved and began taking injections of 5000 mcg. daily because she discovered this was the only dose which would maintain her feeling of well-being. Since learning about hydroxocobalamine (vitamin B_{12b}) from one of my papers, she switched to this form of vitamin B_{12} and discovered she could cut her dose in half.

People suffering from alcoholism would be well advised to have therapeutic trials on vitamin B_{12b} injections, regardless of what their blood levels show. Special attention should also be paid to the folic acid needs of these patients; some need as many as 80 mg. daily of folic acid.

HOW DRUGS AND CHEMICALS DESTROY B_{12}

Vitamin B_{12} absorption is reduced by a number of common chemicals routinely taken by many people. One of my patients came to me in a quite depressed state and was found to be low in serum B_{12}. He responded very well to injections of it, but required enormous doses about every five days to maintain his sense of well-being. Whenever he drinks even a modest amount of alcohol he finds that he begins to build up steam, and requires B_{12b} injections at approximately three- to four-day intervals to calm down. For him, the use of alcohol constitutes a stress factor, which burns up his vitamin B_{12} at an accelerated pace.

As I pointed out in my paper on vitamin B_{12b},[1] a drug called Dilantin, commonly taken by individuals suffering from epilepsy, may also cause a marked depletion in the body's B_{12} stores. Birth control pills lower B_{12} levels. As mentioned, vitamin C helps iron absorption but cuts down on vitamin B_{12} absorption.

Without doubt, many other medications also lower serum B_{12} levels.

It is my strong feeling that all people—especially as they get older—should have periodic tests of their serum B_{12} levels and serum folate levels, since their reduction has profound effects on the central nervous system; it can even induce a form of paralysis. If too-low levels of these two vitamins continue long enough, pernicious anemia may develop, although the anemia may occur after the nervous system damage has been done.

Most physicians mistakenly believe that low serum B_{12} levels and low folic acid levels produce anemia *prior* to causing damage to the central nervous system and producing emotional symptoms. This is absolutely incorrect. I urge you not to let a physician tell you that tests of serum B_{12} levels and serum folic acid levels are unnecessary and only experimental. This may be his way of trying to dismiss a subject on which he has not read up.

I have talked with physicians from all over the world who report that patients, particularly those in advancing years, ask them for B_{12} injections because they make them feel better. Almost invariably, these physicians think that the patients are asking for what amounts to a placebo. Often the doctors give in against their inclination just to pacify the patients. These physicians very rarely check the serum B_{12} levels of such patients to find out whether a deficiency does, in fact, exist. Nor do they consider the distinct possibility that the patient may be suffering from a hereditary vitamin dependency disease, in which case he would require the vitamin in amounts vastly in excess of the so-called average.

THE ESSENTIAL FATTY ACID NEEDS OF ALCOHOLICS

As I explained in the chapter on vitamins, three fatty acids are essential for good health. They can be absorbed in small amounts from various vegetable oils, but the best and safest source is cold-pressed safflower oil. Everyone not allergic to it should have at least two tablespoons a day of safflower oil, in salad dressing or by the spoon if necessary. I consider this particularly important for alcoholics, because laboratory experiments have shown that alcoholic rats reduce their alcohol intake when they consume fatty acids.

THE CALCIUM PANTOTHENATE NEEDS
OF ALCOHOLICS

This substance may be of special help to alcoholics. I suggest from one to five 218-mg. capsules at bedtime, or dispersed throughout the day if you do not find them too relaxing.

SEX AND ALCOHOLISM

The Freudian clichés of several generations ago about alcoholics being orally fixated or having subconscious homosexual tendencies are largely nonsense—psychiatric fairy tales that are being dismissed by the younger generation of scientists.

It is true that use of alcohol can cause liver damage which will make the ratio of female to male sex hormones higher than it should be in men. Always, a person suffering from alcoholism should have his hormone levels studied. If found low in sex hormones, women should be given estrogens. If found deficient in testosterone, men should get injections of testosterone at one- or two-weekly intervals, often for indefinite periods. I might add that thyroid hormone by mouth in the form of desiccated thyroid tablets is also often indicated.

PROPER NUTRITION FOR ALCOHOLICS

Alcoholism is, among other things, a nutritional deficiency disease. Every alcoholic is malnourished. Most people believe that this is a symptom of the disease, but Dr. Roger Williams, among others, believes that malnutrition may be the *cause* of alcoholism; it may be that nutritional and metabolic imbalances are precisely the factor that make one person susceptible to alcohol addiction while another is not. At any rate, he believes that it is impossible to become an alcoholic if you are properly nourished.

Obviously, correcting nutritional deficiencies is one of the first steps an alcoholic must take in recovering from his disease. (Proper nutrition can also help to prevent the potential alcoholic from becoming addicted in the first place.) We have seen that a deranged appetite mechanism is one of the most dangerous symptoms of alcoholism. This usually becomes apparent when the alcoholic no longer desires food at all, and craves only the empty calories of alcohol. But along the way to alcoholism (and the disease usually takes many years to develop), other signals may appear. For instance, alcohol sometimes appears to stimulate the appetite. Alcoholism is often—perhaps always—associated with hypoglycemia (low blood sugar). Therefore an alcoholic may become addicted to both forms of empty calories, alcohol and sugar. He may binge on both alcohol and sweets. The result is an overweight alcoholic who is nevertheless starving to death—and all the while he assures you that he must not be alcoholic because everyone knows alcoholics don't eat.

To break this cycle, either to prevent true alcohol addiction or to recover from it, a high-protein, low-carbohydrate, *no*-sugar diet is essential. Of course, any true alcoholic must give up drinking entirely if he is to recover. But at any stage of the disease, a high-protein diet that acts to keep the blood sugar stable will also act to inhibit the craving for alcohol by preventing the wild swings in blood sugar levels that contribute to the rush he gets from drinking and the drop that makes him need another. Niacin (1000 mg. three times a day) has also been found beneficial to alcoholics, probably because it too acts to keep blood sugar high.

The problem drinker should follow the anti-allergenic, high-protein diet described in earlier chapters and should pay particular attention to a complete range of vitamin supplements. This helps his body (especially his liver and nervous system) to recover from the damage of the disease; as they become healthier he will experience less and less addictive craving.

ALCOHOLICS AND PSYCHIATRISTS

Psychiatrists and alcoholics have not had much use for each other in the past. The psychiatrist was frustrated because he discovered that psychotherapy ("talk treatment") simply did not work, and the alcoholic was frustrated for the same reason. While addiction to alcohol may certainly have emotional consequences for the patient, both he and the psychiatrist must recognize that they are dealing with a basically physical, organic condition, not an emotional trauma. If they can work together on the nutritional aspects of the disease, they will have more success in treating the physical addiction *and* in handling its emotional sequels.

Anyone dealing with alcoholics—and this goes for the patient's family as well as his doctor—should be prepared for some early frustrations. We must all remember that addictions, whether they be to alcohol, drugs, or chocolate cake, are among the strongest forces motivating humans. The behavioral strivings to satisfy addictions can be stronger than the sexual drive, stronger than the drive for food and water, and may even become stronger than the drive for life itself. If those of us without addictions will bear these facts in mind, our patience for dealing with alcoholics will help them—and us.

NOTES

1. H. L. Newbold, "The Use of Vitamin B_{12} in Psychiatric Practice," *Orthomolecular Psychiatry*, Vol. 1, No. 1, 1972.

LIGHT IS NOURISHING!

CHAPTER SEVENTEEN

You're probably wondering why a chapter on light is included in a book on nutrition and emotional health. It's simple: Light, like food, comes to us from the outside—from the environment; like edible substances, it is taken in by our bodies and utilized in a large variety of metabolic processes, which makes it a nutrient every bit as vital as those we take by mouth.

To make the relevance of light even more pointed, let me tell you that the light that most of us city dwellers get is just as inferior as the food that most of us eat, and that it detracts from our physical and emotional well-being quite as much as does our deficient diet.

Before we began civilizing ourselves into semi-invalidism, we received an abundance of *full-spectrum light:* the kind that nature provides for us in the form of sunlight. What we actually get most of the time is a mere *fraction* of the spectrum. Once we are ensconced behind our office desks or in our living room armchairs, science efficiently furnishes us with electric light. If your company is *really* up to date you are probably working under fluorescent light, which may be an industrial

LIGHT IS NOURISHING!   **235**

engineer's dream of perfection—but happens to be the most nutrient-
deficient of all lighting devices. Even ordinary light bulbs are preferable
to the total artificiality of the fluorescent environment.

The full-spectrum light provided by the sun (you also get reflected
full-spectrum light on hazy days or in the shade) extends all the way
from ultraviolet through the visual range into the infrared area. At sea
level, it reaches the earth in a band extending from 290 to 3500
monometers. *All* of this spectrum is necessary for optimum stimulation
of the human organism. Any light source that cuts out some part of the
spectrum diminishes the stimulation you receive, and to that extent
diminishes your well-being. Yet the visible light that lighting engineers
ordinarily think about in the context of light stimulation is a very narrow
band between 380 and 770 monometers. Clearly, this is far from
full-spectrum level, and contains no ultraviolet light at all.

Probably the one function of light that most people are familiar with
is its power to provide our vitamin D needs. This vitamin—also
popularly known as the "sunshine vitamin"—regulates the use of
calcium, magnesium, and phosphorus in our bodies. Because of its role
in the proper formation and functioning of teeth and bones, it is
especially important in infancy, childhood and old age. Its lack during
childhood can cause rickets, retarded growth, and tooth decay; among
the elderly, vitamin D deficiency is partly responsible for a condition
called *osteoporosis* (brittle bones), which causes major fractures, such as
broken hips, as a result of relatively minor falls.

But what about vitamin D deficiency during the middle years?

Obviously, adequate vitamin D intake is one way of helping to
forestall osteoporosis—an affliction that besets a large percentage of
post-menopausal women, and causes no symptoms until it has progressed to a near-irreversible stage. But this function far from exhausts
its usefulness: Vitamin D—and hence, full-spectrum light stimulation—
is just as vital for our emotional health as for our physical well-being,
perhaps most of all during the usually most stressful middle period of our
lives.

THE CASE OF SYBIL

Not long ago a patient visited me who had been to see forty
different doctors over a period of several years. Sybil told me that she

was sure something was wrong with her chemistry, but that no one had been able to discover any such defect during dozens of physical examinations and extensive laboratory work-ups. These had revealed only that she suffered from low blood sugar. The proper diet for this condition had ended her previous propensity for fainting at her desk, but had done nothing whatever for her other complaints. She continued to have muscle cramps and burning sensations throughout her body, often grew very tired, suffered from headaches, and most of the time simply felt ill.

After exhausting their diagnostic means, the other physicians had always come up with the same diagnosis: Her troubles were due to "tension."

This wastebasket (variously labeled "tension syndrome," "hypochondriasis," or "constitutional inferiority") is a favorite depository into which many doctors dump illnesses they can't diagnose. Having read this far, you probably know me well enough by now to realize that the thought of helping a patient on whom forty doctors had given up provided a special, exhilarating challenge.

The additional tests I performed on Sybil revealed a borderline serum B_{12} level and very low vitamin B_3 level. Once these deficiencies were corrected she improved somewhat, but by no means sufficiently. In addition to demonstrable allergies to peanuts, hydrocarbons, cat hair, dust, pasteurized (but not raw) milk, wool, and mold, she was also *clinically* allergic to beef. This means that even though the allergy tests revealed no such sensitivity she now and then had an allergic reaction when she ate beef.

Insofar as her wide-range sensitivities permitted this, we removed all offending substances from her environment. Nonetheless, she continued to have debilitating symptoms, especially fatigue and muscle cramps.

This time, she was sent to one more internist. He hospitalized her, biopsied her muscle tissue, and performed a battery of special tests on it, all of which turned out negative. Once more she was given a diagnosis of "tension," and returned to me.

Psychiatrists have one great advantage over other physicians—they spend more time with their patients. When we see a patient for half an hour or more, week after week, as we do, little bits and pieces of apparently unrelated information tend to crop up and accumulate until, sometimes, they suddenly coalesce into a meaningful pattern. Luckily, that's what happened with Sybil.

One day she said, "You know, it's a funny thing: I can eat all the beef I want without any allergic reaction at home; but every time I eat it for lunch at work I get a reaction."

Time was when I would have dismissed such a comment as the irrelevant observation of a self-absorbed neurotic. But I long ago decided that there is no such thing as a hypochondriac. There are only patients whose ailments resist diagnosis by traditional techniques. Once a doctor comes to this conviction, that doctor is forced to consider every possible lead that the patient supplies.

We had already checked Sybil's place of employment, a very large international corporation. She dealt with computers which, when they were warm, gave off volatile particles of plastic. Amazingly, this very allergy-prone patient was not sensitive to plastics. We also checked the carpeting and air filters in the room where she worked. Some mechanical fiberglass air filters are a source of continual pollution, especially those with fungus growths. Also, some air purifiers use electrostatic screens which put ozone in the air.*

Sybil had checked out satisfactorily to all the substances in her working environment that could possibly be considered allergenic.

What happened next is a good example of how an intelligent patient

* You may be surprised to learn that—effusions of nineteenth-century poets notwithstanding—ozone is highly toxic. It got its undeserved poetic reputation because of the "fresh" odor associated with the purifying effects of thunderstorms. Ozone is, indeed, formed during the course of electrical storms, and occurs on the earth's surface in trace amounts.

But it is an extremely active form of oxygen, containing three molecules as against two in the normal kind we breathe. Proper amounts of oxygen are, of course, not only desirable but vital to life; excessive oxidation leads to death.

Ozone, which is formed by the electrical discharge of oxygen or air, was first discovered in 1785, in the vicinity of an electrical machine running in a laboratory. Since then, our home use of electrical appliances has proliferated almost beyond belief, and any of them may spark and thus produce ozone. An electrostatic filter, for example, whether on an air conditioner, furnace, or—most ironic—on an air purifier, may produce ozone in large quantities. Earthbound biological systems (like humans) have not included ozone in the evolution of their metabolic processes, and their physiology is therefore unable to accommodate it without deleterious effects.

Where ozone does a lot of good is not on earth but fifteen miles above, where nature has created a layer of it to protect us from excess ultraviolet rays of the sun.

can help the doctor, if he will only permit it. Too many of us in the medical profession feel too insecure to accept information tendered by our patients, fearing that our prestige might suffer if we don't appear omniscient. This is a great mistake. An intelligent and observant patient can often be of tremendous help to the doctor, sometimes even when it comes to making a relatively simple diagnosis.

Sybil happened to attend a lecture by John Ott, D.Sc., who talked on full-spectrum light and its importance to human well-being. As a result, she began to study the light conditions in her own environment, and attempted to correlate them with her symptoms. It wasn't long before she discovered that she always felt worse at work, where she was subjected to standard fluorescent lighting. The same type of light illuminated the company cafeteria where she ate lunch.

Impossible as it may seem at first, this turned out to be the correct explanation: She *was* allergic to beef—but only when exposed to fluorescent light while eating it. At the time, this surprised me, too. But not for long. The more one delves into the research on photo stimulation (i.e., exposure to different types of light), the more one realizes that the most common pollution in the civilized world is *light pollution*—a pollution to which we are all subject most of our waking hours.

There is, in scientific research, a basic tenet called the "Law of Parsimony" or "Lord Morgan's Canon" (after its purported promulgator). Roughly translated, Morgan's Canon commands that thou shalt not chase convoluted explanations when a commonsense solution is at hand, because unless and until proved otherwise the simplest (most parsimonious) explanation is the one most likely to be correct.

THE CASE AGAINST LIGHT POLLUTION

From the time life first began on this planet, our primitive ancestors spent their daylight hours in the open, searching for food. Is it surprising that human chemistry came to incorporate light stimulation, and that our body's chemistry evolved with the assumption that full-spectrum light stimulation would always be available? True, certain species have adapted to life without light—for instance, the blind white fish found in the waters of places like Mammoth Cave. Their ancestors have lived in a dark environment for so many generations that they lost their ability to see, since nature tends to eliminate useless organs and chemical reactions and to conserve tissue for utilization in a more productive way.

But we humans have neither retained our old habits nor adapted to our new ones. As short a time as a hundred years ago, seventy-five percent of the people in this country still lived off the soil and spent most of their time outdoors, where they received full-spectrum light stimulation. Now, with the overwhelming population shift from rural areas to cities, most people spend very little time outdoors. They commonly receive from ninety-five to one hundred percent of their light stimulation from artificial sources, which are almost always lacking in some part of the spectrum.

Suppose you went to some foreign country, found a very rare and valuable animal, and brought it back to live in captivity; would you not try to provide it with an environment as similar as possible to its indigenous one? If the animal had been living in a hot, dry desert under perpetual sunshine, would you choose a dark, swampy area as its new habitat and expect it to thrive? Obviously not. You would provide surroundings as similar as possible to its native ones.

Through a process of selective breeding supervised by Mother Nature, animals become uniquely adapted to life in their particular environment—and we tamper with this adaptation at great peril. Eventually, those species that cannot thrive in a given environment simply die off; do not leave offspring; and their genes and genotypes are eliminated from the stream of life.

Yet we blindly take man—a mammal who (yes, I need to emphasize this again) evolved as a hunter of meat and picker of fruits—and chain him to an office by day and an apartment at night, and expect him to thrive in these two little environment cells, neither of which provides the full-spectrum light stimulation under which he evolved.

Ancient civilizations were well aware of the vital importance of full-spectrum light and this is documented by their startling preoccupation with the sun. The Aryans worshipped the sun; they called it "Dyas," a word from which the Latin "Deus" evolved. In Egypt, during the fifth dynasty (2750 B.C.), a sun-oriented theology became the state religion, and sun worship became a central facet of Egyptian life. Ancient Persia's most important god was Ormusza, the god of light; and very close to him in significance stood Mithras, the sun god. The Phoenicians worshipped the sun god Baal, as did the ancient Hebrews, for whom he was also the god of health. Babylon worshipped Marduk, another sun god, whose father was Ea, the supreme healer. In ancient Greece, many healing powers were attributed to Helius, the god of light and sun. Sol, another sun god, was one of the twelve deities of the ancient Romans' religion. In Pompeii, we find many frescoes depicting people stretched out on rooftops, sunbathing. Most Roman houses also had solaria for that purpose.

While these examples might make it appear that glorification of the sun was a characteristic of Mediterranean peoples, the practice actually extended far into the chillier climes—through Central, Eastern, and Northern Europe, all the way to Britain's sun-worshipping Druids.

With the advent of Christianity, Western man's attitude toward the sun changed profoundly. Worship of the sun was condemned, its healing powers ignored, and sunlight itself became associated with paganism. It was to take more than fifteen hundred years before opinion began to change again. The French court physician Theodore Tronchin led the way with his advocacy of walks in the fresh air and sunlight. The impact of Rousseau's back-to-nature philosophy completed the job of restoring sunlight to the lives of the people.

In 1796, the University of Göttingen awarded a prize to J. C. Ebermaier, for his paper on the effects of sunlight on the human body. He was one of the first scientists to recognize that rickets was much more common in low-lying, dark, and damp places than in dry, light-exposed ones.

Sunlight became a popular therapeutic measure and remained so through the first thirty or forty years of this century. Since then physicians have become more preoccupied with chemotherapy at the expense of full-spectrum light. Despite all chemical advances, in the depth of winter most people still feel an instinctive longing for the warm, sunlit spots of the world.

Those who are unable to indulge their inner promptings begin to look for substitutes. Sunlamps have become a popular item, and their manufacture is a lucrative enterprise. Lately the industry has begun to manufacture full-spectrum lights as well, which makes this important source of stimulation available to people on a daily basis and part of the normal lightning in their homes and offices.

Further research is also underway. Two scientific societies have recently been established to further the study of light: the American

Society for Photobiology, whose president is Kendric C. Smith, M.D., of Stanford University's School of Medicine; and the Environmental Health and Light Research Institute in Sarasota, Florida, headed by Dr. Ott. Both these organizations are actively attracting attention to the subject of full-spectrum light, and encouraging research in the field.

WHAT CORRECT LIGHTING CAN DO

Interestingly enough, much current research is being done by a nutritionist, Professor Richard J. Wurtman of the Massachusetts Institute of Technology. One of his experiments was conducted at a home for retired people, and it provides an especially noteworthy illustration of the importance of the subject.

The home's elderly residents were divided into two groups. One group was exposed to full-spectrum light in their day-to-day activities; the other group was not. At the end of the experimental period, the patients in the group exposed to full-spectrum light stimulation showed a marked increase in the absorption of calcium from their food intake.

(Calcium metabolism is an especially important problem in the elderly, because of their aforementioned tendency to osteoporosis, which results from loss of calcium in the bones, making them brittle and highly susceptible to fracture. Osteoporosis is really a two-fold problem. Most of the elderly persons so afflicted tend to have endocrine deficiencies as well. Hormones needed to build strong bones are lacking, which compounds the adverse effect of their defective calcium metabolism.)

In another study, Wurtman placed male and female rats under two types of lights for twenty days. One group was born and raised under the standard "cool-white" fluorescent light tubes. These widely used tubes are very deficient in ultraviolet radiation, and have abnormal ratios of red and yellow emissions, an imbalance which causes a great deal of difficulty in people exposed to it. The second group of animals grew up under the so-called "Vita-Lite," a full-spectrum fluorescent light made to mimic the rays of the sun as closely as possible. Spending a forty-hour week under the Vita-Lite bulbs is roughly equivalent to staying outdoors at noon for thirty minutes once a week in the summer sunshine.

When, at the end of the experiment, the animals were sacrificed, it was found that those raised under full-spectrum light uniformly had smaller spleens, larger hearts, and larger sexual glands than those raised under standard fluorescent light.

It is no accident that this particular study was sponsored by the National Aeronautics and Space Administration, an agency with great interest in light research. Proper light stimulation is obviously of paramount importance for living in the totally artificial environment of space travel, and it will become more important as we penetrate farther into space and stay away from our home planet for longer periods. For similar reasons, the navy already utilizes ultraviolet stimulation for its personnel on submarine duty. This stimulation has not only been found helpful in preventing infections, but also in maintaining the men's emotional health under the stressful, confined conditions of their tours of duty.

Full-spectrum light stimulation is also routinely used in many hospital nurseries for the prevention and treatment of hyperbilirubinemia. Especially prevalent in premature infants, hyperbilirubinemia is a metabolic disorder in which certain bile pigments in the body are abnormally increased so that a baby's skin turns yellow (jaundiced).

ONLY FOOD IS MORE IMPORTANT THAN LIGHT

Dr. Wurtman declares flatly that light is the most important environmental input, after food, in controlling bodily functions. To substantiate this finding he points to the importance of a chemical substance called melatonin, which is regulated by the pineal gland—one of the glands directly stimulated by light. Melatonin circulates in the bloodstream after it is released from the pineal gland. Because it is especially soluble in lipid (fat) solvents, it can pass through the blood-brain barrier without any difficulty. This blood-brain barrier is a very selective gateway; only compounds useful to the brain are allowed to pass through it.

Once inside the brain, melatonin apparently causes an increase of serotonin—one of a group of substances known as neurotransmitters. A neurotransmitter is a chemical that allows one nerve cell to stimulate another nerve cell. Unlike the continuous electrical wiring in a house, the nerve cells of the brain and body are not directly connected with one another; they stimulate each other by releasing minute amounts of chemicals that travel from one nerve fiber to another and thereby activate it.

It is hardly possible to overstress the role played by these neurotransmissions in influencing mood and behavior.

In the February 12, 1970, issue of the *New England Journal of Medicine*, Drs. Wurtman and Robert H. Neer discussed the effects of light stimulation and its two main avenues of influence on the body. The first is the direct effect due to photochemical stimulation of the molecules in the skin, or the tissues immediately beneath the skin; the second is the indirect effect obtained via the light-sensitive cells in the eyes.

The most important known effects of direct light stimulation of the skin are the increase of calcium absorption from the intestines, the decrease in circulating bile pigments, and the well-known tanning effect of ultraviolet light. In all probability, many more biological effects are brought about by such skin stimulation; we just are not yet aware of them.

More germane to the main concern of this book is the effect of light stimulation through the eyes, which seems to be primarily endocrine in nature. Full-spectrum light strikes the retina of the eye and stimulates the optic nerve, which in turn sends out impulses to the hypothalamus—a part of the brain that exercises a profound effect on our emotions. From there, stimulation travels down to the pituitary gland, also called the "master gland," because it regulates the secretions of all other endocrine glands. Such stimulation of the pituitary causes an increase in the size of the sexual and other glands in mammals.

WHAT HAPPENS IN A CITY WITHOUT SUN

The importance of light stimulation to emotional behavior was dramatically illustrated in an article entitled "The Murky Time," published in the January 1, 1973, issue of *Time* Magazine. It tells how the ten thousand inhabitants of Tromso, a Norwegian town 650 air miles and 100 minutes north of Oslo and 200 miles north of the Arctic Circle, spend two months of every year—from November 25 to January 21—without any sunlight whatsoever. During this period, which they call *Mørketiden* (Time of Darkness), the mentally unstable become profoundly disturbed, and even normally well-adjusted people grow increasingly tense, restless, vaguely fearful, and tend to be preoccupied with thoughts of death and suicide.

Even though everything is done to minimize the sense of darkness—lamps on the streets and in gardens burn twenty-four hours a day—the county sheriff of Tromso, Knut Kruse, admits that the townspeople behave very differently during the winter. They spend their time moodily philosophizing about life and tend to become too lackadaisical to pull themselves together for more constructive pursuits. Psychiatrist Harold Reppesgaard of the Asgard Mental Hospital agrees. The entire town changes to a slower pace, he says. People are constantly tired; their powers of concentration are impaired; their work efficiency is drastically reduced.

Some of the citizenry blame lack of proper sleep for their symptoms. But an Oslo physiologist who has researched the emotional problems associated with the annual Tromso blackout has concluded that it is the prolonged absence of light that brings people's undesirable behavior to the surface and accounts for the sudden upsurge in depression, envy, jealousy, suspicion, egotism, and just plain irritability. I think most scientists knowledgeable in the subject would agree that such emotional upheavals are due far more to lack of light stimulation than lack of sleep, which is merely another by-product of full-spectrum light deprivation.

During the period of *Mørketiden* the citizens of Tromso spend much more money on sleeping pills, pep pills, and tranquilizers than at any other time of the year. Their use of hard drugs also increases sharply. People have more accidents and more psychosomatic illnesses. And they share yet another symptom—an instinct to huddle together. Despite their heightened irritability, they desperately need to be with each other. Restaurants, dance halls, and concerts are especially crowded during this time.

What these people want most of all is to escape their sunless world, if only for the briefest vacation in some sunny southern spot. Business firms encourage such vacations as a way of maintaining their workers' stability and efficiency.

The sun's return to Tromso is marked by a special holiday called *Soldag* (Sun Day). On that day, schools and offices are closed. People stream out in the streets to watch the sun rise, shouting and clapping each other on the back ecstatically happy in the knowledge that life will at last return to normal.

What more graphic picture could be drawn to document the effects of proper light stimulation?

Such effects also show up in explorers at the end of long polar expeditions, during which they have had very little full-spectrum light stimulation. These men return suffering from depression, lowered sexual drive, lower blood sugar levels, and lower blood pressure. It would seem that man, despite his almost infinite capacity for adjustment to his environment, has pretty much failed to adjust to a life without full-spectrum light.

Many other observations confirm this. In one radio station, for example, ordinary fluorescent lights were installed as part of a modernization program. Despite the scientifically engineered surroundings, people who worked there soon turned grumpy, began complaining of minor aches and pains, and expressed increasing dissatisfaction with their companions and their working conditions. They did not specifically mention lighting as one of their complaints, and almost certainly were not consciously aware of its deleterious effect. As interpersonal relationships continued to deteriorate, and work efficiency declined spectacularly, experts were consulted and, as a result, full-spectrum light was installed. Almost at once the former spirit of camaraderie returned, and employees settled down to working efficiently together once more.

Such anecdotal evidence is interesting and, in the aggregate, highly meaningful. But to date, most of our hard knowledge concerning full-spectrum light stimulation still comes from research on laboratory animals, just as our knowledge of cancer and cardiovascular disorders continues to expand through laboratory experimentation.

I think it is of great interest that varying light sources can significantly affect the very lifespan of mice. A research strain of mice known as C3H routinely develops tumors at a certain age. The emergence of these tumors has been greatly postponed by exposing these animals to full-spectrum light.

Dr. Ott has also discovered that rats kept under ordinary fluorescent lights develop myocarditis, an inflammation of the heart muscle; whereas rats kept under full-spectrum light do not develop this disease.

Not all animal research is necessarily directly applicable to humans;

but it would seem reasonable to conclude from these experiments that light stimulation has profound biological effects on living creatures, whether they be plants or animals; and we have every reason to believe that mankind's biology is similarly affected.

WHAT HAPPENS WHEN CHILDREN
ARE DEPRIVED OF SUNLIGHT?

W. O. Loomis, M.D., professor of biochemistry at Brandeis University, is convinced that humans lack adequate vitamin D because they do not receive full-spectrum light stimulation. Thus, he says, the deficiency disease known as rickets is in effect the first air pollution disease, because air pollution in the cities cuts down sunlight. He also points out that the disease is far more prevalent in the northern regions of the world than in the southern ones. In New Haven, Connecticut, for example, eighty percent of the children between the ages of two and three years show clinical evidence of rickets; in Puerto Rico, only twelve percent of children in this age group show such signs.

Another interesting study was conducted by Harry S. Hutchinson of Bombay, India, who reports marked differences in the incidence of rickets among Mohammedans, upperclass Hindus, and lowerclass Hindus. Among the rich, well-fed Mohammedans, the incidence of rickets in those under twenty was seventy percent, a fact which Hutchinson attributes to the well-to-do Muslims' custom of remaining indoors, and keeping their children constantly indoors. Among upperclass Hindus, the children are allowed outside more often; in this group, the incidence of rickets among people under the age of twenty was only twenty percent. Among the lowerclass Hindus almost no evidence of rickets was found, despite their very poor diet, presumably because both children and adults spend a great deal of time outdoors.

In 1973 I attended a meeting in Florida devoted to scholarly papers on light stimulation and its relation to biological systems. Eighty-seven universities were represented at the meeting, in addition to scientists from the research departments of major industries such as General Electric.

During a presentation by Dr. Ott we saw a film series on hyperactive children. In the first part, the children were filmed during a routine hour in their classroom. Accustomed as I am to the vagaries of unstable people, I felt that these children were enough to drive a saint to clout them with a Bible. They were totally incapable of paying any attention to the work at hand; they twisted about in their seats like contortionists, kicked each other and the furniture, climbed on top of the desks and crawled under them, raced around the classroom, and in general behaved in the manner typical of the hyperactive-child syndrome, showing their short attention-span and absolute inability to remain in one position long enough to carry out even the simplest task.

At the time when this part of the movie was made, the children's classroom was illuminated by standard fluorescent lights. Subsequently, these fluorescent bulbs were replaced by full-spectrum ones. After the same children had been exposed to the new lights in the same classroom for some months, their activities were again filmed.

The difference was startling. There was no more climbing all over the furniture, no more grotesque body contortions. Now they moved around like normal children, instead of charging about like wild animals. They were markedly less self-centered, more willing and able to interact with each other in a meaningful way. They were also able to sit still in their chairs, and attend to the work before them.

It might be interesting to see what would happen to a classful of normal children after a few months' exposure to full-spectrum light stimulation during school hours. I suspect that their behavior as well as their grades would improve. In fact, a recent study of students, sponsored by the Center for Improvement of Undergraduate Education of Cornell University, seems to confirm it. The study was conducted by James B. Maas, Jill K. Jason, and Douglas A. Kleiber, who report that objective measurements revealed less fatigue and better visual acuity in students studying under full-spectrum rather than the traditional cool-white fluorescent lights.

WHAT SOVIET RESEARCH SHOWS

The Soviet Union has shown great interest in preventive medicine, especially in the area of pediatrics. In one study, M. A. Zamkov and E. I. Krivitskaya of the A. I. Hertsen Pediological Institute in Leningrad reported on the favorable effects of ultraviolet radiation on children. In an experiment lasting from October 1963 through March 1964, two groups of children were housed in their school under similar conditions; the difference was that one group worked under weak overhead ultraviolet radiation and the other group under standard fluorescent lights. The students who had received ultraviolet radiation showed a shorter reaction time to light and sound, which means that their nervous systems were working more efficiently than did those of the children who had not received ultraviolet stimulation. They exhibited less eye strain, and a generally increased working capacity, resulting in significant improvement in their academic standing as compared to the group exposed to standard fluorescent light.

On the basis of these results, the authors advocated ultraviolet radiation for all schoolchildren—a conclusion that certainly sounds reasonable to me, except that I would extend it to the entire population.

There have also been a number of reports from the Soviet Union concerning the beneficial effects of ultraviolet light on arteriosclerosis and arthritis. *Ultraviolet's effect of reducing cholesterol levels has been known for some time.* In this way it offers protection for people prone to high blood pressure, coronary disease, and hardening of the arteries of the brain—often the cause of emotional disorders associated with senility.

In another Soviet study, N. M. Dantsig and his associates established that profound physiological changes occur in human beings deprived of full-spectrum light for long periods.

The same authors also found ultraviolet radiation to be of marked benefit to agricultural animals, with the ideal doses of radiation varying according to the species and the age of the animals. The action of ultraviolet radiation stimulates enzyme reactions and metabolism, increases the activity of the entire endocrine system, and, very significantly, increases immunological responses.

This last benefit is probably largely responsible for the overall improved health of creatures exposed to ultraviolet radiation. They are less likely to fall victim to disease, and are *less prone to suffer from allergies.* Of course, the heightened immunological response is not the whole answer; the endocrine system also affects both susceptibility to infection and to allergic conditions.

SOME INTERESTING FACTS

Some apparently quite unrelated facts converge to add further weight to the mounting evidence concerning the importance of light stimulation. To wit:

- Eskimo women during the long Arctic night do not menstruate and are infertile
- Children in tropical zones mature earlier sexually than do those in more northern latitudes
- Apples grown under glass which cuts out ultraviolet radiation never ripen
- Chinchillas raised under blue colored light produce eighty-five percent female offspring
- Under artificial light, many tropical fish die; others produce offspring with a twenty percent rate of birth defects
- Mice kept under pink light stimulation for up to twelve hours a day develop sores on their tails, and eventually lose them altogether

I once mentioned this last bit of information during an address before the Society of Clinical Ecology in Albuquerque, New Mexico. At the time of my lecture, the participants at the meeting had been indoors for approximately three days, receiving only the usual inadequate light stimulation. I suggested that the assembled physicians might want to check their posterior anatomy upon returning to their rooms. The next day I found an impressive array of my colleagues sunbathing during the lunch recess. I've always wondered what the rear view look into their mirrors had revealed.

Recently, I happened across another provocative item. Employees of the Well of the Sea, a well-known Chicago restaurant located in the Sherman Hotel, were found to have significantly lower rates of illness and absenteeism than people working in other parts of the hotel. I remember eating at the Well of the Sea several times. It is a very dark place, equipped with ultraviolet lights which are, in effect, "black lights." These are used to activate fluorescent decorations, and, quite incidentally, also irradiate the people working in the restaurant.

LIGHT IN MY OWN LIFE

Until a few years ago I knew absolutely nothing about the importance of full-spectrum light stimulation, but since I've learned about it, I have put it to good use. This newly acquired knowledge has certainly not made it possible for me to heal all the emotionally ill persons who consult me. But I firmly believe that by adding full-spectrum light stimulation to the other therapies I employ for emotionally disturbed people I have been of service to a larger percentage of my patients, and that this therapy has helped many of them to achieve a higher level of improvement.

Since I practice what I preach, I have installed Vita-Lites in my office and my home, starting out gingerly with only one or two such lights in the rooms where I spend most of my time. Soon I became quite fond of this type of illumination, and began to find other types of light stimulation annoying. I ended by installing Vita-Lites everywhere. I simply no longer wished to be exposed to ordinary lights.

On my daily walks I now make a point of staying on the sunny side of the street (even though you'll recall that it's not necessary to be in the sun to receive full-spectrum stimulation. Being in the shade is satisfactory too—as long as the light is of the outdoor variety). In addition to living, working, and walking under full-spectrum light, I also regularly employ an ultraviolet sunlamp over my entire body. I use the sunlamp bulb put out by General Electric, and have four of these rigged in an overhead position, so that full body exposure is practical.

I have even had my reading glasses changed to a plastic material that transmits the full light spectrum, including ultraviolet light. Apparently the reflection of light that we receive from the written page is a major source of stimulation to the retina of the eye. Since full-spectrum light stimulation is so important, it is mandatory to wear reading glasses made of this material.

If you wear glasses at all times you should be especially interested in obtaining these full-spectrum lenses. They are also available in dark shades, which reduce the total amount of light stimulation but do not distort the spectrum. The net effect is that you still receive full-spectrum light stimulation, even though the light passes through a dark lens. Nowadays, I wince when I walk down the street and see people wearing ordinary dark glasses, knowing to what an extent they are distorting the amount of light stimulation they receive, thereby almost certainly impairing their health.

My office has been equipped with ultraviolet transmitting plastic windows (quarter-inch) in order that I may get the full-spectrum light blocked out by ordinary window glass. An added benefit is the great reduction of noise entering the office from outside.

Has all this light consciousness improved my life?

This is difficult to answer unequivocally, but I have the definite impression of a heightened sense of well-being, and an increased ability to work effectively for more hours of the day since I have been using full-spectrum lights and reading glasses. Certainly I spend less of the winter daydreaming about a vacation in the Caribbean!

Let me assure you yet another time that I have no financial interests in any of the companies mentioned in this (or any other) chapter. I have records to prove that I paid the full price for all the products which I use and advocate. Whenever I suggest a specific item, it is because I believe that you get more for your money by buying it than by buying any of the competing products.

Vita-Lite is manufactured by the Duro-Test Company of North Bergen, New Jersey. Your electrician can order fluorescent Vita-Lite tubes from them at a price very little higher than that of ordinary fluorescent tubes. These lights should be mounted without any covering whatever, since all coverings necessarily reduce the ultraviolet irradiation. I hope you'll agree that it's more important that your quarters be healthy than decorative.

Your optometrist or ophthalmologist can order the full-spectrum lenses from the Armolite Lens Company, P.O. Box 1038, Burbank, California 91505. Full-spectrum contact lenses may be ordered from the Obrig Laboratories, 1960 Woodfield Ave. East, Bradenton, Florida.

Whether or not you have emotional problems (and who doesn't?), I strongly suggest that you consider looking into the benefits of full-spectrum light stimulation, and ultraviolet light generally, despite warnings to the contrary with which you may have been saturated in the past.

You have surely heard that too much ultraviolet light can cause premature aging of the skin and also skin cancer. True, especially in fair-skinned individuals. You should consult the manufacturer's recommendation for the particular equipment you own, as well as your family physician or dermatologist, to get specific advice for your particular type of skin.

I personally have no concern about taking an ultraviolet treatment once or twice a week. If my skin were unusually dry or very fair, I would certainly consider reducing the frequency. If I had keratoses (dry, precancerous lesions on the skin, which should be removed) or leuko-plakia (precancerous lesions on the lip or other mucous membrane, which should also be removed), I would avoid the use of a sunlamp altogether. Also, its use is contraindicated for persons suffering from porphyria, a rare biochemical disorder characterized by abdominal pain and mental symptoms (and often misdiagnosed by psychiatrists). Some patients who are on medications (the major tranquilizer Thorazine is a common offender) become photosensitive and should avoid ultraviolet treatments altogether.

Almost all the people who have suffered from ultraviolet exposure, let me strongly add, have not been those occasionally basking under sunlamps and tanning themselves at the beach. The people who have suffered skin damages have typically been lifeguards who have made a thirty-year profession of sitting in the sun, Texas farmers who spend their days on a tractor, or seamen working constantly in the open air.

HOW MEGAVITAMINS
FIGHT SCHIZOPHRENIA

CHAPTER EIGHTEEN

The use of vitamins for treating emotional illness goes back over two thousand years. One of the factors in the success of the Romans was their knowledge that scurvy (caused by lack of vitamin C) was often a deadlier foe than the opponents' spears and swords. The Roman army was therefore always supplied with fresh fruits and vegetables. This means of preventing scurvy was forgotten during the Middle Ages, but was rediscovered by James Lind in 1753, and in 1795, lime juice was incorporated into the regular diet of British navy men.

Prior to Lind's rediscovery, the sea captains' manuals, which advised captains on the practical aspects of maintaining a properly run ship, looked upon scurvy as a disease brought on partly by boredom. They advised that seamen have access to amusing conversation, light music, and a cheerful atmosphere, to treat the depression that accompanied scurvy. Since the depression that accompanies scurvy may be of psychotic proportions, one might say that the use of lime juice was the first vitamin treatment for severe emotional illness.

Hans Huber discovered niacin (nicotinic acid) in 1867, but several

253

generations passed before we finally learned that niacin (vitamin B_3) could cure the psychosis of pellagra.

Joseph Goldberger, M.D., of the U.S. Public Health Service, spent much of the second decade of this century wandering through the southern United States, trying to find the cause of pellagra, and at last hit upon a clue in Mississippi. In a mental hospital there he observed that staff members ate a different diet from the patients, and that pellagra was common among the patients but not among the staff. He tested his hunch by placing patients on a restricted diet. They regularly came down with pellagra, which he was able to cure by feeding them foods rich in natural sources of the vitamin B complex.

Still, it was many years before the medical establishment could accept the fact that pellagra was a nutritional disorder, and not an infectious one as had been supposed. It was not until the 1930s that niacin was finally demonstrated to be the specific B vitamin that cured pellagra.

After the introduction of niacin for pellagra, psychiatrists admitted that they could not tell which patients had schizophrenia and which had pellagra, unless the pellagra patients happened to have secondary symptoms other than a mental disorder such as dermatitis and diarrhea. It soon become common practice to administer niacin to all psychotic patients. Those who got better were classified as having suffered from pellagra, and those who did not improve were classified as suffering from schizophrenia.

The situation changed somewhat in 1939 when H. M. Clerkley,[1] M.D., reported that administration of moderately large doses of niacin (0.3 to 1.5 gm. per day) often cleared up psychiatric symptoms in patients who had none of the physical signs associated with pellagra. This raised the question whether or not pellagra or vitamin B_3 deficiency might exist without the classical symptoms of pellagra and, indeed, whether niacin might not be useful in treating the classical symptoms of schizophrenia.

Apparently, A. Hoffer, Ph.D., M.D., and Humphrey Osmond, M.R.C.S., D.P.M.,[2] began their studies on the use of niacin for the treatment of schizophrenia unaware of Clerkley's work. Osmond reports that he and Dr. John Smythies had, early in 1951, begun discussing schizophrenia as a disorder due to the production of an abnormal and toxic form of adrenalin. It is known that solutions of adrenalin left open and exposed to sunlight deteriorate and turn a pinkish color. This form of adrenalin, when injected, causes marked perceptual changes similar to those experienced by the schizophrenic.

Hoffer and Osmond reasoned that, if the production of adrenalin had gone awry in persons suffering from schizophrenia, it might be possible to prevent and cure the disorder. Since niacin and niacinamide (both forms of vitamin B_3) are methyl groups acceptors, they felt that administration of this vitamin in large doses would reduce the body's production of adrenalin, and thus also cut down the abnormal form of adrenalin responsible for causing schizophrenic symptoms.

Early in 1952, Hoffer and Osmond began their clinical studies at Saskatchewan Hospital in Weyburn, Saskatchewan, by giving one patient what they considered a very large amount of niacinamide—500 mg. daily for three days. When the patient did not improve, they tried it on a forty-seven-year-old male patient with many delusions and marked perceptual difficulties, which made his surroundings seem strange and odd causing him great fear. He had previously been in another hospital where he had been noisy and had masturbated openly. At Saskatchewan he had become withdrawn and depressed. There were no overt signs of vitamin deficiency. Beginning on February 14, 1952, he was given one gram of niacinamide daily, plus small amounts of other vitamins. Within two days, he was greatly improved.

Another schizophrenic out-patient, a girl, was treated with niacin with good results. In May of the same year, a seventeen-year-old boy was admitted into the hospital with an acute schizophrenic illness that had only started a few days before admission. He had marked delusions, was excited, overactive, and acted silly. His response to electroconvulsive treatment was not satisfactory. Subsequent insulin therapy had to be stopped when a nerve paralysis appeared during treatment. The boy walked around naked, hallucinated actively, talked incomprehensibly, urinated and defecated in his bed, and generally appeared to be deteriorating by the hour.

He was started on one gram of niacin and one gram of ascorbic acid five times daily. Within twenty-four hours he was practically normal. A Rorschach inkblot test given about three weeks after the initiation of experimental vitamin treatment showed some anxiety but none of the perceptual defects one would expect in a schizophrenic. He maintained his improvement during follow-ups for the next three years.

In a double blind study done by Hoffer and Osmond, one group of patients was treated with standard therapy such as electroshock, sub-coma insulin treatment, barbiturates, tranquilizers, and psychotherapy or combinations of these. This control group which did not receive niacin comprised ninety-seven patients. Over the eight-year follow-up period, there were fifty-six readmissions in this group. The second group, comprising seventy-four patients, received standard psychiatric care plus niacin. There were only twenty-one readmissions among that group, even though these patients did not have proper follow-up administrations of niacin.

In the early days of megavitamin therapy, it was felt that if a patient maintained his feeling of good health for a year, the vitamins could be discontinued. Now, most orthomolecular psychiatrists agree that patients suffering from schizophrenia should be maintained on their vitamins for an indefinite period. Since this practice has been followed the rate of readmissions has been greatly reduced.

Since niacin was first used as the central therapy for schizophrenics, the spectrum of available vitamins and mineral supplements, and the knowledge of nutrition generally, has been greatly expanded. Each addition to niacin therapy has, in my experience and that of others, resulted in a further advance of the improvement rate.

Hoffer's early work stressed that his therapy was primarily beneficial to those who had been suffering from schizophrenia for one year or less. As time has passed, megavitamins have been used more and more on patients who have been sick longer than a year. We often find megavitamins effective for this group of patients but usually therapy must be continued for a long time before results become apparent: one to four years or even more. This is not surprising because profound biological processes must be reversed.

Perhaps the best way to understand the evolution of megavitamin therapy is for me to tell you about my personal experience with it.

While I was still practicing internal medicine, I underwent a nine-hundred-hour psychoanalysis stretching over five years. Then I took a three-year residency in psychiatry and thus qualified as a psychiatrist. Naturally, I was strongly analytically oriented, so during my first few years of practice I stressed the psychoanalytical approach almost to the complete exclusion of any medication. Gradually, I began to realize that there were some patients whom I wasn't helping. Research into the effects of psychotherapy consistently reveals that two-thirds of all patients with emotional illnesses get better no matter what kind of treatment they undergo. Indeed this group also recovers without any treatment at all. The last third seems to be refractory to most forms of treatment.

It began to dawn on me that I was wasting my time and training on a lot of patients who would get better no matter what was done for them. There was, in fact, little point in their seeing me—they were going to get better with or without me. As a result of this insight I began to concentrate more on patients who were not improving, and who were not likely to get better unless some special skills were brought to bear on their problems. It was during this time that I became interested in the biological approach to mental illness. I began using major tranquilizers, anti-depressants and other psychotropic medications, and was pleased with the results that I began to get with some of my chronically ill patients. Quite obviously, I was achieving something with the chemical approach that I had not been able to achieve with the purely psychological one.

In the following years I treated these seriously ill patients by a standard biologically oriented psychiatric approach. I went to great lengths to help these people, changing their medicines back and forth, using combinations of medications, and generally working quite hard to meet the challenge they presented. My practice was in a location with a highly stable population, and I therefore had good follow-up on my patients and knew them well.

At about that time, the parents of one of my patients, a boy suffering from paranoid schizophrenia, requested that he receive megavitamin therapy. As I mentioned in the introduction, I had vaguely heard about the use of niacin in schizophrenia, but knew no details regarding dosage, general management of megavitamin therapy, and possible complications. Nor did I know offhand where I could readily obtain such information. So I pulled the act that nearly all physicians use under such circumstances. I told the parents that megavitamin therapy was still in the experimental stage, with no proof of effectiveness yet available, and that I therefore advised against it.

(I'm telling this story again to help you to call this bluff if you encounter it.)

No physician can possibly know everything about every possible disease. Yet he is forced to maintain his authority-figure image, in order to stay in control of the therapeutic relationship. Inevitably, he learns to trot out certain plausible-sounding phrases whenever he is challenged on something about which he is ignorant. You are still likely to get some variant of this answer when you approach your psychiatrist or family physician for help on nutritional problems or megavitamin therapy.

Megavitamin therapy is compatible with any other treatment for schizophrenia, including tranquilizers, anti-depressants, hormones, and electroconvulsive therapy, as well as psychotherapy of whatever persuasion.

A few patients out of a hundred will experience an exacerbation of schizophrenic symptoms when they begin megavitamin therapy; this usually shows itself in restlessness and perhaps an increase of paranoid notions. This period of increased stimulation usually ends spontaneously by the end of the first month of megavitamin treatment. In most cases the symptoms can be minimized by administration of a minor tranquilizer such as Valium or Librium, but some patients must have their dose of megavitamins reduced and built up gradually. For others, the vitamins may have a sedative effect producing a sense of long-forgotten peace and tranquility.

The next point cannot be emphasized too strongly: A great number of schizophrenics respond faster, more satisfactorily, and reach a higher plane of remission if they receive their megavitamin doses by injection, rather than orally.

Recently I saw a twenty-eight-year-old woman whom I have been treating for over a year. She has multiple food allergies but basically she is schizophrenic. When she first came to me she could not express emotion, was withdrawn, felt that life had nothing to offer her, and was unable to maintain any interpersonal relationships. Men would take her out once or twice, then drop her quickly, or else she would become involved with a man who treated her miserably—and yet she would hang on to him month after month, year after year, because she sought punishment. She felt so full of guilt that she was happier when she was being punished by an unsatisfactory relationship.

This young woman took large doses of the full spectrum of megavitamins and mineral supplements by mouth, and soon improved to the point of functioning somewhat more effectively. But she was still very unhappy, and was unable to form relationships with other people.

Finally I put her on injections of multiple vitamins every other day. Her response became evident within ten days: for the first time, her face was full of life, her eyes had lost their dead, glazed look, and I could feel her reach out to me as another human being instead of giving me the feeling that I confronted a wooden dummy across my desk. She also reported that she had met a new man, that they had had a very satisfactory date, and that she had very real hopes for the future. I have seen such rapid, dramatic changes in many patients.

Another example: One evening I had a desperate phone call from a thirty-four-year-old woman stating that she had been diagnosed as schizophrenic and felt, as a result of her reading on the subject, that megavitamin therapy was the answer to her problem. Her history is so typical of the many misdiagnosed and mistreated schizophrenic patients that it would be useful to tell something of her life.

From childhood on, she had been negativistic, withdrawn, shy, and too quick to show her temper. She was argumentative with her family, especially when attempts were made to control her behavior in some way. In spite of these flaws, she did well in school and got along satisfactorily with authority figures outside her home.

When she reached her teens, she became rather theatrical, and got attention from her peers by her daring behavior. For example, she lost her virginity to a boy she did not really like, much less love, and then told all the girls about the details at school next day, bragging that she was the first in her class to accomplish what she considered to be a feat. There followed scores of sexual encounters with dozens of men, all unsatisfactory. She was unable to achieve orgasm and could not form a close, warm relationship with anyone.

At last she fell in love—this time with a boy who was on the brink of a psychotic break. She ran away from home, and hitchhiked with him all over the world. Later, when he was confined to a mental hospital, she visited him and acted somewhat the martyr. It seemed as though once he was truly psychotic she could afford to love him, because he was entirely unable to return the love and so she had no problem of forming a close interpersonal relationship.

By this time she was deep into the campus drug scene as well, at a time when this was still rather daring. Her family, disgusted with her behavior, withdrew their support, and she struggled her way through a city university.

After graduating she worked for a while on a Master's degree, but was unable to continue intellectual pursuits because of the gradual development of her psychosis. It was difficult for her to concentrate. The men in her life became more numerous and stayed shorter periods of time. She got a job as a waitress and struggled on in this job as long as her strength would allow. Gradually she began to grow weaker, losing not only her intellectual functions but also her physical stamina. When the strenuous work of a waitress became too much for her she took a part-time job and found shelter in a friend's apartment, struggling fiercely to keep herself out of the hospital.

Then she came across Abram Hoffer and Humphrey Osmond's book, *How to Live with Schizophrenia*,[3] and saw her own symptoms reflected on its pages. She had the marked depression and marked perceptual defects that go with schizophrenia, as well as the self-condemnation, the flat affect (feelings), the inability to form interpersonal relationships, and the propensity for misinterpretation of other people's motives, thinking that everyone was hostile and against her.

Her most prominent symptoms were her perceptual defects. When she looked at a photograph, for example, the images seemed to project out toward her and shimmer, making them extremely threatening and frightening. Gradually, the whole world was becoming her torture chamber so that she was fearful of going out on the streets. Not only did the people look strange, but the street itself and everything around her appeared to be destroying her.

The history of her psychiatric treatment is interesting because it demonstrates how often schizophrenia is missed and inappropriate therapy prescribed unless patients are actively hallucinating. For many years she had been under the care of one psychiatrist after another, including a period at a prominent university clinic. Her last therapist, an orthodox Freudian, had had her lie on the couch and just talk.

All the psychiatrists had missed the diagnosis of schizophrenia. She had even specifically asked them whether she was schizophrenic and had been told that she was not. The misdiagnosis is confirmed by the treatment she received, because it is decidedly contraindicated to have a schizophrenic patient lie on a couch and free-associate. These patients bring up material that they are unable to resolve, and fling themselves further and further out into left field. If any psychotherapy at all is indicated for them, most psychiatrists agree that reality-oriented, face-to-face therapy is best. Such patients need to talk about their here-and-now problems in concrete ways, to a therapist who is supportive, often directive, and who sets limits for them. (In my opinion this applies to nearly all patients in psychotherapy—not just to schizophrenics.) Certainly she should have had one of the major tranquilizers and anti-depressants to offset her marked depression and to reduce her developing psychosis.

When she first came to me she was in such a bad state that I did not do my usual biochemical work-up but began treatment right away, because I felt she was too close to requiring hospitalization to tolerate any delays. I assumed that she had hypoglycemia, because ninety percent of schizophrenics suffer from it. She was therefore put on a sugar-free diet with reduced carbohydrates and emphasis on meats, fats, and multiple feedings. She was given an intravenous injection of adrenal cortical extract and 1000 mcg. of vitamin B_{12b} intramuscularly. At the same time, she was put on 1000 mg. of niacin, 1000 mg. of ascorbic acid, and 100 mg. of pyridoxin three times daily. On this regimen, she experienced almost immediate relief from the most pressing of her symptoms.

Make no mistake: this woman was not magically cured after this one visit. It would be a great disservice to give the public the impression that we can deliver more than we can in reality. We are physicians, not magicians, and reversing profound biochemical changes takes hard work for a long period of time. When I say that this patient improved greatly almost immediately, I mean that there was no longer a question of her requiring hospitalization. Her symptoms were reduced in severity by perhaps twenty percent, and this is a significant percentage when it occurs at the point of desperation, where the patient is almost ready to give up the fight for sanity.

During the next six months, the struggle to keep this woman afloat continued. Her dosage of vitamins was gradually increased. In order to discover a particular patient's tolerance level, many of us who use niacin increase the dosage to the point where the patient is nauseated, and then cut back somewhat. It is very important in treating these patients to bear in mind that many are nauseated by ordinary niacin tablets because of the binders they contain. Many more can take a starch-free, sugar-free niacin tablet without being nauseated. This particular patient was put on pure niacin powder, because she could take more of this without becoming nauseated.

During the next six months she improved only slowly. Fortunately, I became interested in food allergies around that time and began checking her. She was particularly allergic to sugar, corn, wheat, and milk products—a typical pattern among schizophrenics. Once these conditions were eliminated, she began to feel markedly better. She had a return of energy that she had not felt for several years, and much of her depression lifted. Her perceptual defects almost disappeared; when she looked at photographs they no longer appeared to be jumping out at her. She also lost much of the fear that she had experienced when walking on the street with other people. She began working full time and related much better to other people.

Then followed a period of about six months during which many variations in her vitamin levels were tried.

At the end of that period, she was taking the following vitamin supplements:

Natural vitamin A	10,000 units daily
Natural vitamin D	400 units daily
Glutamine	Five 200 mg. capsules three times daily
Ascorbic acid (vitamin C) powder	3 gms. four times daily (this is the same as 3000 mg. four times daily, for a total of 12,000 mg. daily)
Thiamin (vitamin B_1)	Three 500 mg. tablets three times daily
Riboflavin (60 mg. tablet)	2 tablets three times daily
Niacin powder	3 gms. four times daily
Pyridoxine (vitamin B_6)	100 mg. four times daily
Calcium pantothenate (218 mg. capsules)	2 capsules at bedtime
Dolomite powder	1 teaspoon dissolved in a glass of water at bedtime
Choline capsules (650 mg.)	1 capsule three times daily

Inositol tablets (650 mg.)	1 daily
Biotine tablets (50 mg.)	1 daily
Folic acid tablets (1 mg.)	1 tablet three times daily
Crude liver capsules	2 capsules three times daily
Acidophilus capsules with pectin	2 capsules three times daily
Sea salt used freely on food	

In addition, she still receives the following injections:

Hydroxocobalamin (vitamin B_{12b})	1000 micrograms intramuscularly daily
Berocca-C	2 cc. intramuscularly every other day

This is a mixture of vitamins; 2 cc. contains 10 mg. of thiamin, 10 mg. of riboflavin, 80 mg. of niacinamide, 20 mg. of pyridoxine, 23 mg. of calcium pantothenate, 0.2 mg. biotine, and 100 mg. of ascorbic acid.

Also, once a week she receives an injection containing 100 mg. thiamine, 150 mg. riboflavin, 200 mg. niacinamide, 50 mg. of pyridoxine, and 125 mg. of ascorbic acid.

It may seem extraordinary to give such doses of injected vitamins along with the massive doses she was taking by mouth. But the proof is in the practice: There has been a definite and sustained improvement in her condition since she has been taught to administer her additional vitamins intramuscularly. Attempts have been made to reduce these intramuscular vitamins, but with each attempt she loses her feeling of well-being and experiences a return of her symptoms.

The above regimen advanced her to a third plateau much higher than any of the others she had reached during her one and a quarter year of treatment with me. She then was put on the anti-depressant Tofranil (50 mg. three times daily). We had tried many different anti-psychotic medications with her but the results were not good. Finally we found that 50 mg. of Thorazine at bedtime caused another improvement in her condition. With these additions of the Tofranil and Thorazine, the patient reached a fourth plateau—the highest yet—and began to regain her ability to concentrate. She could now read books; previously she had been entirely unable to engage in any intellectual pursuits.

After several months a thyroid compound, cytomel, 25 micrograms daily, was added to her regimen. Within three days, she improved again and reached a fifth plateau. Now she is completely independent, and is leading a worthwhile life as a high school teacher, free of most of her former symptoms. An up-to-date psychological test shows that she is still basically schizophrenic, but that most of the disease's manifestations are in remission.

Her hard-core schizophrenic personality will probably keep her isolated from other people to a significant emotional degree all of her life, but she has improved to the point where she can lead a reasonably satisfactory, self-sufficient life. The transformation has been marked, though she must continue her strenuous diet, vitamin program, and medication indefinitely to prevent a relapse.

THREE STUDIES IN MEGAVITAMIN THERAPY

As with every form of therapy, disputes exist about the efficacy of megavitamin therapy. Greenbaum[4] reported that he was unable to find evidence that niacinamide was helpful in a double blind study involving seventeen children who received niacinamide at a rate of 1000 mg. per 50 mg. of body weight, and twenty-four children who received a placebo. Improvement of observed behavior was used as the criterion for efficacy. He reported no significant difference in the two groups that could be attributed to niacinamide.

The mathematics of his report do not bear out his conclusion. The facts are that the improvement score for those on niacinamide was 4.0 units and for the placebo group only 2.6 units. This researcher considers the difference between 4.0 and 2.6 statistically not significant, yet he found fifty-four percent greater improvement in the niacinamide group than in the placebo group. If he wishes to support his conclusions, he must therefore perform the research project again, with a much larger number of children.

In another study, Ananeth[5] performed an experiment in which methionine was given in large daily doses to exacerbate the symptoms of schizophrenia. You will recall that one of the theories of the action of niacin and niacinamide is that it is a methyl acceptor; by accepting the methyl groups of toxic molecules it detoxifies them so they are unable to work adversely on the nervous system. These schizophrenic patients were given methionine and niacinamide at the same time in order to study whether or not the niacinamide was in fact able to accept the methyl groups from the methionine and protect the patient from increased mental symptoms.

The niacinamide did not protect the schizophrenic patients from an increase of symptoms upon administration of methionine, but there was a serious defect in the design of the experiment. Patients were given 20 gm. of methionine daily, but only 3 gm. of niacinamide. To accept the methyl groups donated by such a large dose of methionine would require at least 16 gm. of niacinamide daily. The 3 gm. administered were clearly inadequate to protect the patient. Here again, the conclusions were entirely false.

In a recent experimental study at Rutgers University, Richard J. Wittenborn, M.D.,[6] found niacin was not useful for the treatment of schizophrenia. He used one control group receiving small amounts of niacin, and one experimental group receiving 3000 mg. of niacin daily. But a very large percentage of patients dropped out of the experimental group, so I do not feel that this study represents a valid test of niacin. One can assume that the patients who dropped out were either much improved or much sicker. Since no one knows what happened to them, it is not possible to draw a conclusion about the entire group tested.

The experiment suffered from other flaws. A large number of the patients on niacin developed a darkening of the skin. This is a very rare complication, which I and other orthomolecular psychiatrists have seen only a few times in the course of treating many hundreds of patients with niacin and megavitamins. I do not know why Wittenborn, *et al.*, had such a high percentage of skin complications, but it suggests that something was wrong with their vitamin preparation. The second major flaw is that the patients were restricted to taking niacin alone. Today, I think there is no orthomolecular psychiatrist who does not employ multiple megavitamins. At the very least, patients are almost all uniformly treated with large doses of ascorbic acid and pyridoxine as well as niacin, besides being placed on a low-carbohydrate, sugar-free diet, since about ninety percent of schizophrenics have defects in their carbohydrate metabolism.

In the experiment at Rutgers University a niacin preparation was used that was not starch-free and not sugar-free. Such tablets are usually poorly tolerated by patients. This may account for some of the skin changes. Also, it is my own observation that niacin given alone may bring about a deficiency in another vitamin in some people. I have seen it produce cracks in the corners of the mouth which are typical of certain B vitamin deficiencies. As soon as I add pyridoxine (vitamin B$_6$) and riboflavin (vitamin B$_2$) the cracks cleared up.

The greatest mistake made in the research project headed by Wittenborn was to throw schizophrenics who had recently become ill into the same category as those who had been ill much longer. If you look at his clinical results in terms of how long the patient had been ill, you do find that those on niacin showed a significant improvement rate over those who did not receive it. Hoffer and his colleagues always indicated that their treatment was much more effective for patients who had only recently become ill.

Also the Rutgers project made the very grave mistake of giving the same dose of niacin to each patient. They should have increased the dose for each patient until the point of nausea and then dropped back down a gram or two a day for maintenance.

I need hardly tell you how foolish I think it is to give only one of the B vitamins in any therapeutic endeavor. In my experience, that is ineffective medical practice.

I personally have had considerable experience in the field of psychiatry. I have used psychotherapy, I have used traditional chemical therapy and I have combined both with megavitamin therapy. I simply find my results far and away more satisfactory by adding megavitamin therapy. It is not surprising therefore that I advocate it and employ it. Any physician wishing to evaluate it properly should work with a pyschiatrist experienced in this sub-specialty.

I have long felt that research methods to test the effect of megavitamins has been incorrect. Attempts have been made to select two groups of patients, so-called matched pairs. Then one group is given the vitamin (unfortunately the single vitamin niacin) and the vitamin is withheld from the other group. The progress of both groups is then observed.

Such a research plan is shot through with many faults, most prominent among them that schizophrenia is only a symptom, not a disease. Perhaps we will eventually find as many as fifty different biological defects producing the symptom complex we call schizophrenia.

If you think you can talk with people and then place them in matched pairs, try grafting the skin from one matched pair to the other and you will soon learn that the grafts will not "take" for the elementary reason that the chemistry of the so-called matched pairs is very dissimilar.

For a long time I have been advocating a research design in which patients suffering from schizophrenia would be placed on megavitamins and whatever other medication they might require. Exhaustive psychological tests should be performed before the start of megavitamin therapy, and at regular intervals thereafter. Patients who register improvement should then have the vitamins withdrawn. The psychological tests should then be repeated. I feel that this would be the clearest way of demonstrating the efficacy of megavitamins. Many times, I have seen well-controlled schizophrenics go into the hospital for an appendectomy or some other procedure and be taken off their megavitamins. These people often become psychotic in a few days and can be brought under control again only by restoring their vitamins once more.

Being in private practice, I am only able to earn a living because I produce positive results. A university professor has an assured supply of patients coming his way because of his position in the university. He may or may not be a good clinician; he may or may not get good results with his patients. It really does not make any difference, because of the prestige of his position. I don't mean to imply that professors in universities are necessarily inadequate clinicians, but the pressure on them to get results is certainly much less than that of someone in private practice.

WHY GOOD DIET IS VITAL FOR SCHIZOPHRENICS

Schizophrenics should be placed on a natural diet of fruits, nuts, roots, and meats, which our ancestors ate for millions of years and for which our enzyme systems have evolved through a long evolutionary process. I look upon persons suffering from schizophrenia as suffering from enzyme defects. Many people in our population can handle enzyme strains produced by the relatively new foods, such as wheat and sugar, to which we expose ourselves. But many others cannot, and schizophrenia may be one of the consequences.

What about the theory that patients suffering from schizophrenia often have increased needs for vitamin and mineral supplements? We have known for some time that certain people do not have vitamin deficiencies but, rather, what some scientists call vitamin-dependency disorders; their enzyme systems require much larger amounts of vitamins than do those of the average person.

Leon E. Rosenberg, M.D.,[7] of Yale University has done a great deal of work on vitamin dependent people. In a talk sponsored by the Jackson Laboratories, Johns Hopkins University, and the National Foundation of the March of Dimes, he discussed people with vitamin dependency disorders. Among these were several hundred children who were subject to convulsions unless given pyridoxine (vitamin B_6) in very large amounts. No other substance was found that could control this convulsive disorder. When the children were given pyridoxine the convulsions ceased; when pyridoxine was taken away the convulsions returned. There could be no question about the relationship between the eradication of the symptom of convulsion and the administration of the vitamin pyridoxine.

In my opinion, many persons suffering from schizophrenia do have one or more vitamin dependency disorders. I have several patients, for example, who require injections of hydroxocobalamin (vitamin B_{12b}) in amounts of 2000 micrograms daily in order to feel well.

MAY VITAMIN DEPENDENCY BE INHERITED OR ACQUIRED?

Prisoners of war who were held for long periods in Japanese internment camps suffered from severe vitamin deficiencies for many months. Following their return home, they were given vitamins in normal amounts, but they did not respond to them. They required extremely large doses in order to function properly because, apparently, some permanent change had taken place in their enzyme systems. Abram Hoffer, Ph.D., M.D., has told me in personal communications that when the massive amounts of vitamins were reduced in these patients, the symptoms of vitamin deficiency returned. It has been necessary to maintain the ex-prisoners on very large doses of multiple vitamins for indefinite periods of time.

All life, whether simple bacterium or man, shares certain common biochemical processes. Enzyme systems must break down foods for all living creatures, and enzyme systems must burn this food and manage to take away the waste products of metabolism. Since brain cells *are* cells, and part of the living organism, a malfunction of enzymes is reflected in the working of the mind. We sometimes forget that complex mammals such as man are a collection of cells interacting with each other. A single malfunction can set off a chain of others, in a domino effect. In the last analysis, all of life hinges on the chemistry of each single cell.

Not only may the genetic enzyme machinery of schizophrenics require greater vitamin and mineral concentrations to function properly, but there may also be a tissue deficiency of any of these substances. Let me remind you again that if a patient lacks the particular protein molecule needed to carry the B_{12} vitamin from the blood into the tissue, he may require many times more vitamin B_{12} than the person with normal amounts of this special carrier-protein. Or persons suffering from schizophrenia may have abnormal blood/brain barriers that prevent nutrients from passing into the brain. It is quite possible that the brain cells are more sensitive to deficiencies in nutrients than other cells in the body. We already know they are very sensitive to changes in the concentration of blood sugar. These postulated local vitamin deficiencies in the brain have been called "localized cerebral deficiency diseases" by Linus Pauling.

In sum, a person suffering from schizophrenia is probably vitamin dependent in many cases and requires much larger doses of vitamins than the average person.

Not all schizophrenics improve on megavitamin therapy. But there is no question at all in my mind that a great many do improve on it.

More and more people accept this view as time goes on.

If you had asked the people at the National Institute of Health about megavitamin therapy ten years ago, they would have said that it was nonsense. If you had asked them a year or two ago, they would have said that some people suffering from schizophrenia might benefit from megavitamin therapy.

While giving a talk in London in September 1971, I had an

opportunity to converse with Loren Mosher, M.D., at that time in charge
of research for the National Institute of Health. He told me then that in
his opinion about five percent of schizophrenics could benefit from
megavitamin therapy, which was an enormous concession on the part of
the establishment. In my opinion, the percentage is much much larger. I
hesitate to name a figure, but I'd guess that, given an ideal complete
orthomolecular regimen (including a sugar-free, wheat-free, low-
carbohydrate, high-meat, high-fat diet, and injectable vitamins and
supplementary minerals with certain crude sources of vitamins such as
crude liver extract) between fifty and seventy-five percent of schizophrenic patients can benefit. As we learn more about the subject, this
percentage is likely to go even higher. But even now, we do not have such
a wealth of effective therapies against psychosis that we can afford to
ignore the orthomolecular approach.

NOTES

1. H. M. Clerkley et al., "Nictinic Acid in Treatment of Atypical Psychotic
States Associated with Malnutrition," Jrnl. of the Amer. Med. Assn., Vol. 112,
May 22, 1939, pp. 2107–2110.
2. Abram Hoffer, Niacin Therapy in Psychiatry (Springfield, Ill.: Charles C.
Thomas & Co., 1962).
3. Abram Hoffer and Humphrey Osmond, How to Live with Schizophrenia (New
Hyde Park, N.Y.: University Books, Inc., 1966).
4. G. H. Greenbaum, "An Evaluation of Niacinamide in the Treatment of
Childhood Schizophrenia," Amer. Jrnl. of Psychiatry, Vol. 127, July 1970, pp.
89–92.
5. J. Ananeth et al., Canadian Psychiatric Assn. Journal, Vol. 15, 170, p. 15.
6. Richard J. Wittenborn et al., "Niacin in the Long-term Treatment of
Schizophrenia," Archives of General Psychiatry, Vol. 28, March 1973, pp.
308–315.
7. Leon E. Rosenberg, "Inherited Defects of B_{12} Metabolism," Science News of
the Week, Vol. 98, August 22, 1970, pp. 157–158.

GOOD SEX
FROM GOOD NUTRITION

CHAPTER NINETEEN

At the turn of the century, Sigmund Freud determined that good sexual adjustment is important for mental health. In fact, he went further, and hypothesized that emotional illnesses were essentially sexual in origin. This idea seized and held the imagination of the psychiatric profession for nearly half a century. In retrospect it seems hardly surprising that Freud should attach such importance to sex. He was a virgin until thirty and became impotent in his early forties, which must have greatly contributed to his intellectual preoccupation with sex.

I often find that seriously disturbed patients report that their sex lives are unsatisfactory. But it is a great mistake, in my opinion, to attribute their emotional illnesses to poor sexual adjustment; they usually have unsatisfactory sex lives *because* they are emotionally disturbed. When we correct the biological defects that are causing their emotional problems, by administering vitamins, minerals, and hormones and by treating their allergies, their emotional condition improves and their sex lives usually become satisfactory. You improve your sex life by improving your emotional health; not the other way around.

271

IS MORE SEX BETTER SEX?

Many people equate more sex with better sex. That is like saying that a five-pound steak is better than a one-pound steak, that a Pontiac is better than a Porsche, or that a king-size bed is better than a double bed. One of my patients is a prostitute who has intercourse several dozens of times each week; yet she is completely frigid and does not enjoy sex at all. Another of my patients, a vigorous seventy-eight-year-old man who owns an insurance company, jets to Chicago once a month to visit his girlfriend. When he returns to New York and tells me about each sexual encounter, his face dissolves into a saintly expression of glory as if he were speaking of a wonderful miracle. Sex may not come to him as frequently as in the old days, but it is beautiful and endearing when it does.

When we are happy and secure, we may not feel as much need for sex as when we are tense and frightened. It may be the same way with money. The insecure man may be forever trying to make another dollar to put with all his other dollars in the hope he will somehow find security through his wealth. He desperately runs from business deal to business deal and stores away his money, but no amount of savings will produce the inner peace he seeks.

This restless man may have a great need for sex and may indulge in it frequently (especially if it is free), but it may not give him satisfaction. Indeed, each encounter may leave him less satisfied than before. This man frequently uses sex in an attempt to relax himself. We all know that orgasms tend to be followed by a period of relaxation. He, or a woman like him, may use sex the last thing at night in an attempt to fall asleep. Sex may have nothing to do with love for a person, and may not even have anything to do with sex itself. Rather, it becomes a mechanism by which he tries to reduce tensions. Such a person does not derive great satisfaction and pleasure from the act.

So before you answer the question, "How good is my sex life?", be sure to ask yourself what you mean by good sex. Do you mean a wonderful experience that leaves you feeling fulfilled? Or are you talking about relieving a nervous itch? In the Freudian view, with which we are so familiar, anxieties, depressions, and emotional problems of all kinds are supposed to stem from unresolved sexual feelings. But the opposite is just as likely to be true. For many people, sex becomes the mechanism by which they try frantically to relieve feelings (restlessness, anxiety, depression, etc.) that are not sexual at all.

Poorly nourished people tend to have more sex—but not more fun.

To carry this observation to its logical conclusion, let me point out that populations explode in areas of the world where malnutrition and even starvation are chronic problems. Examine the birth statistics of the poorer South American countries and you will discover that their populations are rising at a staggering rate. Study the population figures for a country such as India, where semi-starvation stalks the whole nation, and you will discover the birth rate to be enormous when compared with that of such stable and relatively well-fed countries as Denmark and Sweden.

Why this seeming paradox?

Eventually, I suppose Mother Nature explains everything. Apparently the increased sex drive among the semi-starved and poorly nourished is an attempt on nature's part to preserve the species. Nature seems to realize when an individual weakens, and, so wherever premature death raises its head, sex flourishes. Nature seems to want an individual to reproduce before fading away and it therefore encourages a frenzy of sexual activities, never mind whether there will be enough food to feed the offspring. Some of them will probably live to carry on; certainly none will live if there is no sex, and hence no new life.

HOW THE PROSPECT OF DEATH STIMULATES SEX

Men as well as women are noted for their increased sexual drives in their forties. Again, we see nature pushing them for sexual activity and reproduction before sexual death overtakes them. By "sexual death" I refer to the inability of women to have children after the menopause and to the waning sexual desires of many (though by no means all) men in their fifties and, more especially, even later in life.

We all know that wartime stirs up sexual activities. Soldiers ready to go overseas or into battle experience a strong need for sexual relations and women tend to be particularly receptive to these men in uniform. Again, this is sex being prodded to the foreground by death—even by the prospect and contemplation of it.

One of the most interesting stories I heard from physicians who served overseas during World War II was told to me by a surgeon who was operating in a tent not far from the front lines. Returning casualties were divided into two groups. The first group consisted of soldiers with not very serious wounds. It was judged possible to save them. The second group were so seriously injured that it was unlikely that surgery would save their lives. The largest number of patients could be saved by first treating those who had a good possibility of living. The surgeon who told me this story was walking past the number two group, the men so badly injured that there was little hope of saving them. As the surgeon walked by, accompanied by his operating nurse, one of these nearly-dead men reached out, grabbed the nurse's leg, and ran his hand up toward a part of her anatomy that interested him very much.

"Let's take that soldier next," the surgeon said. If there was that much will to live, then he was certainly going to give the man every chance. In fact, what the surgeon saw was a dying man's natural reaction to sexual stimulation.

Those of us physicians who have spent years of apprenticeship as interns and residents in hospitals know that it is the rule for people to die with their hands clutching their genitalia, a last desperate expression of their sexual drive as they fade away.

Such activation of sex by the threat of extinction happens throughout the animal and even in the plant kingdom. For example, we know that when grass is poorly nourished it goes to seed, puts its last strength into the formation of seeds that can produce new life and hence preserve the species.

It is hardly necessary to say that if malnutrition goes beyond a certain point, sexual activity ceases. Sex increases only through the gray band that extends from good nutrition to true starvation. After true starvation begins, all sexual interest quickly wanes. By starvation I mean a total lack not only of calorie intake but a prolonged lack of adequate vitamins and minerals.

If frequency of sexual activity is your goal, and each one of us must decide for ourselves exactly what our goals are in life, then the remainder of this chapter should give you some new ideas for increasing the frequency of your sex.

The first obvious conclusion from these remarks is that, to have frequent sex, it is best to be malnourished. I don't advocate this road since being malnourished is not desirable for your general health. If you are malnourished you will be more susceptible to infections such as the common cold, pneumonia, and tuberculosis. It is quite possible that malnutrition will increase your chances of getting hardening of the arteries, heart disease, senility, and even cancer.

After the malnourished pass through their period of sexual frenzy, sexual desires rapidly fade away.

To be obsessed with sex is not a sign of good health, physical or mental. Quite the contrary. This is true for societies as well as individuals. Some people have decried the similarity between the decadence of ancient Rome and the peep shows and porno movies in Times Square, and in one way, they are correct. A society responds to the threat of disintegration, just as an individual does. Never have the American people been under more biochemical stress from inadequate diets, air and noise pollution, and toxic and allergenic substances in their food and water—and never have Americans been so overtly obsessed with sex.

YOUR PRESCRIPTION FOR THE GOOD LIFE

Many people who feel less than their best hope against hope that if they can find some magic to improve their sex lives the rest of their problems will melt away. You should know by now that this is not true. There is no magic cure for an ailing sex life, and if there were, it would not cure all your misery. To have a truly fulfilling sex life, it is necessary to be physically and mentally healthy. This is necessary for healthy sexual desire and satisfactory performance, and it is also necessary if you are to recognize a good sex life when you achieve it.

The most responsible advice I can give you is: Apply what you have already learned in this book about achieving your own best nutritional program. Once you have eliminated depression, fatigue, anxiety and other emotional symptoms caused by deficiencies, allergies and poor diet, your energy and zest for living will increase—and so will your sex life. Or you may find that your sex life was quite adequate in the first place if only you had been together enough to enjoy it!

HOW NUTRITION AFFECTS IMPOTENCE

There has been a lot of talk about vitamin E as a cure for impotence. It has come to be known as the sex vitamin, probably because it was found to prevent spontaneous abortions in many animals. While the claims are almost surely exaggerated, I think it important that anyone with an impotence problem pay attention to vitamin E; it often helps to increase energy levels, and this is a boon whether you are impotent or not. Vitamin E probably produces this effect because it helps to detoxify environmental pollutions that slow us down. It also supplies more oxygen to each cell, so that they burn their metabolic fuels more efficiently.

Fatigue and depression are the great enemies of sexual desire and performance. Therefore, the nutritional factors that most often counteract depression are the ones most likely to help a sexual problem. These are thiamin and niacin, which often give people a lift, and vitamin C, which is also a detoxifying agent and will help you to deal with pollutants and allergens. For a lift, you might also include a trial on glutamine (see the chapter on alcoholism for discussion of this nutrient).

HOW SEXUAL WISHES COME TRUE

I should point out that while none of these substances alone can cure impotence, your confidence in their value could have a very positive effect.

Let me tell you an anecdote about the effect of belief on sexual performance. I once had a patient, a college student who was quite religious but was able to reconcile sex with his girlfriend with his fundamentalist religion. At one time, her period was late and he was certain that she was pregnant. He was not able to marry her at that time because his father had told him that he would cut off the allowance if the boy married while in college.

The boy got down on his knees and prayed to God for the girl not to be pregnant. If God would only not let the girl be pregnant, the boy promised, he would never have intercourse again. He pointed out to God that he was aware that he had offended Him with his sexual behavior, but that he was now a new person and had seen the light. He requested that God reciprocate by allowing the girl to menstruate.

A week later, the girlfriend did get her period. As you might guess, the boy began to have second thoughts about his vow of chastity. Unhappily, the next time he visited his girlfriend and wanted to have intercourse he discovered that he was completely impotent and he remained so for over a year.

Sex is between the ears as well as between the legs.

WHAT ABOUT APHRODISIACS?

In ancient Egypt radishes were advocated as a sex-stimulating food. The Romans sang the praises of onions. The French believe that eating frog's legs makes them passionate. Catherine de Medici swore by artichokes. Others praise mushrooms, carrots, spinach, turnips, celery, and even asparagus. Caviar and oysters have their advocates, and a great authority on love, Casanova, and the ribald physician Rabelais both reported good results from truffles.

I cannot attribute aphrodisiacal qualities to any of these foods, but it might be a pleasant pastime for you to try them for yourself. Conceivably, your findings just possibly might agree with those of Casanova and Catherine de Medici. Hardly anything is impossible.

Perfumes would not seem to fall under the classification of foods—not when you first think about them. And yet, in a larger sense I suppose anything we take into our body is a food or nourishment. Since I have included light as a part of this book on nourishment, I see no reason why I cannot include perfumes just because they happen to be inhaled.

Perfumes are often used as sexual stimulants. I suspect scientific studies would show that they are effective. Perfumes could also probably act as an allergic agent, and if a perfume happened to depress someone, then certainly it would be counterproductive. But if a perfume-sensitive individual happened to feel slightly confused or excited by an odor, then it is quite possible that sexual appetites would be increased.

In any case, most people get the cue that a perfume means that the wearer is trying to appear sexually attractive. Effort and enthusiasm alone are certainly turn-ons. The ugly man who courts energetically often beats out the handsome man who pouts in the corner.

Let me re-emphasize: Whatever anyone believes will increase one's sexual appetites is likely to do so. If a girl loves a $50 perfume in which she has absolute faith, she will certainly be more bewitching and she herself will be turned on from her efforts and her faith in the new product. If a man swallows 1200 units of vitamin E before taking off his trousers and believes with all his heart and soul that the vitamin E is going to put vim where it counts, then it will almost surely do so, too.

HOW MEGA-NUTRIENTS
HELP YOUR HEALTH,
BEAUTY AND WEIGHT CONTROL

CHAPTER TWENTY

When I was a high school student and dating the girl who I was then certain was the great love of my life and would command my every attention forever, I brought her by my home one afternoon to meet my family. The next day, we were talking about her. After bragging about her, I turned to my grandmother and asked her if she didn't think Dorothy was the most beautiful girl she had ever seen.

My gnarled grandmother gave a highpitched laugh and said that all sixteen-year-old girls were beautiful.

At the time I thought my grandmother was being rather inconsiderate and not giving me due credit for having discovered such an extraordinary girl. Now that I am older I can appreciate her wisdom. She was saying that youth in itself is a kind of beauty, for youth represents good health, happiness, lack of cares and responsibilities, and a time in life when the pleasures of the body are at their height. Youth is not the only kind of beauty, but it is an important category of beauty and one to be seriously considered in this book that deals with nutrition and emotional problems; it is especially appropriate to talk about beauty

following the chapter dealing with sex and nutrition, for beauty has
forever been and will forever be tied in with sexual attraction.

Consider first the many kinds of beauty: the beauty of the body, the
beauty of the intellect, the qualities in a personality that can in some
people be called "a kind of beauty." Even a station in life may be
beautiful—witness the "beautiful people." They may be charming to
look at or behave in an interesting way, and their social position and
wealth enable them to lead the "beautiful life."

At its most basic, beauty is tied in with reproduction. A man is
inevitably drawn to a woman whom he considers beautiful for whatever
reason. Perhaps the woman has fine, delicate features and skin like
moonlight, so that the man is attracted to her, wants to be close to
her—closeness that he wants to increase until he is engulfed by her very
body in the act of closeness that in its ultimate state becomes sexual.

Not only does he want to be ultimately close to her; he wants her to
be a part of him so that their selves join together and form another being.
He wants her to mother their children and thereby pass on some of his
own flesh with her beauty into the future of the race; for, ultimately,
what we seek as "beauty" is nature's way of deciding who shall
reproduce and who shall not. In the dance of life, we are marionettes
moved hither and yonder by the unseen strings of our inherited genetic
programming and our biochemistry.

Consider a debutante ball at an elegant hotel. The girls wear lace
and chiffon designed by the leading couturiers of two continents. They
look over their escorts in black tails, white ties. Watch the girls come
forward one by one and then all join in their dance.

What, you might ask, could be a more civilized scene? In biological
fact, this is but another mating dance, very similar to mating dances of
Amazon natives covered with mud and bright feathers, and not too
different from the mating dances of bees. Each of these living beings is
engaging in a biological drama to assure the future of the species.

If youth in itself is a high form of sexual attraction, so is wealth
(there is a certain beauty about a woman of any age who wears mink and
diamonds) and so is power.

Hardly anyone would call Henry Kissinger either young or handsome, and yet women tell me they feel very much sexually attracted to
him. I am sure some of this attraction is tied up with the station he
reached in life. Almost anyone who is famous finds himself sexually

attractive. I know several movie queens, none youthful or beautiful, yet they always attract men.

If a person has charm, vivaciousness, and gives out vibes that strike a chord, then this person is beautiful regardless of his physical appearance, station in life, or age. I am certain Sammy Davis, Jr. was attractive to women long before he became famous. The sheer biological force of his personality would be attraction enough.

I have known some women who seemed to lack all qualities of beauty; yet when I sat down and talked with them I could feel their intellects working and I would find them fascinating simply because of the quickness and the range of their minds.

But all the forms of beauty I have mentioned depend on good health. To have a youthful appearance, a pleasing personality, success, and an intact intellect you must be in good health. Most of you who want to maintain your youth should read the chapter in this book on aging and follow the suggestions given there. If you follow the general directions throughout this book, you may even advance your station in life. If you feel better, you may earn more money. No one ever has given, or ever will give you a better recipe for success. If you follow my directions on nutrition, it is quite possible that your intellect will improve. Almost certainly, your personality will improve because you will lose much of your free-floating anger and begin to realize yourself as a person and stop short-circuiting your natural attributes.

A NEW ANSWER TO WEIGHT PROBLEMS

Beautiful people can come in any size: tall, short, fat, thin. But unless you are an unusually appealing person like Twiggy or Winston Churchill, you are likely to be more beautiful with a good figure, neither too fat nor too thin.

Slender people have another advantage besides the social or sexual: fat people die young.

If one of your goals is to be physically more attractive and to live longer, then you should be concerned with your weight, as I am with mine. Many people attempt to live without facing the realities of the world, but, as a physician, for many decades I have been forced to live my life chest-deep in the most important realities we humans face. Since

I graduated from medical school, almost a third of a century ago, almost every day of my life has been spent doing battle with Death and Insanity. For almost longer than I care to remember, I have spent my life in my office and in hospital rooms where patients come to me with their problems, and, for a fee, I hire myself out to help them in their battle. Yes, I know about reality.

I repeat: Fat people die young. They die from high blood pressure, diabetes, coronary artery disease, and if they escape these killers their mortality rate is also very high in case they need surgery for a broken leg or appendicitis.

I understand fat people, because I too am a fat person even though I am six-foot-one-inch tall and weigh 175 pounds.

Let me explain: As I approached the boredom of middle age, I was certain that my enzyme system was beginning to fail me. Having always been used to the kind of energy that allowed me to work fourteen hours a day, I found myself tiring easily. I had reached a stage in life with a large practice, and a comfortable humdrum philosophy of life. The excitement, the challenge, the struggle, had all but disappeared. I was only another psychiatrist sitting behind a desk, listening to stories I'd heard a thousand times.

Lacking the challenges and struggles that I had been used to in my early life, I had little outlet for my aggressions. By "aggressions" I do not mean anger, but rather the kind of go-get'em spirit that enabled man to cross the Atlantic Ocean in a sailboat, to turn the prairies of this continent into tillable land and to build cities such as the world has never known before.

When you catch an animal, confine him to a zoo, feed him the wrong food, and let him live out his weeks with boredom as his chief companion, then that animal, its aggressive impulses frustrated, begins to tear and bite even at its own flesh.

I turned to food: ice-cream with chocolate topping piled high with whipped cream; garlic bread; hotcakes dripping with maple syrup—and all the other foods embraced by carbohydrate freaks. My weight skipped from an already pudgy 190 to 230. I was beginning to huff and puff and look like Orson Welles, but I became adjusted to my new shape. Being fat myself, I began to see fat as beautiful. I knew fat people died young, but for a time I managed to shove this unpleasant fact on the back burner, by telling myself that not *all* fat people die young.

Then I discovered my cholesterol hovering at 312 and decided that, being a sane person who enjoyed life and wanted to hang around to see a few more reels of the show, I'd better get on the ball and do something about my weight, my cholesterol and my nutrition generally. I began to buy books on weight reduction by the shelf-full and to try different systems on myself. Later, after I had mastered the subject and applied it to myself, I applied it to my patients.

The first step toward weight reduction is to put yourself on the proper nutritional supplements—at least the basic program mentioned in this book: natural vitamin A, 10,000 units daily; natural vitamin D, 400 units daily; 1 heaping tablespoon of brewers' yeast twice daily; vitamin C, 5 to 10,000 mg. daily; vitamin E, 200 units two times a day; lecithin, 2 heaping tablespoons daily. Also, safflower oil, 2 tablespoons daily, in addition to one kelp tablet twice a day, seasalt used on food and 2 teaspoons daily of dolomite.

Ideally, everybody should have a hair test for minerals so that additional minerals may be taken if needed, and some people do not require the dolomite I have repeatedly mentioned.

If this regimen of nutritional supplements does not control and reduce the cholesterol levels (and it almost always does), then, assuming that your doctor approves, you should take 1000 mg. of niacin three times daily as outlined in other chapters in this book.

In the back of my mind I have a new theory about obesity. One of the reasons people overeat, I believe, is that this gives them a feeling of strength and power. As an overweight opera star once told me, "Unless I have a full belly I can't belt out the notes." The added strength of more food, more food than this patient needed for normal weight, gave her strength to project her voice better. (I pointed out in the chapter on food allergies that eating foods to which we have an allergic addiction keeps us from getting weak and allows us to avoid the withdrawal symptoms.)

But eating large quantities of food does more. When people speak of large quantities of food they almost always mean carbohydrates. One of the effects of eating large amounts of carbohydrates, I suspect, is that it increases the blood volume. People's weight goes up markedly after eating carbohydrates, because they are thirsty and are able to store the fluids. It would be interesting to do blood volume studies on obese patients. I suspect that the studies would show that when people are hungry the blood volume is reduced and that after eating carbohydrates the blood volume is increased. I suspect that this problem of volume is also strongly connected with body levels of sodium and potassium. In my hair studies on hundreds of patients I frequently find patients are low in sodium, or in sodium as well as potassium, and this is particularly true of overweight patients.

HOW VITAMINS HELP WEIGHT CONTROL

You can probably gain the added strength of which my opera singer patient spoke when the proper diet is combined with the above mentioned supplements. I know that when I cut out certain vitamins from my own diet it is much harder for me to control my appetite. When I have my vitamins and minerals in near balance, food is not necessary in large quantities to give me a feeling of force and strength. Incidentally, my opera singer patient experienced the same feeling after her nutritional supplements were properly organized.

I find that most people with allergic conditions generally enjoy greatly reduced sensitivity to food once their nutritional supplements are balanced properly. Apparently the body is able to handle allergenic material and detoxify it effectively if the body cells are working at optimal level.

I have already discussed ideal diets in this book and am able to state without question that people who are underweight almost universally gain weight on this diet, and those who are overweight lose weight. To summarize: The diet consists of omitting all sugar, sweets, wheat, barley, oats, corn, milk, and products made of any of these foods. This means no sugar, no honey, no bread, pastries, or cheese.

In addition, omit all processed foods such as hot dogs, salami, bottled drinks, and so forth. People losing weight should also cut out nuts. After reaching ideal weight, the nuts are allowed except for cashews. Only nuts in the shell should be used. Have fresh fruit, but no fruit juices.

You are to eat all the fresh meat *(including the fat),* fresh vegetables, fresh poultry, fresh fish and eggs you want. One fruit is allowed three times a day as dessert. I also allow a modest serving of baked potato or brown rice with meals if desired, and do encourage patients to have between-meal and bedtime snacks.

Basically, the only thing you should drink is water or herb tea. Distilled water is best; the distillation takes out chlorine, fluorides, and all the factory waste products that are found in public water supplies. You may have heard about the cancer-producing city water in New Orleans. Already such dangerous water has been discovered in other large cities. True, when water is distilled, the minerals are also removed, but with the program I have given you there should be no problem to get adequate minerals; you will be getting them from dolomite, kelp, and yeast as well as from the fruits and the many vegetables you will be eating.

Again: A high fat intake is desirable. You need not worry about your cholesterol because the vitamins and lecithin will take care of that without difficulty. When I followed a high-carbohydrate diet my cholesterol was 313, but on a high-fat, high-protein diet with nutritional supplements my cholesterol stays at about 165. Triglycerides (another kind of blood fat) will also fall to desirable levels.

For a change of pace you might drink a natural sparkling mineral water such as Saratoga water or Perrier or Vichy with a twist of lemon or lime in it. Some patients can get away with drinking black coffee. You can only discover through trial and error whether you are in that category or not. I would not advise coffee substitutes such as Postum, which contains molasses. You should definitely not have artificial sweeteners nor the calorie-free bottled drinks, to which many people are sensitive. Many people are allergic to the low-caffeine coffees, and the solvents used in making them have recently come under suspicion.

Alcoholic drinks should be cut out while you are trying to lose weight. Not only does alcohol increase allergic reactions; it also decreases the will to lose weight. We all have mixed feelings about gaining good health. Part of our personality desires it and part of our personality says, "The hell with it, so I'm fat and I'll die young, and who cares?" I am trying to get you to let the health-oriented part of your personality take over. If you use alcohol, the health-oriented part of your personality will quickly melt away.

If you feel compelled to cheat with the alcohol, avoid all sweetened alcoholic drinks and drink the alcohol straight or with water or lemon or lime. It is best to use the alcoholic drink that you like least; that is the one you are least likely to be allergic to and it will therefore be easier for you to stop drinking. (Some alcoholics who have allergic-alcohol addictions will be completely alcoholic on Scotch, but if they change to vodka they may find that they can drink it without overindulging.)

While you are losing weight, it is absolutely necessary that you stick with your diet every day of the year, though in most cases it will not take that long to lose the weight you need to shed. Losing at the rate of one-half to one pound a week is ideal.

After you reach your desired weight, you can begin to relax a little. I suggest that you weigh yourself every morning for the rest of your life; if you are above the figure you have set for yourself, you must cut back your food intake.

If you feel you must cheat, cheating should be confined to one day a week. After you have reached your ideal weight, you just *might* get by with using alcohol one day a week. Don't quote me as saying this is permissible, but I have been in practice long enough to know that people are human, and many of them need to let their heads come out and play now and then.

People who have difficulty losing weight should also have their thyroid activity and sex hormones checked. If either of these is low or if the morning underarm temperatures are below 98.2 degrees, when measured for ten minutes by the clock before getting out of bed in the morning (either an oral or rectal thermometer under the arm), then a thyroid supplement should be considered. If the sex hormones are low, it is essential to correct them.

THE BEST WAY TO GAIN WEIGHT

If you wish to gain weight, it is absolutely necessary that you stop smoking, and under no circumstances drink any coffee. You should follow the same nutritional supplements outlined above, and the same diet. Only you may have all the fruits, brown rice, and baked potatoes you wish and may include nuts in your diet. Use untreated nuts. Be sure to read the container to make certain the nuts do not contain MSG or other added chemicals. Attention to hormones may be important for people who are trying to gain weight as well as those who are trying to lose it.

HOW TO NOURISH YOUR HAIR

As you know, I dislike thinking in terms of one vitamin or mineral or hormone, or for that matter, of one physical effect. For example, you always hear that vitamin C is good for bleeding gums. It is true that if gums are bleeding because of scurvy, vitamin C will correct the problem. But vitamin C, as all other vitamins and minerals, is used by every cell in the body. If you have scurvy you will have much more to worry about than bleeding gums. You will be tired and depressed. Wounds will heal poorly. If the condition lasts long enough (and to a profound enough degree) you will die.

Every cell in the body must have proper nourishment. If the cells are nourished properly, then each will reach full potential. In this section I will write about hair, nails, and skin separately, but I must repeat that it is impossible to isolate these tissues from the rest of the body. You cannot have beautiful hair and have the rest of your body sick.

Not long ago a Korean girl consulted me. She had a timid, mousy look about her. Her skin, instead of being a beautiful orange-yellow Oriental, was a dull brown. Her face was puffy. Her black straight hair could have been a cheap wig. Her eyes looked as dull as a cloudy December morning. Her husband was an important artist, a man of taste and intelligence. When I first saw the woman I wondered why he ever married her; she seemed to have nothing to offer in looks, youth, or personality.

Then he told me what his wife had been like when he had met her several years previously and how she had deteriorated into the woman sitting across the desk from me.

Laboratory studies showed that she had a low NAD (Nicotinamide Adenine Dinucleotide). She was suffering from hypoglycemia. She was somewhat anemic from an iron deficiency. She was also low in zinc, potassium, and sodium. Her thyroid function was slightly below normal. She was deficient in folic acid. The allergy test revealed she was allergic to dust, tomatoes, corn, cigarettes, and rice.

She was given my basic supplements. Her diet was corrected, and large doses of folic acid were prescribed. She was given a trial injection of vitamin B_{12b}, which made her feel a great deal better even though her blood serum had shown that she had a normal B_{12} level.

Her injections were repeated at weekly intervals for a few weeks, then the length between her visits was gradually increased.

You have never seen such beauty unfold. It was like watching a time-lapse photograph of a flower opening its petals to the sun. Gradually she became vivacious, her eyes shone, her hair developed a sleek black beauty, and her skin lost its puffiness and took on life once more.

She reminded me very much of a black woman who consulted me a number of months ago because of tiredness. She visited me again the other week. Her only complaint now is that her looks have improved so much that young men annoy her. The patient is almost fifty years old but men at work, men she meets at cocktail parties, and even old friends, have made a nuisance of themselves trying to seduce her. After telling me about her new complaint, she laughed and said her new looks might be a problem but she wouldn't trade places with her former tired, dragged-down self.

Let me also tell you another story about myself. There is no end to what one can learn about nutrition and dietary supplements. For years I have been starting, stopping, increasing, decreasing, adding, substracting supplements to my own diet, and I am still learning how to try and hone my supplements to the best possible level for me. A few months ago I decided to try torula yeast. This is a yeast rich in minerals and in vitamin B_1 and vitamin B_2. After going on torula yeast (and this was the only change in my supplements), my hair began changing. I had always had a slight wave in front, but gradually I noticed the wave increased in depth and other waves began coming into my hair, so much so that I complained to my barber who said that he had never seen hair change so much as mine and that my old cut would not be satisfactory any longer. Accordingly he gave me a "poodle cut." His parting instructions were that all I needed to do was towel-dry it every morning.

Now that my hair is cut in a different way I find that it is full of curls. My old friends have joked with me about having had a permanent, though they know me well enough to realize that getting permanent waves is not my thing. At any rate, I feel that torula yeast has made my hair curly. Will one or two tablespoons of torula yeast do the same for your hair? I don't know, but one way to answer that question: Try, but don't desert your primary or brewers' yeast.

Just to illustrate how complicated the harmonics of nutrition are:

my hair is now losing its curl in spite of the continued use of torula yeast.

HOW HAIR IS AFFECTED BY THYROID

Since thyroid supplements were first discovered in the last century, physicians have been aware that the physiology of the hair is greatly affected by the thyroid hormones. If the thyroid activity is low, your hair will be dry, brittle, dull, and uninteresting. Blood tests should be done for thyroid activity; but even if the blood tests are normal you may require thyroid hormone.

One reason why there are so many different thyroid tests is that none is wholly satisfactory. Broda O. Barnes, Ph.D., M.D., has reported in an article in the *Journal of the American Medical Association* that the most accurate single test for thyroid function is the underarm temperature method (mentioned earlier) taken with either an oral or rectal thermometer placed in the armpit for ten minutes by the clock before getting out of bed in the morning. If this is below 98.2 degrees then a thyroid preparation should be taken. Of course this must be done under your doctor's supervision.

Generally, the simple desiccated thyroid tablet is the best to use and it is usually started in half-grain doses for people under forty-five. The dose is increased every three or four weeks. Generally two or three grains daily is the top dose. For people older than forty-five, it would probably be best to start at one-quarter grain and build up every two or three weeks by one-quarter grain intervals.

Incidentally, Dr. Barnes has written a book entitled *Heart Attack Rareness in Thyroid-Treated Patients*, published by Charles C. Thomas & Co., Springfield, Ill., in 1972, in which he convincingly builds up an argument for the use of thyroid extract to prevent heart attacks. So, while improving the beauty of your hair, you just may be saving your life.

HOW TO PREVENT GRAY HAIR

To prevent grayness of the hair or to help it return to its natural color when it is already gray, most nutritionists tend to agree that para-aminobenzoic acid, PABA, is the most important vitamin. Once, when I was appearing on a TV talk show with Carlton Fredericks, he told me that he took 500 mg. daily of PABA and attributed his scarcity of gray hairs to this vitamin supplement. But of course he does not neglect the rest of his vitamin-mineral intake.

PABA is available in health food stores over the counter in small tablets (about 30 mg.) which are probably not enough to help much. Because of the filler that they contain it would not be a good idea to take the number needed to give you 500 mg. daily. PABA is available by prescription (trade name: Potaba) in 500 mg. tablets (I have already discussed the injectable use of PABA in the form of Dr. Aslan's H_3). I have seen many patients whose hair became darker and much of it returned to its original color after adding PABA to the nutritional regimen. In my own case, it is difficult for me to evaluate the results. The hair on my head contains only a very few strands of gray, even though I am fifty-three years old. However, my beard is quite gray and the use of PABA does not seem to have any striking effect on returning it to a darker color.

Folic acid is usually considered an important vitamin in the prevention and cure of gray hair.

A folic acid deficiency tends to make hair fall out more rapidly than normal, resulting in thin hair. This may even extend to the eyebrows and eyelashes. Folic acid is available in this country only by prescription in 1 mg. doses. It can be bought in Canada without a prescription in 5 mg. tablets. I, as you know, test all my patients for their folic acid blood levels and find many are improved by taking folic acid: 5 mg. three or four times a day. Recently I markedly increased some dosages of folic acid to 10 to 20 mg. three or four times daily; a number of patients who were not improving have gotten better at this dose level.

Tests have indicated that some of my patients do not absorb folic acid well. These patients are given folic acid by injection. One word of caution: It is a good idea to have occasional injections of vitamin $B_{12}b$, say 1000 micrograms every three months, if you are going to be taking folic acid by prescription.

Calcium pantothenate is generally considered another vitamin that is especially important in the prevention and cure of gray hair. It is available in sugar-free, starch-free tablets and capsules of 218 mg. Take one to five of these a day, usually at bedtime because they tend to have a relaxing effect.

Do not forget that iodine is very important in the proper function of the thyroid gland. A very good source of iodine is kelp tablets that are readily available in health food stores. Also, kelp is a very good source of potassium and trace minerals. Minerals are most important for proper hair, but you should have your physician do a hair test on you to see what your present mineral levels are before you take any supplements.

HOW PROTEIN HELPS HAIR

Remember that hair and nails are largely protein in composition and it is therefore imperative that you have a good protein intake if these two tissues are to be healthy, beautiful, and strong.

Some people find that hair is improved if they use a protein-oil treatment. Probably the best is the special mayonnaise to be mentioned under the section on skin care. Work the mayonnaise into your hair, wrap a towel around your head, and let it stay for about half an hour. Then shampoo.

Many people are afraid to wash their hair frequently. Dermatologists tell me there is no reason not to wash the hair every day if you so desire. My clinical experience agrees with them. A daily wash is especially desirable if you have a tendency toward skin blemishes or acne.

One important point to consider: The normal scalp (and all the rest of the skin, for that matter) is covered by an acid mantle, an invisible acid surface that discourages the growth of bacteria and fungi. Most shampoos and soaps are alkaline. They neutralize and wash away the protective acid mantle and replace it with an alkaline mantle that not only fails to give protection against germs but actually encourages their growth.

Acidity and alkalinity are measured by what is called the pH. The pH scale runs from 1 to 14. Half-way down the scale is neutrality, pH 7. Any pH above this figure (7–14) is alkaline; any pH below 7 (1–7) is acid.

If you would like to test the pH of any of your shampoos, soaps, or skin lotions, ask your druggist for a roll of Nitrazine paper, made by E. R. Squibb & Sons, Inc., Princeton, N.J. 08540 and available without a prescription. Simply dip the end of a strip of this tape into the product (if testing soap, moisten soap first) and observe the color change in the tape. Compare it to the scale illustrated on the Nitrazine paper carton and you have the pH of your product.

We would certainly be more in tune with the natural chemistry of our bodies if we used only acid (low pH) products on our skin, including shampoos, soaps, creams, and lotions. The use of these products would be especially useful if your skin is sensitive, dry, or oily or if you have a tendency to get blemishes or acne.

In general, such products are labeled "acid balance." Although such products are available at the cosmetic counter in department stores or in drug stores, I have not had an opportunity to test them all. I have found the following products satisfactory and have personally tested their pH: Earth Born Shampoo (The Gillette Company, Personal Care Division, Boston, Massachusetts 02199), and Amino-Pon Shampoo (Redkin Laboratories, Inc., Van Nuys, California 91401). The latter company also makes a low pH bar soap called Amino-Pon Beauty Bar.

If you use an ordinary alkaline shampoo, it should be followed with a lemon rinse to restore the acid mantle: Add the juice of one lemon to a pint of (preferably) distilled water.

I would like to take this opportunity to condemn pressure spray cans in general. Many preparations for the hair are sold in such containers. Dr. F. Sherwood Rowland of the University of California has developed strong evidence that chemicals from pressure cans are reducing the ozone level in the upper atmosphere. If this ozone level continues to be reduced, it will allow harmful amounts of ultraviolet rays to bombard the earth. I feel that it behooves all of us to avoid all pressure cans.

Many people are also allergic to the chemicals in pressure cans.

BEWARE OF DYES

I think that hair dyes are generally dangerous. They are usually made from aniline chemicals that often cause allergies such as red, itching scalp, puffy eyes, and swollen ears. This aniline dye is absorbed through the scalp and excreted in part through the urine. Urinary bladder cancer has been reported to be high in workers in aniline dye plants in the United States, Australia, and Europe.

The slowly darkening hair formulas (clear solutions that are added to the hair daily at first, then at gradually lengthening intervals) contain large amounts of lead. I have not had enough experience with these preparations to know how much lead is absorbed from their formulas into the body, but I feel they should be used with caution. If you use such a preparation regularly, I would suggest that you have hair on other parts of your body analyzed (pubic hair for example) to discover whether or not your body is in fact absorbing lead from the hair darkener.

Laboratory research shows that lack of magnesium may cause hair loss, as may an under-supply of proteins. The biotin and inositol found in lecithin is apparently important, as are all the B vitamins. In laboratory mice, biotin, inositol, and calcium pantothenate have all been demonstrated to prevent falling hair. Vitamin B_6 (pyridoxin) seems to be particularly important in maintaining proper hair texture and amount.

WHY SERIOUS ILLNESS CAN HURT YOUR HAIR

We have all heard of hair falling out following a debilitating illness such as typhoid fever. In all probability the hair falls out because stress caused by the fever and the disease have depleted the body of vitamins and minerals; what we are seeing is a vitamin-mineral deficiency, as well as a protein deficiency, particularly since some debilitating diseases such as typhoid fever often are accompanied by diarrhea that robs the body of nutrients.

NO MORE DANDRUFF

If you are worried about dandruff, I think it is quite safe to say that you can forget about it if you will follow the nutritional program outlined in this book. Even the minimal program should eliminate your dandruff if you will use both the diet and the regimen of dietary supplements as well as the acid shampoos. Don't forget that lecithin granules contain not only inositol and biotin but the kind of fatty oils that are good for your hair. Also, the two tablespoonfuls a day of safflower oil will be a great help to your hair.

HOW COPPER HELPS YOUR HAIR

A proper amount of copper is needed in experimental animals to maintain dark color to the hair. Copper is readily available in the yeast I have recommended.

VITAMIN E FOR HAIR AND SKIN

Some people have found it beneficial to add extra vitamin E oil to the mayonnaise-protein hair conditioner. The special mayonnaise to be mentioned under the section on skin is mixed with an additional amount of vitamin E oil from several 200 IU capsules. Pierce the capsules with a pin, squeeze the contents into the mayonnaise, and stir.

HOW TO GET HEALTHY, ATTRACTIVE NAILS

Fingernails have much in common with hair. Proper hormone levels are necessary, especially thyroid, in order to have healthy nails.

Since nails are made almost entirely of protein, you must eat adequate amounts of protein. Beauty experts often recommend that you drink unflavored powdered gelatin dissolved in fruit juice in order to strengthen your nails. This is a perfectly legitimate way to increase protein intake. But remember that gelatin is an incomplete protein and requires, in addition, the complete kind of protein that you find in eggs, fish, fowl, and meat so the body will utilize it properly.

MINERALS FOR YOUR NAILS

Nails contain a small amount of minerals. Patients deficient in iron develop koilonyehia (longitudinal ridging and flattening of the fingernails) and there have been reports of patients' fingernails improving after taking kelp. There is some controversy as to whether or not calcium is beneficial to nails. It is my clinical impression that patients who take calcium, magnesium, and any other deficient minerals grow much stronger and better nails when these substances are added to the diet.

VITAMINS FOR NAILS

Just as vitamin A and vitamin C are very important for good hair, so they are important for proper nail health, though I must say again that I dislike speaking of specific vitamins and minerals for specific organs or diseases. Each cell in the body requires each nutrient to function properly, but certain tissues show deficiencies in certain vitamins sooner than others. So if you lack vitamin C or A, your nails may reflect this condition early.

ARTIFICIAL NAILS

Nail hardeners contain formaldehyde and should be avoided at all cost, and so should the artificial nails that can be cemented onto your nails. These products create many difficulties for some people. I feel they do not get at the source of any nail problem and should be avoided except in extreme circumstances where good nails are required immediately in order for you to earn a living (for example if you're a model or in the theater). Even in these instances, the artificial nails should be done away with as soon as possible.

Until nails become strong they should be kept short; the best thing to use is an emery file. I recommend that you file in one direction only; filing in a back and forth motion with an emery board tends to split the nails.

A good treatment at night for nails is beauty mayonnaise (see page 296) containing a small amount of lemon juice for acidity. Apply this beauty treatment to your hands before going to bed, and wear white, well-washed cotton gloves over the mayonnaise to keep it in place while it is working.

Don't forget that nails, like skin and hair, require an acid atmosphere. This means you should keep your hands out of alkaline detergent or other chemicals. Interesting enough, people who work with their hands have better nails than those who do not use their hands in their occupations. Apparently the use of the hands stimulates the circulation and makes the nails grow better. Nails also grow better in warmer climates.

Serious illnesses may cause defects in nails just as they may cause defects in hair growth. For example, many people may develop Beau's lines (longitudinal lines) in their nails if they have a certain South American hemorrhagic fever. Nails may become lined and flat with a B-complex or iron deficiency. Excessive hang nails may indicate low protein, vitamin C, or folic acid.

YOUR SKIN MAYONNAISE RECIPE

Before talking about the skin, let me give you my recipe for the mayonnaise pack for your skin, nails, and hair.

Place one egg in a blender or a bowl suitable for mixing. Add the juice of one lemon. As your ingredients are mixed, either with the blender or by hand, slowly add safflower oil, a pinch of seasalt, and the oil from three 400 IU pearls of vitamin E. Continue adding the safflower oil slowly until you get a thick mixture with the consistency of mayonnaise. Of course, this should be stored in the refrigerator. If you need larger amounts, simply use the same proportions and double or triple the recipe.

Some skin packs are made with the addition of vitamin A and D oils. However, since vitamins are absorbed from the skin surfaces and since vitamins A and D are both fat-soluble vitamins which are stored in the body and can accumulate to abnormal levels, I feel it is best not to apply them directly to the skin surfaces.

HOW TO TREAT DRY SKIN

Like hair, good skin tone and health depend on the body's health. In general, therefore, the best advice for healthy skin is that you follow the diet and diet supplement recommendations I've outlined elsewhere.

Dry skin should be treated for half an hour daily with the mayonnaise pack; this should be applied to the face and hands and left in place; ideally it should be removed with olive oil or coconut oil. The less soap that is used on dry skin the better, especially in the wintertime. As a further precaution in winter, consider using a vaporizer indoors (at least in your bedroom at night) to maintain a relatively high level of humidity. Your diet should especially emphasize fats, both saturated as found in meats and unsaturated such as safflower oil.

If you have dry skin, you should realize that this can be a symptom of thyroid trouble. You would probably be well advised to take a kelp tablet three times a day for iodine, and you should ask your physician for thyroid tests. Repeat: Multiple thyroid tests should be taken since no one thyroid test is wholly satisfactory. Take your underarm morning temperature. If this temperature is consistently below 98.2 degrees for ten days and if there is no reason for the physician to withhold thyroid medication, then thyroid medication should be prescribed up to 2 or 3 grains daily. It should be started at a low dose and gradually built up.

After three or four months' trial on thyroid, if there is no improvement in general feeling of well-being or improvement in the skin texture and disappearance of any dryness of the skin, then this thyroid hormone probably has nothing to offer you.

People with dry skin tend to get eczema easily. Many people with eczema have food allergies that lead to the skin lesions. People with eczema should pay particular attention to my chapter on food allergies. Most physicians (even most allergists and dermatologists) have only limited knowledge of food allergies and seem to lack the patience required to discover whether food allergies are affecting their patients and, if so, precisely what these allergies are.

Although everyone needs good nutritional supplements, some people with eczema have specific needs for large doses of vitamins. I have one patient who is able to maintain himself free of eczema as long as he takes 3000 mg. of niacinamide daily. Until this was discovered, it was almost impossible to control his eczema, even with the use of cortical steroids. Other patients may require high doses of other vitamins or minerals to maintain their skin in good condition.

HOW TO TREAT OILY SKIN

Although anyone can develop skin difficulties as a result of taking a nutritional supplement (this allergy to supplements appears in the form of skin blemishes), people with oily skin are particularly prone to develop blemishes from iodine compounds. Iodine is found in iodine salt and in kelp tablets. Anyone with a tendency toward acne or any kind of blemishes, especially those in oily skins, should check out his or her sensitivity to iodines. People with oily skin usually do not need thyroid preparations; indeed, their skin may be made worse by thyroid preparations.

Cleanliness is the key to blemish-free skin. Ideally I think a person with oily skin should shampoo his hair daily, bathe daily, and wash his face three or four times a day. After washing the face and hair it is a very good idea to rinse off the skin and scalp with an acid solution such as the juice of one lemon in one pint of water. Oily skins are easily infected. Alkaline soaps tend to take away the normal acidity of the skin but this acidity (which has a bacterial-killing effect) can be replaced by the use of this mildly acid lemon juice rinse. Better: Use acid soaps and shampoos.

Those with oily skin should take care to steam their faces regularly to remove blackheads. Vitamin A in rather large amounts is important for some people to maintain their skin in good condition. I have recommended 10,000 units of vitamin A daily as a minimum intake. If your physician agrees, and if you find it is helping, I think it would be perfectly safe for you to run your vitamin A dosage up to 25,000 to 50,000 IU daily—but no more. It is important that a natural source of vitamin A be used, since the natural products seem to be much less toxic than the synthetic form.

WHAT ABOUT PROFESSIONAL SKIN CARE?

I have referred some of my patients with problem skins to Georgette Klinger, who runs a facial salon on Madison Avenue in New York (212-838-3200). In general, the technicians there do a good job of helping patients with their skin. You can learn good skin hygiene from them.

(Unfortunately, I am not sufficiently familiar with similar establishments in other cities to be able to make additional recommendations.)

It may seem strange to hear a physician say that he refers patients with skin problems to a cosmetics salon. However, I have had very disappointing results when I send patients with acne and other *uncomplicated* cosmetic problems to dermatologists. Many dermatologists seem unable to resist giving patients antibiotics for acne. True, antibiotics help oily skin problems such as acne but they do so at a great price. Antibiotics cut down vitamin absorption from the gastrointestinal tract. I have seen several patients who came to me severely disturbed after taking antibiotics, until their vitamin levels became depleted. Dermatologists also seem to neglect proper cleansing and proper nutrition. It's the same old story: Some physicians tend to regard medications as the solution to every problem.

Vitamin E squeezed from capsules may be applied directly to the skin. It is said to prevent scar formation following wounds. Tradition also has it that vitamin E helps retard wrinkling of the skin. However, I have not had enough first-hand experience to verify this claim.

HOW SUNSHINE HELPS YOUR SKIN

You should be aware that excessive suntanning causes wrinkling of the skin; if carried to great lengths, it may even lead to skin cancer in susceptible people, especially those with pale skin. But do not make the mistake of feeling that your skin does not need sunshine (see pages 234–252). Sunshine is extremely important for skin, especially for oily skin or acne. Many people with acne should keep their skin dry even to the point of peeling. This is helped by the use of sunlamps which you can use under your physician's supervision.

HOW SMOKING HURTS YOUR SKIN

Compelling evidence says that smoking increases wrinkling of the skin. Possibly this happens because each cigarette uses up 25 mg. of vitamin C from your body—which means that most smokers inevitably are deficient in vitamin C. One of the functions of vitamin C is to maintain integrity of the connective tissue which lies just underneath the skin and supports it. When this support wastes away, the skin on top is left baggy and wrinkled.

Whether you smoke or not, an adequate intake of vitamin C is, as I have stressed before, essential if you want to maintain your good looks. But a high vitamin C intake is especially important if you smoke.

WHAT TO DO ABOUT LIVER SPOTS

All of you have noticed brown spots on the backs of the hands of middle-aged and older people. These spots have the romantic-sounding name of *fleur-de-cimetière* (flower of the cemetery), implying that death has his/her eye on you.

Many preparations are recommended for local application to do away with these brown spots. To me, there seems little point in making them disappear unless you get to work on the basic chemistry of aging. Why put a finger in the dyke when it is easier to build a new dyke?

Again, I recommend full vitamin dietary supplements; in addition, special emphasis should be given to vitamins E and C. In my experience, these two vitamins are particularly important in doing away with the brown spots which occur with aging.

Vitamin B_6 (pyridoxin) is also important for maintaining healthy skin. Many people have a puffiness which is really a water-sogged condition of the skin which can be cleared up by taking 50 or 100 mg. of pyridoxin three times a day.

For healthy-looking skin, allergies must be attended to, since they can also cause the puffy, unhealthy appearance of skin with pale, sickly texture.

Any discussion of skin health and beauty must include mention of sex hormone therapy. Today many women are given estrogens at the time of menopause and continue on them indefinitely. A very high percentage of women in the upper income brackets who can afford so-called luxury medicine take estrogens these days. Not only do they prevent coronary heart attacks and help stabilize them emotionally but I, along with many authorities, also feel that estrogens keep the skin more pliable, more youthful and vigorous and allow fewer wrinkles.

The same applies to men and testosterone, although men are, as pointed out in other parts of the book, badly neglected in the field of hormone therapy.

Local application of hormones to the skin are probably of no value.

I have discussed reports on the youth-maintaining effects of para-aminobenzoic acid (PABA) or the H_3 preparation of Asa Aslan, M.D., in the chapters on vitamins and aging. Anyone interested in maintaining a youthful appearance must maintain youthful-looking skin. To this end, you might consider having your physician give you a prescription for Protaba, 500 mg. to be taken daily as a source of para-aminobenzoic acid; or, have him periodically give you a series of injections of H_3. I suspect, when all the data is collected, this will prove to be important. My policy is that, if a preparation has a good chance of being helpful and no chance of doing harm, it should be tried promptly.

HOW TENSION AFFECTS YOUR BEAUTY

People who are so tense they are about to snap at their wires are not attractive. No matter how beautiful the hair and skin, extreme tenseness turns other people off. I don't know why this is so, but the indisputable fact is that it gets on people's nerves to be around someone who is uptight. You cannot be truly beautiful and be emotionally disturbed.

The same applies to people who are depressed. No matter how romantically a case of stoic misery may be portrayed in a novel or movie, in real life sadness is rarely appealing. It is boring and oppressive to be around someone who focuses mainly on the misery of life. Real beauty requires mental health as well as physical health.

I have discussed sex in terms of mental health and physical beauty, because, in our society at least, the two are closely connected. It is nearly impossible truly to look your best unless you are mentally and physically healthy, yet very few people can feel really happy about themselves when they think they look unattractive. And people who do not feel good about themselves do not usually have satisfactory sex lives, as we have seen. Our society tends to identify sexual beauty with the beauty of youth, although this is by no means the only kind of beauty, or even the most important.

Youth does have its attractions, of course, but so does wisdom, experience, intelligence, and good nature. I think the reason we put so much emphasis on the beauty of youth is that we associate aging with illness, loss of energy and vitality, and with death. This association is not inevitable. If we pay attention to proper nutrition, hormone therapy and especially to food allergies, energy, vitality, and freedom from illness will no longer be the special province of youth. Perhaps then we will be able to re-examine our rather irrational prejudice in favor of one period of life, and come to appreciate each stage of life for its own special qualities. With good physical and emotional health you can maintain a very real kind of beauty throughout your life, and with it a fulfilling sex life.

AGING: HOW TO PREVENT TIME FROM DESTROYING YOUR MIND

Although aging is an invariably fatal disease that afflicts us all, its complications—the mental disorders of senility—can be dealt with far more readily than most people realize.

So far, medicine's frequently applauded success in prolonging man's average lifespan is largely illusory. We have greatly reduced the rate of infant mortality, which makes the statistics for average life expectancy look better. We have also decreased early deaths from infectious diseases so that the second largest killer of young adults, after accidents, is suicide. That suicide should be a major cause of death poignantly illustrates that, while medical science has improved our chances of living, it has done little to improve the quality of those extra years.

In 1850, the average human lifespan was 38.7 years. In 1900 it was 49.2, and now that figure has been extended by some twenty additional years. Unfortunately, the quality of life over the age of forty is almost exactly what it was three hundred years ago. Indeed, as our civilization continues to mechanize the food industry, resulting in the removal of more and more essential elements from the diet and the addition of

303

chemicals, the sum total of man's modern ecology may already have caused a shortening of our potential life span all over again. Current indications suggest that even if our leading killers—cancer, heart and circulatory disease, kidney and respiratory disease—were all eliminated, but no further progress were made in retarding the fundamental aging process or delaying its onset, very little additional time would accrue to man.

In nature, death is not necessarily an inevitable part of life. Single-celled creatures, for example, reproduce by subdividing. One cell simply splits into two halves, creating two living creatures where there had been only one. Such cells have no particular pre-programmed lifespan and can theoretically subdivide indefinitely, except when environmental circumstances over which they have very little control cause their demise. Only when such cells gather together, each specializing in a particular function, and form a more complex animal, does the prospect of death enter into the process of life.

Man, of course, is a collection of cells living together in an enormously complex symbiosis which arrived at the present advanced state through a series of adaptive evolutionary modifications that were technically a marvel of success but produced complicated side-effects.

The one-celled animal's splitting in two is known as asexual reproduction. Sexual reproduction through mating is reserved for complex animals; only when we have sexual reproduction do we have death. In the most basic biological sense, then, death is the price we pay for sex. I leave it to you to decide whether the barter was worth while. In any case, I'm afraid you and I have little say in the matter.

Young people have only a vague conception of death, which is one reason why they are so often quick to rush into dangerous, even life-threatening situations. Once in our twenties, we tend to take the world about us a bit more seriously and look at it more realistically. Still, thoughts of death are far away. Not until the thirties do we begin to lose our omnipotent delusions of youth. This is the decade that brings the knowledge that very few of us are going to become Nobel Prize-winners, movie stars, or president of the United States. Vague notions of physical decay and death begin to stir in us occasionally when we look in the mirror and view our spreading midriffs and thinning hair with growing distaste.

In the forties, many people experience a relative lessening of zest for life. Sexual interest may wane, stairs may become a bit more difficult to climb. Reflections concerning old age, the loss of mental faculties, and the reality of ultimate death come to occupy a more prominent place in our thinking. These reflections proliferate with increasing momentum during our fifties, sixties, and seventies.

AGE THIRTY: THE TURNING POINT

Archeologists tell us that fifty thousand years ago man was a very short-lived mammal. Only five percent of primitive men lived past the age of thirty, and only one percent past forty-five. Was man designed to die at about age thirty? Quite possibly. Old age even for us begins at that time. That may seem like a very startling statement today, but if you will contemplate it for a moment, perhaps you will agree with me.

We all know, for example, that the most taxing sports are always dominated by young people. Teenage girls are often at the peak of their achievement in speed swimming contests. Boxers are at their best during their twenties, as are long distance runners. This is why, at about age thirty, the hope that helped carry us forward during difficult times in our teens and twenties often begins to fade. Experience, as well as the subconscious knowledge of our waning powers, cause an onset of half-cynical, half-wistful resignation.

If you contemplate your life, chances are you can detect a sort of natural turning point around the age of thirty. Karl Gustav Jung, the noted Swiss psychiatrist, wrote about the "two halves" of life, and believed firmly that the problems of the first part of life and those of the latter part were totally different, and had to be approached psychotherapeutically in entirely different ways.

WHY CHEMISTRY IS CRUCIAL

I agree with the end result of his findings, though not with his theoretical underpinnings. Jung was, of course, a psychoanalyst, and remained one even after his break with Freud. His explanation of the emotional turmoil of the second half of life is therefore strictly psychoanalytic. Once I might have shared that view, but today I feel very differently. During the decades I have spent trying to help emotionally ill people, I have come to a belief that psychological problems are largely chemical problems.

As you know, I treat patients with psychological means as well as with chemical ones. The fact is that I have been able to help many more people achieve much higher levels of performance and happiness by biological means than by psychotherapy. Once we normalize the chemistry of the central nervous system, problems that appeared to be psychological have a habit of melting away. Patients become emotionally stronger once we correct their chemistry. Then they gain the strength needed to deal with the slings and arrows of outrageous fortune that come to all of us.

Gradually—too gradually—the chemical approach to emotional illness is taking over the field of psychiatry. Even conventional psychiatrists are moving away from psychoanalysis. The analysts have had their day. Time was when psychoanalysts had waiting lists of people anxious to be seen five times a week for five years or more. Today these analysts spend a great percentage of their time doing eclectic psychotherapy, often even using chemotherapy. Freud himself anticipated this state of affairs when he wrote: "We must recollect that all our provisional ideas in psychology will some day be based on organic structure. This makes it probable that special substances and special chemical processes control the operation." [1]

Since the advent of the major anti-psychotic medications of the mid-1950s, we have been rapidly approaching the very era of psychochemistry predicted by Freud. And since chemistry, for all living creatures, also involves nutrition, it is particularly appropriate to pay more attention to nourishment in all its forms; for unless the cells of the body are properly nourished, they cannot achieve or maintain their full efficiency.

As I discussed earlier, all chemical reactions in the body depend on enzyme systems to carry out their work. These enzyme systems are very efficient in youth, but gradually, as part of the aging process, they lose their efficiency. The girl swimmer who broke records at sixteen achieved championship status partly because she had the good luck of being born with efficient enzyme systems, so that her muscles could work effectively and her nervous system could coordinate the muscular activity with great precision. The longer she is properly nourished, the longer her enzymes will work effectively. Up to a point, that is. Gradually, no matter how well nourished she may be, her enzyme systems will begin to deteriorate and at some point she cannot help but lose her championship status.

The purpose of proper nutrition is to furnish ideal substances for our enzyme systems so that they can reach whatever inborn potentials they possess, and remain at their ideal level for as long as possible. It goes without saying that, no matter how well nourished a person may be, he will eventually reach a period of senility and old age. The question is: when?

The point of this chapter is to discuss how you can avoid the emotional illnesses that normally beset the later years, or at least postpone them as long as possible.

TO POSTPONE AGING—START NOW

It is never too early to begin a program of adequate nutrition. *Now* is the time to stop drinking soda pop, eating hot dogs and french fries, and going on ice-cream sprees. If you are a mother-to-be, let me remind you also that the food you eat and the nutritional supplements you take affect not only you, but, to an equal extent, the child within you. Remember also that what your baby eats even during the very first months after birth will influence him until the day he dies.

Although periodic depressions frequently occur during the first half of life, these are usually shortlived and relatively mild. A profound, long-term depression in a young person is relatively rare, and often indicates severe trouble.

In the second half of life, depressions are so frequent as to be almost normal. Together with receding energy levels, they are perhaps the most important difficulties associated with the aging process.

In fact, since loss of energy and a feeling of depression are so very common in middle-aged and elderly people, we must consider that these are themselves symptoms of the condition we call aging—that is, of the growing inefficiency of our enzyme systems. Uncorrected, these enzyme systems deteriorate at an ever-increasing pace, and the symptoms escalate until they reach the dreaded end point of senility, with its loss of memory, disorientation, misperceptions, and degeneration of all intellectual life. To treat the disease we must find out how to delay or prevent the breakdown of enzyme systems that causes it.

HOW YOUR BODY CAN ATTACK ITSELF

Roy L. Walford, a professor of pathology at the University of California School of Medicine, has spent much of his life investigating the immunological aspects of aging.[2] He presents a convincing argument for the theory that in part, old age is caused by abnormalities in people's immunological system. This is the system that produces antibodies to fight infections, and to control substances to which one is allergic; it is also the system that forms so-called auto-immune antibodies. Forming auto-immune or "self-immune" antibodies is what the German bacteriologist Paul Ehrlich called "the horror reaction"—the immunological reaction in which the body forms antibodies against its own organs and thereby destroys them.

Hashimoto's disease is the classic "horror reaction" and the one most studied. In this disease, the body forms antibodies against its own thyroid tissue and eventually destroys it as if it were a foreign invader like a germ. We now know that such auto-immune reactions are quite common and that they increase with advancing age. There is a growing medical belief, for example, that the inflammatory, crippling type of arthritis is in fact an auto-immune reaction. Also, when a person has a heart attack and part of the heart muscle is destroyed, the body often forms antibodies against the heart muscle, and may go on to destroy more of the heart muscle than was originally damaged.

The work of L. Robert[3] suggests that arteriosclerosis (hardening of the arteries) is in part an auto-immune phenomenon. It is even possible that such failure may be involved in cancer. Much evidence points to the possibility that cancer may be caused by a virus to which certain people are susceptible. Since cancer is most common in the older age groups, the question of whether immunological failure plays a part is obviously most significant.

Just as proper intake of vitamins, minerals, and proteins greatly improves your ability to fight disease, immunological response is much better in persons who receive full spectrum light stimulation (see Chapter

17). All these factors suggest that nutrition is a vital element in *maintaining* normal immunological functions, thereby providing one possible way of delaying the onset of old age.

Another theory of aging holds that its primary cause is the cross-linking between certain large molecules in the body, such as proteins and nucleic acid. "Cross-linking" refers to the abnormal joining of proteins, and could involve genetic materials such as DNA, thus interfering with the cells' metabolism and their ability to divide. Or the cross-linked connective tissue might be less permeable to the body chemicals. In that case, aging would cause a choking off of cells, rendering them unable to receive essential nutrients.

This is why anti-oxidants are in all probability very important to our bodies. They help prevent cross-linking of molecules, and thus help prevent the choking of the tissue cells. Both vitamin E and vitamin C are thought to be highly effective anti-oxidants. In all likelihood they delay the aging process, and therewith the onset of the emotional illnesses associated with age.

CAN VITAMIN E SLOW DOWN AGING?

Vitamin E, like all vitamins, is still a controversial issue, despite years of reliably reported therapeutic successes in many areas. The very experienced Dr. Shute in Canada has used it over several decades, and is particularly impressed by its ability to spare and even repair blood vessel damage.

Drs. Lester Packer and James R. Smith[4] of the University of California extended the hayflick limit of human lung cells by adding vitamin E to the media in which they were grown. The "hayflick limit"—the end of their normal reproductive life—of fifty reproductions passed the one hundred twentieth reproduction and was still going strong.

The verbal gyrations of some people who are supposed to be authorities on vitamins never cease to amaze me: A few years ago, the New York Academy of Science held a symposium on vitamin E. At its end, spokesmen for the attending members told newspapers that the scientists had no concrete evidence that vitamin E plays an important role in human disease. A year later (1972) the academy published the results of that symposium in book form. Entitled *Vitamin E and Its Role in Cellular Metabolism,*[5] the volume is composed of papers presented at the symposium, and is full of information on the vital importance of vitamin E and its use by every cell in the body. Some of the papers even discussed its specific therapeutic uses favorably!

The book repeatedly refers to vitamin E as an anti-oxidant, and speaks of its role in hydrogen ion transportation. The fact that it is an anti-oxidant means that, in all probability, it *does* slow down the aging process. The fact that it is active in the transfer of hydrogen ions means that a high level of vitamin E might well enable the cells which are partly choked off by a cross-molecule to function better than they would without this vitamin.

THE MOST IMPORTANT VITAMINS
TO SLOW AGING

Let me remind you once again that the intake of any single vitamin is of limited usefulness. To get the maximum possible benefit from vitamins you must maintain a proper diet, and take all the vitamins and minerals you need, since they work in unison like the members of an orchestra.

Specifically to prevent aging, several vitamins are of extra importance: vitamin E, vitamin C, niacin, and vitamin B_{12}. In addition we should (but as yet cannot) concern ourselves with vitamin B_{15}, which is a new vitamin not yet available on the American market.

VITAMIN B_{12} IN THE AGING PROCESS

The auto-immune reactions discussed above are particularly evident in people with low serum B_{12} levels. For vitamin B_{12} to be absorbed, a special enzyme is required: the *intrinsic factor.* Auto-immune reactions may block or bind the intrinsic factor in the stomach, preventing vitamin B_{12} from being absorbed. Also, auto-immune reactions may be directed against the parietal cells in the stomach, and thus destroy the cell's ability to *produce* the vital intrinsic factor. As we grow older, we may develop stronger and stronger auto-immune reactions, so that less and less of the intrinsic factor is produced by the stomach, until we reach the point of not absorbing sufficient vitamin B_{12} to satisfy the body's needs. Further, proper blood levels of B_{12} also require an extrinsic factor, which is found largely in meat. Vegetarians therefore run a special risk of receiving too little of that factor, and therefore too little vitamin B_{12}. If you eat little meat, watch B_{12} closely.

THE PATIENT WHO WEPT FOR SIX MONTHS

Several years ago a seventy-six-year-old woman was brought to my office by her daughter, who stated that the mother had been weeping uncontrollably for the past six months and had recently become so incapacitated that she was unable to do her housework. She had been to see five physicians who had treated her in five different ways, mostly with anti-depressants and tranquilizers. One doctor had given her injections of multiple vitamins, which had not helped either.

In spite of her normal B_{12} level, I gave her an injection of 1000 micrograms of vitamin B_{12b}, but no anti-depressants or any other medication. I told her quite frankly that we might or might not be able to help her with nutritional supplements; if not, we would have to use electroconvulsive therapy. Although I did not say so to her or to the family, I suspected that she would require electroshock treatment. Yet when she returned to my office three days later, she was considerably improved. She was no longer crying, and reported that she felt much stronger and had slept throughout the night for the first time in many months. When she returned again after three more days, she looked happy and told me she could keep house again.

During subsequent visits the daughter was taught to administer the injections to her mother twice a week, or more frequently if she seemed in greater need of the vitamin.

When she returned several weeks later, the elderly lady told me that she could feel herself becoming depleted of the vitamin about every three or four days, and always felt completely restored after receiving another injection. At the time of that visit she was feeling the way she had felt ten years earlier, and was busy with all the household chores which she, like so many good German housewives of her generation, immensely enjoyed.

This woman represents as good an example as I can recall of a vitamin-dependent individual. I am sure we raised her vitamin B_{12} level to enormous heights. It would have been a waste of money to have retested her to see what her new level of functioning was. But I would judge from my experience in testing other patients that it must have been rather high, anywhere between 1200 and 2500 mg/ml, since she had received several injections of vitamin B_{12} already. Perhaps she was one of those persons whose enzyme functions gradually fade with age, but can be restored to normal performance by providing massive amounts of vitamins. It is even possible that certain metabolic pathways, not normally employing vitamin B_{12}, switched pathways, and made use of this invigorated set of enzymes. At any rate, a few injections of B_{12b} turned a crying, shuffling old woman into a bright-eyed, merry elderly housewife who could once more take an active role in life, be a useful member of society and enjoy her remaining years. Such transformations are what chemistry and nutrition are all about.

SPECIAL NUTRITION NEEDS OF OLDER PEOPLE

One of the reasons the old have more emotional disorders than the young is that they tend to skimp on their diets. They often have no family to cook for, and don't consider it worthwhile to prepare good food just for themselves. Their reduced energy levels incline them toward shortcuts in food preparation. Too often they subsist on processed foods like TV dinners, rather than shopping for fresh vegetables daily and cooking them in small quantities for each meal.

Financial problems also play a part. Since most retired people must live on severely curtailed incomes and because they value some of the diversions of life more than sound food, they tend to save money by living on cheap, non-nutritious foods.

Yesterday, while lunching in a restaurant, I observed an elderly lady sitting at a nearby table. Her lunch consisted of a tiny hamburger lost in a large bun, an anemic slice of tomato atop a dollar-sized lettuce leaf, and a generous helping of mashed potatoes with gravy. For dessert she had a vanilla ice-cream sundae. From her tired movements and the sad look on her face I suspected that this was a rather typical meal for her.

When I see people eating such food, especially when they also appear depressed or otherwise emotionally disturbed, it always makes me feel depressed, too. I have an intense urge to engage them in a discussion about food, to implore them to pay more attention to their diets. I always restrain myself because people would naturally consider it presumptuous for a stranger to tell them how to conduct their affairs. But I hope this book will reach such people and find them in a receptive mood.

SPECIAL NIACIN NEEDS OF THE ELDERLY

I also greatly favor the routine administration of niacin to most elderly people. Aside from its other benefits, discussed in an earlier chapter, this fascinating vitamin has an additional effect that has nothing directly to do with its action as a vitamin. Niacin counteracts blood clotting tendencies and is therefore of special interest for the older age group that is more prone to blood clots in the brain (stroke). Niacin is also thought to give protection against blood clots in the blood vessels of the heart—the condition known as coronary thrombosis (or heart attack).

One cause of heart attacks might be the fact that blood platelets begin to stick to the vessel walls, and constitute the nucleus around which the clot is formed. You may already be familiar with · the anti-clotting drugs administered to patients who have suffered a heart attack or phlebitis. If the post-coronary patient is on some medication that makes his blood clot less easily and he begins to take niacin too, *the dosage of the medication must be very carefully adjusted, because niacin will increase the drug's effect.*

This effect of niacin has been known for some time. As early as 1938, T. D. Spies[6] found that the abnormal electrocardiograms of cardiac patients reverted to normal after these patients were given the vitamin. Luigi Condorelli, writing in a book entitled *Niacin in Vascular Disorders and Hyperlipemia*,[7] states that he considers niacin a "most efficacious drug for the treatment of cerebral thrombosis."

In another chapter of that volume, Elaine Bossak Feldman[8] describes her use of niacin in the management of severe disorders of fat metabolism, in which large fatty deposits were visible in the skin. The photographs of these lesions, taken before and after treatment with niacin, are spectacular, and should be seen by all doubting Thomases. They make it easy to imagine the cholesterol deposits in one's own arteries disappearing in a like manner.

The same volume also contains an article by Drs. Ernst Ost Stenson and Svend Stenson, entitled "Regression of Atherosclerosis During Nicotinic Acid Therapy: A Study in Man by Means of Repeated Arteriographies." [9] They present graphs of pulsations in the arteries of the leg which clearly demonstrate that circulation is vastly improved by treatment with niacin.

Anyone concerned with hardening of the arteries should consider niacin therapy at the dose level of 3000 mg. or more a day. As we grow older, hardening of the arteries is a universal problem. If you are fortunate enough to avoid death from diseases secondary to the hardening of the arteries, such as thrombosis (heart attack), or cerebral thrombosis (stroke), then you will probably live long enough to develop the type of hardening of the brain arteries which leads to, or contributes to, senility.

Niacin, when taken in adequate doses, puts a negative electrical charge on the red blood cells which affects their oxygen-carrying ability. As we grow older, our red blood cells develop a tendency toward "sludging": the red blood cells stick together and go through the blood vessels in clumps like grapes. This has been observed by studying the small blood vessels in the eye through a microscope. These sludged red blood cells obviously cannot travel through the finer arteries of the body, and thus do not deliver adequate blood supplies to their ultimate destination: the tissues of the body.

Also, since these blood cells touch each other, the surfaces of the red blood cells exposed to oxygen are reduced so gas exchange is no longer rapid and efficient. Once the sludging is broken up with niacin, the red blood cells' full surface area is again exposed to the oxygen in the lungs, so that it can quickly and efficiently receive their full saturation of oxygen.

Not only does such breaking up of the sludged red blood cells help the circulation in the brain and therefore forestall senility in its early stages; it is also of obvious aid to people suffering from narrowing of the heart arteries, and in disorders where the blood vessels of the legs are narrowed and insufficient blood supply is the result.

Linus Pauling has reportedly said that if one could only get enough oxygen to the brain cells, depression could be altogether avoided. It is easy to see how niacin would enter into the picture of supplying more oxygen to the brain cells.

HOW OVERFEEDING HASTENS DEATH

More than a generation ago, C. M. McCay and his associates[10] described an experiment in which they prolonged the life of laboratory animals by about a third merely by underfeeding them from birth. Only the total calorie intake was reduced. In all other respects, the animals' diet was kept entirely normal.

I can imagine how many mothers will react to the suggestion that they underfeed their babies! Although pediatricians are beginning to get the message, such a proposal is not only anti-motherhood to most women; it is downright un-American, almost godless. Mothers seem to have a strong instinct to overfeed their babies.

This may have been a useful instinct in the past, when the regular availability of food supply was in doubt. I suspect that our modern views about keeping babies fat is a holdover of the time when a relatively well-fed baby meant that a baby had a better chance of living. Today, it is not only useless; it is dangerous.

Babies are fed formulas containing table sugar. Canned baby foods similarly contain table sugar. The more sugar the foods contain, the better the babies like them. The better they like them, the more they eat, and the richer the manufacturers grow. Given the composition of present-day babies' food, if you cater to Junior's appetite, in all likelihood you shorten his life. So if you want your children to live longer, to ward off for as long as possible the senility that comes with old age, underfeed them from birth, and keep on underfeeding them for as long as their food intake is under your control.

This means: A baby should be at (or better still, slightly below) the weight that is "normal" for his age. Many pediatricians are aware that scientifically it is best for babies not to be overweight, but there is so much pressure from the mothers that often the pediatricians do not pay sufficient attention to overweight conditions.

Although each of us has an inherited pre-programmed time to die, our lifespan probably can be influenced for the better by correct nutrition. McCay's laboratory animals, like us, also had a pre-programmed life span, and yet their lives were increased by a third through low-calorie diets. Translated into human terms, such an increase would mean that a person biologically programmed to die at sixty-six, and underfed from birth, could increase his lifespan to ninety-nine.

HOW PANTOTHENIC ACID HELPS LONGEVITY

Some years ago, Roger Williams, Ph.D., of the University of Texas, grew interested in royal bee jelly because of its extraordinary effect on longevity. If female larva of a bee is fed in the usual way, the result is a drone, an infertile worker bee, whose life as a rule lasts only for a few short weeks in the summer. But if the same larva is fed royal jelly, the result is a fertile queen bee with a lifespan of six to eight years. Williams traced this effect to the royal jelly's high pantothenic acid content.[11]

He took two groups of laboratory mice and fed them the standard laboratory diet (which, I might add, is far superior to the diets of humans. I think we are the only civilization in which laboratory mice and the family dog eat better than man). The diet contained all essential nutritive elements, including some pantothenic acid. But one group of mice had additional pantothenic acid added to their drinking water, so that they averaged 0.3 mg. of extra pantothenic acid daily. The mice in both groups were then observed over their entire lifespan. The forty-one mice on the standard laboratory diet lived for an average of 550 days; the thirty-three mice that were fed the standard chow plus the pantothenic acid in the drinking water lived for an average of 635 days.

Translated into human terms, the first group would have died at age seventy-five; the second group would have lived to be eighty-nine. This strikes me as a sufficiently significant extension to make one consider adding a few pennies' worth of pantothenic acid to one's diet. It seems a relatively cheap way of buying a possible postponement of the old age and senility that haunts us all.

LIVER SPOTS AND AGING

A poignant hallmark of aging is the appearance of brown pigmentation (as mentioned in the chapter on health and beauty) not only on the skin but also in the internal organs and most visibly on the backs of the hands.

Before I became interested in nutritional supplements, these brown spots were regularly appearing on my own hands. After I began taking at least 3000 mg. of niacin, and a like dosage of ascorbic acid in order to lower my serum cholesterol, I gradually observed a marked regression in these brown spots. Today, a number of years later, I can only find two very small ones.

In London, while delivering a paper at the Academy of Orthomolecular Psychiatry, I had an opportunity to discuss this phenomenon with Mark Altschul, M.D., of the Harvard University School of Medicine. He expressed the opinion that this disappearance of pigmentation was probably due to my large intake of vitamin C. Apparently in at least one individual, this particular aspect of aging was reversed by megadoses of this vitamin. While full substantiation of such a statement would require control studies, there is little doubt in my mind that my observations would be proved accurate because I have often observed the same phenomenon in my patients.

HOW INOSITOL AND CHOLINE HELP

Two additional helpers in the battle against aging are the B vitamins inositol and choline, which assist the body to form lecithin (the important emulsifying agent which also reduces blood cholesterol levels). Little is known about inositol. We have not yet been able to establish for certain that it is an essential nutrient, just as a great many other findings in the field of nutrition are not yet established beyond all doubt. I think it would be foolish to assume that inositol is unessential.

In my own dietary planning certainly inositol is essential. Experiments on rats have shown that it is important for the phospholipids, a prominent compound found in brain tissue. It has also been shown to reduce cholesterol in rabbits. Like choline, inositol also prevents fatty infiltration of the liver. And perhaps the most interesting discovery regarding inositol is that human cells grown in a tissue culture have been found to thrive much better when inositol is added to the broth in which they live.[12]

It is therefore probably a good idea to take supplements of choline and inositol in the form of lecithin granules, two heaping tablespoons twice a day.

PABA AND AGING

What about the provocative substance para-aminobenzoic acid (PABA)? [Many years ago, Ansbacher[13] produced achromotricia (gray hair) in rats on a diet deficient in PABA. He then reversed the process and restored their hair color by administering PABA. Since graying of the hair is one of the most ubiquitous characteristics of aging in humans, I thought you might be interested.]

One of the most intriguing facets of the relationship of PABA and aging revolves around Ana Aslan, M.D., who as I mentioned earlier, has been an advocate of a special type of procaine injection (H_3 or Gerovital, an acidified form of procaine buffered with potassium) as a device to retard aging, and even to reverse some of its effects. Procaine is the local anesthetic commonly known in this country as novocaine. You have probably made its acquaintance in the dentist's chair.

For years a violent dispute has been raging through the international medical community regarding Dr. Aslan's findings. They have been rejected by the American medical establishment, though I am far from convinced that this was wise.

You may well ask what a local anesthetic could possibly have to do with aging. The answer is quite simple. The B vitamin PABA makes up part of the molecule of procaine. The procaine, or novocaine, molecule is broken down in the body to release PABA, a fact that seems to have escaped some American observers.

Nutritionist Herman Goldman, M.D., has visited Dr. Aslan's clinic in Romania on several widely-spaced occasions, and reports that some of the patients who appeared to be vegetating when they went into treatment in their sixties became actively engaged in useful pursuits, and were full of life and vigor, ten years later. Perhaps this isn't very conclusive proof of the efficacy of procaine injections, but certainly it is enough to deserve some attention. In addition, H_3 is supposed to have a rejuvenating effect on the glands, especially the pituitary, thyroid, and sex glands.

All the material in this chapter really deals with fighting a battle against premature exit from life. In a battle of little consequence, pop guns may be satisfactory, but in a life-and-death battle I personally prefer a cannon. That's why I favor using any substance that offers hope of helping our enzyme systems to work more effectively and to last longer—especially when the risks involved in the treatment are slight.

Accordingly, some time ago I decided to include H_3 in my own personal therapy. I began using small intramuscular doses to make certain I tolerated it well, and gradually built up to Dr. Aslan's recommended dose of 6 cc. three times weekly for twelve weeks.

Since I felt good when I started the injections it has been difficult for me to judge their effects. Do I have more energy? Is my beard less gray? Probably, but I'm not certain. Will I live longer because of the injections? I hope so!

CELL THERAPY AND AGING

No discussion of the aging process and its retardation would be complete without mentioning cell therapy. Although this form of therapy does not involve a nutritional supplement taken by mouth, it is a form of nutrition, because it uses a substance of biological origins, even though it is administered as an injection. As such, it is not essentially different from crude liver extract, or any of the vitamins that may also be given by injection.

Cell therapy rests on the assumption that "like cures like," and consists of the injection of the cells of various organs of unborn animal fetuses, for the purpose of rejuvenating the corresponding organ in the human patient.

The man who brought it to prominence in Europe was the Swiss physician Paul Niehans. Though Niehans himself died some years ago at the age of 88, his method continues to be used by thousands of physicians all over Euope. Some of the injections still consist of fresh animal fetus cells; but the great majority by now consists of dry frozen material, the result of a cell-preserving process known as lyophilization. In West Germany, for example, the preparation of the cell therapy substance is in the hands of the Hygiene Institute of the University of Heidelberg, and is controlled by the West German Ministry of Health.

Patients undergoing the treatment, which consists of a series of injections, are required to be in residence at the treatment facility, and to avoid all alcohol and tobacco during the course of treatment.

I have not yet been convinced of the benefits of Niehans' cell therapy, but I am keeping an open mind on the subject. Not so the FDA, which has prohibited the use of cell therapy, and the import of lyophilized cell-therapy material into this country. Hence, people who are interested in such treatment must travel to Europe, where their purses are considerably lightened by many practitioners of the technique. I can see no really sound reason why the FDA should not allow cell therapy to be administered in this country, since there appears to be very little danger associated with it, and it is not possible to say with certainty that it is *not* helpful.

In the prestigious scientific journal *Nature*,[14] Drs. Karl R. Merril and Mark I. Greier reported that genetic material had been successfully transferred from bacteria to human cells, and that this genetic material was capable of activating enzymes that could be used by cells grown under artificial conditions and cannot metabolize milk sugars properly. This successful transfer of genetic material from one cell to another suggests that cell therapy deserves more scrutiny by serious scientists, who can now use the more sophisticated apparatus and techniques available for research in cellular enzyme chemistry.

We might write an entire volume on the aging process, its possible causes, and its mental disorders. We might investigate, for example, the reasons for the "pockets of longevity" such as exist in remote rural areas of Russia, Tibet, and South America, where people are said to live active lives to ages 150, 160, and even beyond. We might look at the intriguing phenomena presented by many schizophrenic patients who often appear much younger than their chronological age (and, incidentally, have an exceedingly low rate of cancer).

But such discussions would exceed the practical limits of this book. I therefore bring the topic to a close, with the sincere hope and belief that this, along with the preceeding chapters, will help all of you to lead healthier, happier, more productive, and, yes, longer lives.

NOTES

1. Sigmund Freud.
2. R. L. Walford, *The Immunologic Theory of Aging* (Baltimore, Md.: Williams & Wilkins Co., 1969).

3. L. Robert *et al.*, "Constituants macromoléculaires de la paroi artérille; antigéniticité et role dans l'atherosclérose," *Nat. Rech. Sci.*, Vol. 169, 1968, p. 395.
4. Lester Packer and James R. Smith, "Vitamin E Extends Cells' Life Span," *Medical World News*, October 25, 1974, p. 47.
5. N.Y. Academy of Sciences, "Vitamin E and Its Role in Cellular Metabolism," *Annals of the New York Academy of Sciences*, Vol. 203, December 15, 1972.
6. T. D. Spies in "Nicotinic Acid in the Therapy of Cardiovascular Apparatus," *Niacin in Vascular Disorders and Hyperlipemia*, Rudolf Altschul, ed. (Springfield, Ill.: Charles C Thomas & Co., 1964), p. 167.
7. Luigi Condorelli, *in* Rudolf Altschul, ed., *Niacin in Vascular Disorders* (Springfield, Ill.: Charles C Thomas & Co., 1964), 156–169.
8. E. B. Feldman, *ibid.*, p. 208.
9. E. O. Stenson and S. Stenson, "Regression of Atherosclerosis During Nicotinic Acid Therapy: A Study in Man by Means of Repeated Arteriographs," *in* Rudolf Altschul, ed., *op. cit.*, p. 245.
10. C. M. McCay *et al.*, "Growth, Aging, Chronic Diseases, and Life Span in Rats," *Archives of Biochem.*, Vol. 2, 1943, p. 469.
11. R. B. Pelton and R. J. Williams, "Effect of Pantothenic Acid on Longevity in Mice," *Proceedings of the Society for Experimental and Biological Medicine*, Vol. 99, 1958, p. 632.
12. H. Eagle *et al.*, "Myo-Inositol as an Essential Growth Factor for Normal and Malignant Human Cells in Tissue Culture," *Jrnl. of Biolog. Chem.*, Vol. 226, 1957, p. 191.
13. S. Ansbacher, "P-Aminobenzoic Acid, a Vitamin," *Science*, Vol. 93, 1931, p. 94.
14. Karl R. Merril *et al.*, "Bacterial Virus: Gene Expression in Human Cells," *Nature*, Vol. 233, October 8, 1971, pp. 398–400.

HOW TO SAVE MONEY ON
YOUR NUTRITIONAL NEEDS

In these times most people prune budgets and question every purchase. Although this economy is usually brought on by necessity, the world's resources are limited and waste is always unbecoming. I was shook up the other day to learn that the world's total food supply in storage is enough for only twenty-seven days. Viewed in the great ebb and flow of life in the universe, we occupy a very vulnerable position.

Before giving directions on how to save money on nutrition, let me give you several examples from my practice on how to make money from nutrition.

About seven months ago a twenty-four-year-old woman (I'll call her Joan) visited my office for the first time. She had been holding an important behind-the-scenes job in television until three months previously, when she was demoted to routine office duties with a sixty percent cut in salary. She had been called in by the manager who told her as kindly as possible that her work was no longer adequate. She had missed one or two days of work every few weeks and seemed to have lost her intelligence and her enthusiasm. The company vice president hoped that the reduction in salary and job responsibility would "shake you up enough to bring you back to your former good senses."

The young woman sitting across the desk from me wept as she told her embarrassing story. Her face was puffy. Her skin was so pale she looked as if she had been chained in a dungeon.

She had had hepatitis a year and a half ago and had never recovered her energy. She was so weak that she drank a pot of coffee a day and still could barely drag herself to the office. Saturdays and Sundays she spent in bed, partly because she was too weak to do anything else and partly because she was trying in the only way she knew to regain enough strength to go to work for another week.

She had had a good marriage for four years before her slump began. Finally her husband had decided she was lazy, inadequate, and anything but the energetic, interesting girl he had married. After she had been exhausted for a year, he insisted that her doctor consult with another internist for a complete work-up. Both physicians agreed she was in good health, but depressed and should see a psychiatrist.

She then visited a psychiatrist several times who also thought she was depressed and began probing into her marriage and past life to explain her lack of enthusiasm for life. When this tack did not produce results, she stopped "therapy."

At this point her husband became thoroughly disgusted and left her.

When she saw me, one and a half years had passed since the beginning of her hepatitis. She still complained of all the difficulties I have mentioned plus weak legs, eyes that burned, and a puffiness and swelling not only of her face but of her hands and ankles. Her hair was dry and she said that she was excessively sensitive to cold. The history revealed that she was taking multiple vitamin tablets, lecithin, and vitamin E.

I require all my new patients to have a physical examination. In the case of Joan, because of her history of hepatitis, I felt that a work-up for possible chronic liver disease was indicated. I sent her to a liver specialist at Mount Sinai Hospital in New York. He hospitalized her for a thorough examination, including a liver biopsy. He concluded that she had no liver disease and felt her symptoms were due to a psychoneurosis.

Here is what I found on a routine clinical work-up: Her six-hour glucose tolerance test was abnormal; a sharp drop (87 mg. percent) in her blood sugar level during a one-hour period indicated hypoglycemia.

At the time of the sharp drop, she became nauseated, weak, and sweaty. A hair test for minerals revealed that she had a tissue deficiency of sodium, potassium, magnesium, and calcium. Her estrogen and serum folic acid levels were also abnormally low.

Blood tests showed that she was also low in vitamin B_1, B_6, and nicotinamide adenine dinucleotide. Sublingual tests showed that she was allergic to twenty-one out of twenty-four substances for which she was tested. She fell asleep when tested for mold. She became very tired when tested for fish. When tested for cats she became flushed in the face, began sweating, and fell asleep for about fifteen minutes. She felt excessively tired after being tested for corn, and developed a headache and pains in both knees after being tested for milk.

I put Joan on a diet that eliminated the foods to which she was most sensitive. Other foods to which she was only mildly allergic were rotated so that she ate them only every four or five days, a technique that helps reduce all-over sensitivity reactions to foods in those patients who are allergic to so many nutrients that it is impossible to eliminate them all.

I gave her a vitamin-mineral regimen to correct her deficiencies, and, because of her history of sensitivity to cold, her dry skin ahd hair, and her low morning temperatures, I prescribed thyroid tablets even though her thyroid tests were normal.

I gave her a trial on vitamin B_{12b}, even though she had a normal vitamin B_{12} level. She felt a great deal more energy after having B_{12b}, and now gets an injection every week from a neighborhood nurse.

During the first two months of therapy, this patient made slow but quite definite progress. Her energy increased and her taste for life began to return. But we noticed that sometimes she became depressed and tired after visiting a cottage on Long Island in which she owned a share. Then we discovered that she had trouble only on rainy weekends. We concluded this was due to her mold allergies, since the cottage would be moldier on wet weekends and she would stay inside more. When we eliminated her visits on rainy weekends, her painful bouts of fatigue and depression faded away.

Incidentally, when Joan went into her mold allergy slump, her face, ankles and hands became swollen. This swelling (edema) is a typical allergic reaction. A traditional physician would prescribe a diuretic to promote water loss—exactly the wrong treatment for a person like Joan: it does nothing to treat the allergy that caused the problem, and it drains the system of sodium. (In common with many depressed people Joan had an abnormally low sodium level in the first place.)

After three months Joan was greatly improved. She had a sparkle to her personality again. Her face had lost its sallow puffiness. She was able to think clearly and her memory returned. She had regained her old efficiency at work, and with it her old job. Her lost interest in sex returned and she began dating. I did not retest her estrogen level and did not give her estrogens because I felt that her hormone levels would return to normal after her biochemistry was corrected. Her periods, which had stopped altogether, did return. At first they were painful and unpleasant but soon they became quite normal.

When Joan visited me this week she reported a $3,000 raise in salary. She now earns more money because she has the energy, the will to work, the intelligence and enthusiasm that she had lost while sick. In plain dollars and cents, many people who follow the directions in this book will earn more money like this patient who is back in the swing of life again after having languished for a year and a half.

As I so frequently tell patients, an investment in good health is a capital investment that will pay off; it is not money down the drain as is spending money for a night on the town. The catch is that the money must be spent for good medical care, not the inadequate care that most people had received prior to being studied from a nutritional standpoint.

Let me tell you next about Ann, an honors college graduate who came to me while barely holding on to a three-day-a-week clerical job because she was almost incapacitated by schizophrenia, which had not been helped by psychotherapy at a famous private clinic or by any of the three private psychiatrists she had seen. After six months of nutritional therapy she took a full-time job and now has moved up to a very gratifying position in one of New York's major industries. Now that she is healthy again, she not only earns more money but has gotten back her self-respect and is alive once more.

Two months ago I saw a patient from Philadelphia who had been in severe depression for more than a year. He had made two serious suicide attempts. He had been admitted to Silver Springs Psychiatric Hospital in Maryland on two occasions and was receiving psychotherapy when I first saw him. Tests revealed low tissue calcium, magnesium, and iron.

He was also borderline low in testosterone (male sex hormone). I put him on injections of testosterone and mineral vitamin supplements.

After about two weeks his depression began to lift, and now, eight weeks later, he is prepared to return to work. When he first visited me he was about to lose a very responsible position because he simply had not been able to function at work. He will soon be returning to full responsibility and I have every reason to think that he will be even more effective than in the past.*

The economic advantages gained by these three patients are obvious. Because they feel better, they can earn more money. Before they corrected their nutritional and hormonal deficiencies they were disorganized, depressed, and used up most of their low energy reserves merely to hold themselves together. They had little left to give to their employers. Now they are on the ball, full of vim, enthusiastic, and imaginative: assets to their employers.

Protein, in the long run, costs less than sugar and macaroni. Buying vitamins is cheaper than skipping vitamins. All I advise is: Give nutrition a fair trial. In the long haul I truly believe preventive medicine pays for itself many times over, not only with improved income, but with better health, more happiness, and a longer life. Only you can be the judge of that, but you can't judge until you try it.

HOW TO WATCH YOUR STEP
IN HEALTH FOOD STORES

A word of caution: Like supermarkets, most health food stores are carefully arranged to parade you past shelves of frivolous junk before you get to the nutritional supplements of solid value that you seek. We are a nation of impulse buyers; don't be deceived into thinking that Wholesome Wheat Crunchies or Pure Unrefined Honey Buns are any less harmful because you find them in the same store as the yeast and the organic meat. If you are sensitive to wheat and carbohydrates, their relative purity may make little difference.

Similarly, beware of the strawberry face-creams and other "organic"

* Six months have passed. He's working better than ever before and earning more money. Also, his sex life is great and his sick marriage has recovered.

goos and cosmetics. Probably more people are allergic to strawberries than to any inexpensive unscented cold cream. Ice-creams, Granola, processed soups and other food mixes and snacks cost much more in health food stores than elsewhere. The only advantage of the health food products is that they are probably (but not always) free of chemical additives. You still should not have them.

WHAT TO BUY AT THE HEALTH FOOD STORE

Of the foods you can buy either here or at a supermarket, you should opt for organically produced nuts, seeds, nut butters, and cooking oils. The fact that these foods are naturally produced, without chemicals, food coloring, heat processing, or hydrogenation makes a difference worth paying more for.

HOW VALUABLE ARE HEALTH BOOKS?

To spare yourself expense and a wealth of confusing misinformation, resist crackpot health fad books on sale at most health food stores. If you want a sound basic book on nutrition for yourself (or to give to your doctor) I recommend *Nutrition Against Disease* by Roger Williams, Ph.D. Books by nutritionist Carlton Fredericks are also sound, and Adelle Davis' books are often useful, though dated.

I mention Adelle Davis because her work has been so popular that her opinions have been read like the Bible. I appreciate that she has done as much as anyone to popularize pure foods and the importance of adequate vitamin intake, but her work reflects none of the more recent advances in the field of food allergies, and I strongly disagree with her advocacy of whole wheat, milk, cheese, and yogurt for all. In fact I know of no book, other than this one, in the nutrition field that takes adequate account of food allergies.

FORM A CO-OP FOR ORGANIC FOOD

If you have reason to believe that sensitivity to food additives is causing you emotional problems, it will be important for you to find a source of pure or "organically grown" meats and vegetables. Many health food stores supply produce and frozen meat and poultry, but it does tend to be expensive. The best solution I know to this problem is to form or join a food cooperative; members pool time and resources, buying food wholesale to divide among themselves at no mark-up.

Food co-ops report that they can save their members from forty to sixty percent on their food bills every week, which is clearly an admirable saving whether you want organic food or not. The important thing will be for you to join with members who share your attitudes toward food since they buy in bulk for everyone in the group. You cannot pick and choose the way you do in a retail store.

Not every food co-op is interested in organic food. Many buy from the same sources as the supermarkets. Others rely heavily on grains and dairy products. If you would like to start your own cooperative of like-minded people, I recommend *How to Start Your Own Food Cooperative,* by Gloria Stern, published by Walker & Co.

Your co-op can also get help from your city government or from the U.S. Department of Agriculture. In New York, the New York Community Training Institute, 225 Lafayette Street, New York, N.Y. (212-431-6964) will give you advice about organizing. You can also receive a market newsletter published three times a week with news of the best local food buys, by writing to the U.S. Department of Agriculture Market News, Room 4A, Hunts Point Market, Bronx, N.Y. (212-542-2225). Elsewhere, too, local offices of the U.S. Department of Agriculture provide similar services.

THE CHEAPEST POSSIBLE PURE FOODS DIET

As you know, I believe most people do best on a diet of meat protein. As you also know, meat is the most expensive item in your budget and not everyone can afford to eat the diet I recommend, no matter how they stretch their budgets. Chicken, turkey, and fish are less expensive sources of high quality protein, although they provide less fat than beef, lamb, or pork, and fat is important to those who need to keep their blood sugar stable. When you eat poultry, do eat the skin, which is fatty, and when you eat canned fish, don't let the oil get away. In the vegetable kingdom many foods contain some amino acids, although only soybeans contain all eight. Soybeans are excellent and inexpensive. Anyone on a limited budget should eat them frequently.

When you use vegetables as a source of protein, it's important to learn how to combine foods so that the missing acids in one vegetable will be supplied by another in the same dish or at least at the same meal. The main foods in such a regimen are seeds, legumes (peas, beans, lentils, and the like) and grains, principally rice. Agrarian cultures throughout history have evolved peasant dishes that supply complete proteins in this way; brown rice and beans is one such combination; Middle Eastern tahine sauce, which combines chick peas and sesame seed paste, is another. Many Oriental vegetable dishes combining rice, sesame seeds, and soybean curd are also good sources of protein.

Remember: the key to vegetable protein benefits is to eat the right foods *at the same time.* If you eat kidney beans at one meal and rice at the next, you supply your body with substantially less usable protein than if you ate exactly the same amount of each food in the same meal.

Incidentally, yeast contains a very high grade of protein. Vegetable proteins have become a source of increasing interest because of the world food crisis. Ecologically, it is far more extravagant to raise a cow on grains and fodder than to eat the grains and fodder yourself. This is called eating lower on the food chain, and if the world population keeps growing at its present rate, we may all be forced to eat this way eventually. This is a form of starvation. We were ontologically designed to eat meat.

Some people oppose eating meat on moral grounds. They feel it is wrong to slaughter animals for feed. Some people even believe meat-eating increases their aggressive tendencies. I personally suspect that being properly nourished has more to do with the control of aggressions than anything else, but of course there *are* people who are allergic to meat. Perhaps their moral distaste for meat eating is a result of a sensitivity to meat that does indeed make them depressed or hostile.

In any case, it would be foolish to pretend that everyone will rush out and eat steak three times a day, no matter how persuasive I am. If you don't like it, are morally opposed to it, or can't afford it, I might as well shout down a well. So if you want to learn more about vegetable protein read *Diet for a Small Planet*, by Frances Moore Lappe. It is available in paperback from Ballantine Books.

A LOW-PRICED WAY TO RAISE BLOOD SUGAR

For those who can't afford meat every day but must control their blood sugar, try adding a piece of fatback to your vegetable dishes. This very inexpensive source of fat will help stabilize your blood sugar while your beans and brewers' yeast supply you with protein. If you cannot afford both a high-meat diet and vitamin supplements, you would be much better off to eat this way and to spend your last dime on the rock-bottom basic nutritional supplements I am about to describe.

STRETCHING YOUR MEAT WAY OUT

Many supermarkets are now offering a form of ground beef that has been stretched with vegetable protein—principally ground soybeans. If you are not allergic to soybeans (and it is not a common allergy) this is an excellent way to keep meat in your diet. Read the label carefully to be sure no chemical preservatives or wheat have been added.

If you want to be even more economical you can make your own ground meat and soybean mixture. Soak soybeans overnight in water or soup stock. They will increase to almost double in bulk. You can grind up the soaked beans in a blender or food mill and add them to practically anything for extra protein at very little cost, or simply toss them into beef patties or meatloaf as is. After soaking they have the consistency of a raw peanut (rather crunchy).

Remember: a peanut is a legume, not a nut. If you prefer a more mushy, bean-like consistency, cook the soybeans in water or stock for several hours before adding them to the meat. Incidentally you can use peanuts (caution: many people are allergic to peanuts) in exactly the same way, although they are more expensive and less complete than soybeans.

To stretch the meat even further, add seeds (see *Diet for a Small Planet* to learn which ones to use for the best protein). Add cooked brown rice, and chunks of steamed potato, sweet potato, winter squash, or eggplant—or all of them—to meat for a nourishing, filling, high-protein low-cost meatloaf or casserole.

Bean curd from any Oriental specialty store is also an extremely inexpensive high-protein meal stretcher. Orientals, who eat no dairy products, often use bean curd to complete seed or rice proteins, much as a Western cook would add cheese. Remember also that eggs are still an excellent and relatively inexpensive source of protein and essential nutrients. An egg or two in any meatloaf or casserole boosts the value and makes a low-fat mixture hang together better.

African, Near Eastern, and Far Eastern cookery also make good use of peanut butter and sesame paste. Don't imagine that peanut butter is just for kids. The supermarket variety of peanut butter is hydrogenated, robbed of lecithin and essential fatty acids, and laced with sugar (dextrose) and preservatives. Avoid it. Buy non-processed peanut butter from a health food store or make your own. Seed and nut butters from a health food store can form the basis for delicious sauces and dips which combine with beans or rice to make a valuable protein.

Chinese Vegetarian Cooking by Kenneth H. C. Lo (Pantheon Books, cloth or paperback) is an excellent introduction to this kind of cooking. In addition to providing unusually good recipes, it will teach you the correct way to steam or stir-fry a vegetable without cooking out all the food value. It also gives instructions for adding meat to the recipes if you prefer.

HERE'S FREE PROTEIN!

Many people avoid inexpensive cuts of meat because they contain bones, which they consider waste. Bones are a valuable food. Don't throw bones away. Bones contain mineral deposits of calcium held together by a matrix of protein. Even save the bones left on people's plates after dinner (they're going to be boiled, so don't worry about germs).

You should also save the hearts and gizzards of poultry that you ordinarily throw away. If the butcher trims meat or bones for you after weighing, be sure he gives you everything you paid for. (Some butchers will also let you have other people's unwanted bones free, or at very low cost.)

After you have saved a pot full of bone and meat scraps, add water, cover, and simmer for three or four hours. The resulting stock will turn into a jelly that is nearly pure protein. You can use it in soups, sauces, or casseroles, or whenever a recipe calls for soaking or cooking in water. And if you still want to use the calcium left in the bones, you can cook them to death in a pressure cooker and eat them. Very good protein. Very good calcium. The information in this paragraph will save you the price of this book at least once a week.

PET FOOD—A NOBLE EXPERIMENT

I have said several times that the average American dog is better nourished than his owner. According to recent estimates, as much as forty percent of the pet food sold in America is being bought by people who don't have pets. I reasoned that some dog foods are animal protein, and that thirty cents' worth of protein is better for you than thirty cents' worth of macaroni. I decided to try a meal with dog food to test it myself.

I chose Thanksgiving Day so I would have time to recover in case I got sick. I selected cans of Alpo, Ken-L Ration, and Carnations' Mighty Dog. The first two contained preservatives, so I rejected them. I ate parts of a can of Mighty Dog Beef and Chicken, and Mighty Dog London Broil. They tasted very much alike. Both needed salt and pepper. I am happy to report no unpleasant side-effects whatever. That's the good news.

The bad news is that dog food isn't really cheaper. A six-and-a-half-ounce can costs thirty-one cents at this writing. That works out to nearly eighty cents a pound. You can buy beef and soy bean pattie mix for less, or make your own beef and soy mix. On the whole, I must conclude that dog food probably won't kill you, but there are better solutions to the problem.

If my budget were strained to the limit, there are certain basic items of nutrition I would buy if it meant limiting my diet to rice, beans, and fatback. The first of these is yeast.

CHOOSING YEAST THE LOW-BUDGET WAY

As you learned in the chapter on planning your vitamin regimen, yeast is fifty percent protein, thus providing important amino acids that enable the body to use its other food better and to manufacture certain essential nutrients. It is also a rich source of the known B vitamins, and quite possibly contains others as yet undiscovered.

By far the least expensive source of B vitamins you can buy is torula yeast. In my health food store, one pound of torula yeast costs $1.65 as against $2.10 for the cheapest brewers' yeast. Eight grams, or one heaping teaspoon, contains 7 mg. of thiamin as against 4 mg. in *fourteen* grams, or a heaping tablespoon, of brewers' yeast. It contains more of the other B vitamins in roughly the same proportion. Thus it costs less, and you need only half as much to do the same job. Note well: nutritional research has revealed that brewers' and primary yeast contain small amounts of nutritional essentials *not* found in torula yeast. Torula yeast is excellent, but should not make up more than fifty percent of your yeast intake.

You will probably find various doctored types of yeast on health food shelves. Some contain added vitamins, notably B_{12}. Some yeasts are flavored or "instant" to dissolve more easily. Read the labels carefully. In yeast, as in any food, you want as little processing as possible. In any case, the more it has been tampered with, the more it will cost.

GETTING VITAMIN C (ASCORBIC ACID) THE LOW-BUDGET WAY

The next essential basic is vitamin C. Ascorbic acid powder is much less expensive than buying vitamin C tablets or capsules. It is also better tolerated, provided you take it well diluted. Remember to buy powder rather than crystals. Some crystals are mistakenly labeled "powder." The powder looks like baby powder, the crystals like sugar. The crystals are often poorly tolerated. Be sure the powder contains no filler. You may be offered a powdered form of vitamin C that costs less per bottle than pure ascorbic acid. If the strength is not close to 4000 mg. per teaspoon, then the powder has been cut and is no bargain. Some hot-shot vitamin pushers have begun to copy heroin pushers.

Beans can easily be sprouted at home. They offer an excellent source of vitamin C, as do all other types of sprouts.

GETTING VITAMINS A AND D
THE LOW-BUDGET WAY

The third essential is a pearl (natural source) containing both vitamin A (10,000 units) and of vitamin D (400 units). The larger the jar, the more you are likely to save. Combining the two vitamins in one pearl is less expensive than buying the vitamins separately.

VITAMIN E ON A TIGHT BUDGET

Vitamin E is expensive. Nevertheless, I consider it an essential source of natural Alpha-tocopherol to counteract the effects of stress and pollution, and to combat aging. If you can possibly afford it, take a 200 I.U. capsule a day; if not, cut down to 100 I.U.'s daily.

These are the nutrients I consider basic. In an emergency, I would cut down on solid food before cutting these out. Only slightly lower on the priority list stands lecithin. If you have any history of high blood pressure or heart disease in your family; if you are a man in your thirties or older or a woman past menopause—I would recommend two tablespoons of lecithin granules daily. Since you are leaving out milk, you must add a teaspoon of dolomite powder at bedtime, to insure an adequate intake of calcium and magnesium.

HOW TO FIND
MEDICAL HELP FOR
YOUR NUTRITIONAL PROBLEMS

CHAPTER TWENTY-THREE

We all harbor delusions. A wife may be deluded into thinking her husband is the most brilliant man in his field. If he is a certified public accountant, she may hear night after night about the clever little twists that he has discovered during his working day to save his clients' money, convincing her time and time again that no one can really touch him in the field of accounting.

In some ways, physicians are perhaps the most deluded people of all. Each physician, if pressed, will admit that other physicians might be well-trained and have proper qualifications, but he also believes that none has his great learning and innate talent—the unique combination of qualities that make him the greatest healer in his particular field. Perhaps physicians must have this delusion, if only because they do deal every day in life-or-death decisions. What other person, minute after minute, hour after hour, day after day, year after year, makes decisions in which the stake is as important as human sanity or life? Does not anyone who lives out his years with this responsibility need the delusion that he is a god, that he is unsurpassed as a decision-maker? Otherwise how could he possibly handle so much responsibility?

As a physician, I also entertain the delusion that I am a great healer. And when you ask great healers to recommend other healers, you ask them to perform a difficult task. What would Mohammed say if someone had asked him what spiritual leader to consult in his absence?

No two conventional physicians practice exactly alike, although today there is a tendency for more standardization of medical practice, what is referred to in some quarters as "cookbook medicine." Among physicians who are interested in nutrition, there is much more variation in their approach and techniques than among physicians who confine themselves to helping the sick through the use of standard medications.

I have all the qualifications for using standard medical approaches to treat illness and frequently do use these approaches in combination with nutritional approaches. What I do to help sick people get better has gradually evolved into the system set forth in this book. The reason why a physician's activities are referred to as "practicing medicine" is because no physician can ever learn all the intricacies of the science and art of healing. And so my system still grows. I use the approaches that I have described here only because they give me the best results in my practice. You should not expect my approach to treatment to be like anyone else's approach in his own practice.

Other physicians know more than I about psychiatry. Others know more than I about the effect of allergies, vitamins, minerals, and hormones on the central nervous system. But I do have a good knowledge of these subjects and, more important, I have integrated them in a system to help people, especially those with emotional difficulties. Using the foregoing as my perspective, let me tell you about other sources of medical help for nutritional problems:

1. *William H. Philpott, M.D., psychiatrist, 33915 Del Obispo, Dana Point, California 92629, (714) 496-3911.*

Dr. Philpott is the psychiatrist whose approach is the closest to mine. Naturally, I think he is a very good psychiatrist.

Dr. Philpott, unlike me, takes care of children as well as adults. He treats hospitalized patients as well as office patients, whereas I usually see patients only in my office.

2. *Marshall Mendell, M.D., 160 East Avenue, Norwalk, Connecticut, (203) 838-4706.*

Dr. Mendell is an allergist—a rare one because he has a deep knowledge of food and environmental allergies. He does sublingual testing for foods the same as I. If I had any kind of allergy, I would certainly consult Dr. Mendell. Note, however, that he is not a psychiatrist.

3. *Theron G. Randolph, M.D., 720 North Michigan Avenue, Chicago, Illinois, (312) 828-9481.*

I hope Dr. Randolph will not be offended if I refer to him as the "Grand Old Man" of food and environmental allergies. He is a creative and gifted physician who has not been sufficiently appreciated by his generation. Dr. Randolph does food allergy tests primarily by admitting patients to a hospital for several weeks where they fast and are then given food-provocative tests. Dr. Randolph is an internist, not a psychiatrist.

4. For general health information, I suggest that you study several authors. As I have mentioned earlier, I particularly fond of Roger Williams' book entitled *Nutrition Against Disease*. This professor of biochemistry at the University of Texas has had a long and brilliant career in the field of nutrition. His book is a great first book for everyone to read. It would be difficult for you to choose a better gift for your physician than *Nutrition Against Disease*. Quietly and without trying to jolt the reader with fear or in any way being spectacular, Dr. Williams builds a great case against the way American medicine is practiced today, and presents the plain facts of the importance of nutrition in any therapeutic program.

He also has written several other books, and you will find them all in your health food store in soft cover editions.

5. *Carlton Fredericks, Ph.D.*, is the author of several books on nutrition that I have already recommended. I have in mind particularly his books *Low Blood Sugar And You*, New York, Grosset & Dunlap 1970, and *Eating Right For You*, New York, Grosset & Dunlap, 1972. Dr. Fredericks has a lecture course in nutrition at Fairleigh Dickinson University in Rutherford, New Jersey (near New York City). Some of

these courses are taught in the evening, so they are easily available to adults.

I know of no other adequate nutrition course being taught today. If you want to learn more about the subject, reading his books and attending his courses would be a great step forward for almost anyone.

6. *Abram Hoffer, M.D., Ph.D., 1201 CN Towers, First Avenue South, Saskatoon, Saskatchewan, Canada (306) 165-4933*, is a psychiatrist who became famous for advocating niacin in the treatment of schizophrenia. To his great credit, Dr. Hoffer has expanded his interests to include general nutrition in the treatment of emotional disorders and has even recently become interested in allergies as they affect schizophrenia and the central nervous system. I know of no one in the world who knows more about the treatment of schizophrenia than Dr. Hoffer. I can recommend him without reservation.

7. *David R. Hawkins, M.D., 1355 Northern Boulevard, Manhasset, New York, 11030, (516) 627-7530.*

Dr. Hawkins, is, along with Linus Pauling, the co-editor of the book *Orthomolecular Psychiatry*, published by W. H. Freeman & Co., San Francisco, California. This book is a collection of technical articles on the vitamin approach to the treatment of schizophrenia. It is aimed primarily at professional audiences. Some of the articles are only fair and others are quite good.

Dr. Hawkins is a psychiatrist with a wide knowledge of vitamin therapy for emotional illnesses, especially for the treatment of schizophrenia and alcoholism. He is also beginning to take an interest in food allergies as they affect emotional illnesses, and has started to incorporate these new ideas in his practice.

Dr. Hawkins runs a private clinic. During my contacts with other members of the clinic, I found that their knowledge of nutritional therapy is less than Dr. Hawkins'.

8. *The North Nassau Mental Health Center, at 1691 Northern Boulevard, Manhasset, New York 11030, (516) 627-7550* will furnish you with the names and addresses of members of the Academy of Orthomolecular Psychiatry. There are perhaps two hundred members scattered throughout the world. Like any relatively large organization, it consists

of individuals with widely varying talents and training. The interest of members tends to concentrate on the treatment of schizophrenia with large doses of synthetic vitamins. A number of members also have good knowledge of hypoglycemia. Some are becoming interested in the effects of food allergies. Hopefully this trend will gain momentum because I believe it is not possible to treat emotional illnesses adequately unless food and environmental allergies are tested for and taken into consideration in the therapeutic program. Most of the members of this organization are psychiatrists.

9. A list of the members of another professional organization, the *International College of Applied Nutrition*, can be obtained from the office of the secretary, P.O. Box 386, LaHabra, California 90631. ICAN has a large membership of physicians from various specialties who are interested in nutrition. I am not personally acquainted with many of them and the exact caliber of their work. However, from attending their meetings I would say that their heart is in the right place and they are certainly trying to help the public and physicians to become more interested in nutritional approaches to all medical problems.

10. *Lawrence Dickey, M.D., 109 W. Olive St., Fort Collins, Colorado, (303) 482-6001* is a former surgeon who has become interested in allergies, especially food and environmental allergies, and has become an expert in the field. No one with an allergy problem would go wrong seeing him.

11. *Fred Klenner, M.D.*, is a general practitioner in Reidsville, North Carolina. (919) 349-5432. As I have said earlier, he probably knows more about ascorbic acid than anyone in the world and has a great knowledge about the use of vitamins and minerals for physical illnesses. If I were suffering from Parkinsonism, multiple sclerosis, or amyotrophic lateral sclerosis, I would be especially anxious to consult Dr. Klenner. Incidentally, he has a son in medical school who will soon be joining him, and Dr. Klenner has taught his son well.

12. *The International Academy of Metabology, Inc.*, with headquarters at 2236 Suree Ellen Lane, Altadena, California 91001, (213) 798-0409, will give you a list of members, all of whom are interested in

nutrition. Only a few of the members are psychiatrists. Again I agree with some members' approaches to treatment and disagree with others'.

13. *Warren Levine, M.D., 140 Joralemon St., Brooklyn, New York 11201 (212) 624-1975,* is a family doctor with a wide knowledge of nutrition.

14. *Prevention Magazine,* available from Rodale Press Inc., 33 East Minor St., Emmaus, Pennsylvania, 18049.

The field of psychiatry, in particular, is in a state of flux. More and more psychiatrists are beginning to question the traditions and clichés of the past. They are becoming more eclectic in their choice of treatment. More and more of them are becoming dissatisfied with the results that their efforts are producing in their patients. Patients are becoming increasingly sophisticated and demanding, and I think it's high time that they expect more and get more from their therapists.

If your search for a doctor who is experienced in up-to-date nutrition is unsuccessful, let me urge you again to show this book to an open-minded physician who is within your reach; urge him to read the literature to which I refer throughout; and do your best to persuade him to treat you accordingly. You deserve it.

VITAMINS AT A GLANCE:
WHAT'S WHAT AND WHICH IS WHICH

Although this is primarily a book about mental health, it should be clear by now that the reason vitamins do affect your emotions is that they affect the physical environment in which your emotions work; that is, you body. So here, for quick reference, is what each vitamin does physically. This is to help you see at a glance what physical symptoms may indicate a deficiency in a certain vitamin; what factors may cause you to need more of a certain vitamin than your neighbor (or than your cave-dwelling ancestors); and what amount of each vitamin is officially recommended. (My own recommendations are different and are discussed in the text.)

I have included entries on which vitamins work together. This is to remind you that even when you have an apparently adequate intake of one vitamin, it may not be able to do its job if you are low in one of the elements it combines with.

I have also included a brief list of the chief dietary sources of each vitamin, because natural crude sources of vitamins are always important. I have not attempted to report exactly how much of each vitamin is contained in each food, because, as you know, this fluctuates wildly according to where the food was produced, how long it has been stored, and how it is cooked. And I repeat, you should not rely on food sources alone to provide an adequate intake of vitamins.

I have omitted the B vitamins choline, inositol, and PABA, because I consider research on them to be very incomplete. And while accepted medical practice is to group vitamins according to whether they are fat- or water-soluble, I have chosen to list them here in alphabetical order for the sake of clarity.

VITAMIN A. Fat-soluble.

Chief Functions: When adequately supplied, vitamin A helps maintain normal growth and bone development; it helps to provide protective sheathing around nerve fibres; and it helps to maintain healthy skin and hair and nails. It is especially crucial to healthy vision. Vitamin A is present in the eyes themselves and is used up in the process of seeing. When it is deficient the eye has trouble processing light, particularly bright or artificial light. It helps to maintain healthy mucous in the respiratory system, and thus helps to fight infection and allergic symptoms.

Symptoms of Deficiency: Impaired vision, particularly "night blindness" and sensitivity to bright lights; poor growth and bone development, especially in children; impaired hormone production; dandruff, or other dryness or itching of skin and scalp; dry brittle nails; susceptibility to colds and allergies; tooth decay.

Works With: Vitamins B_2, B_{12}, C, D, and especially E.

Factors Affecting Need: Exposure to bright or artificial lights, and to movies and television; exposure to environmental pollutants including air pollution, cigarette smoke, and toxic food additives such as sodium benzoate; insufficient proteins, fats, and liver bile (impairs absorption); liver damage.

Best Dietary Sources: Yellow fruits and vegetables such as carrots, yams, winter squash, peaches, and apricots; also spinach, parsley, turnip greens and other dark green leafy vegetables; liver, including fish liver and fish liver oils.

Minimum Daily Intake: 5,000 I.U.'s.

Overdose Symptoms: (Produced by a daily intake of 50,000 to 100,000 I.U.'s over several months); headaches, nerve damage (with attendant nervous symptoms); fatigue, insomnia, loss of appetite, pain in bones and joints, jaundice, loss of hair.

Where It is Stored: In the liver and kidneys. It is believed that vitamin A helps the liver to purify the blood of environmental poisons.

How Long It is Stored: Long term storage.

VITAMIN B_1 (Thiamin). Water-soluble.

Chief Functions: Helps in carbohydrate metabolism, growth, maintaining appetite and good digestion, and in nerve function.

Symptoms of Deficiency: Beri-beri; heart pain or failure; nerve death; depression, tension, insomnia, forgetfulness; weight loss; numbness in extremities; swelling in ankles and elsewhere.

Works With: Vitamins B_2, B_3, B_6, B_{12}, C, D, and pantothenic acid.

Factors Affecting Need: While it is present in many foods it is easily destroyed by soaking and cooking; older people may fail to absorb it adequately.

Best Dietary Sources: Wheat germ, yeast, rice bran, soy flour, ham, beans, eggs, beef, pork, lamb, turkey, mushrooms.

Minimum Daily Intake: 1.5 milligrams.

Overdose Symptoms: Edema, restlessness, sweating, rapid heart beat, cold sores; trembling, low blood pressure, liver disorders; vitamin B_6 deficiency.

Where It is Stored: Heart, liver, kidney, brain.

How Long It is Stored: Short term storage.

VITAMIN B_2 (Riboflavin). Water-soluble.

Chief Functions: Necessary in every cell in body; especially helps maintain respiratory system mucous membranes; necessary to healthy skin and eye tissue.

Symptoms of Deficiency: Dandruff; skin lesions, cracks in the corners of the mouth; inflamed tongue and mouth; nerve degeneration; hormonal defects; sensitivity to bright light, and other visual difficulty.

Works With: Vitamins A, B_1, B_3, B_6, B_{12}, folic acid, pantothenic acid, and biotin.

Factors Affecting Need: Riboflavin is easily lost in urine (i.e. your need may be increased if you drink and pass a lot of liquid); it is destroyed by light.

Best Dietary Sources: Yeast, kidney, liver, heart, avacados, beans, green vegetables, wheat germ.

Minimum Daily Intake: 1.7 milligrams.

Overdose Symptoms: Tingling in extremities; itching.

Where It is Stored: Heart, liver, kidney.

How Long It is Stored: Short term storage.

VITAMIN B_3 (Niacin, Niacinamide, Nicotinic acid). Water-soluble.

Chief Functions: Co-enzyme in your fat metabolism (important in controlling blood fat levels); principally significant in complex chemical interactions affecting the working of the nervous system. For this reason, niacin has been critically important in the nutritional treatment of mental illness.

Symptoms of Deficiency: Pellegra; depression, nervousness, weakness, insomnia, headache; loss of appetite; skin disorders; diarrhea.

Works With: Vitamins B_1, B_2, B_6, B_{12}, D, pantothenic acid, and folic acid.

Factors Affecting Need: While much may be lost in cooking, or through impaired absorption caused by illness, it is likely that one of the greatest thieves of niacin stores is emotional stress, which is also the most typical symptom of niacin deficiency.

Best Dietary Sources: Yeast, liver, heart, turkey, chicken, peanuts, tuna, halibut, swordfish.

Minimum Daily Intake: 20 milligrams.

Overdose Symptoms: Nausea; vomiting; activation of peptic ulcer.

Where It is Stored: Liver, heart, muscle.

How Long It is Stored: Short term storage.

VITAMIN B_6 (Pyridoxine). Water-soluble.

Chief Functions: Important in red blood cell formation and in production of hormones in the central nervous system. Used in metabolism of carbohydrates, fats, and all proteins.

Deficiency Symptoms: Nervous disorders; convulsions, tension, rashes; blood disorders; hardening of the arteries; edema.

Works With: Vitamins B_1, B_2, B_3, folic acid, biotin, C, E, and adrenalin.

Factors Affecting Need: B_6 is rapidly destroyed by heat (i.e. lost in cooking); also easily lost in water, through soaking food or frequent urination; B_6 is affected by estrogen levels. Nausea or morning sickness caused by pregnancy or the Pill is often helped by additional B_6. Since B_6 is used in protein metabolism, a high protein diet often causes an elevated need for B_6.

Best Dietary Sources: Yeast, beef and pork liver, salmon, herring, brown rice, bananas, and pears.

Minimum Daily Intake: 2.5 milligrams.

Overdose Symptoms: Virtually unknown.

Where It is Stored: Skeletal muscles.

How Long It is Stored: Short term storage.

VITAMIN B_{12} (Cobalamin). Water-soluble.

Chief Function: Used in production of nucleic acid (therefore important to health of all body cells); affects protein and fat cells, including production of genetic material DNA and RNA; used to maintain sheaths on nerve tissue; important in blood formation.

Deficiency Symptoms: Poor growth; inflamed tongue; disturbed carbohydrate metabolism; fatigue; anemia, including pernicious anemia; spinal cord degeneration; brain degeneration; any emotional disorder up to and including insanity.

Works With: Vitamins A, C, E, B_1, folic acid, biotin, and pantothenic acid.

Factors Affecting Need: Vegetarian diet or any diet low in animal protein may cause B_{12} deficiency. Many people cannot absorb B_{12} when taken orally, so that their B_{12} levels can only be maintained by injections.

Best Dietary Sources: Lamb and beef kidney; lamb, beef and pork liver; beef brain; egg yolk; clams, sardines, oysters, crabs, salmon, herring.

Minimum Daily Intake: 6–8 micrograms per day.

Overdose Symptoms: Generally unknown except for a possible high hemoglobin count.

Where Stored: Liver, lungs, kidney, spleen.

How Long Stored: Long term storage.

FOLIC ACID. Water-soluble.

Chief Functions: Many complex metabolic functions; important in production of nucleic acid, thus necessary to all body cells; important to maintaining healthy blood count.

Deficiency Symptoms: Intestinal disorders; fatigue; low white blood count; pernicious anemia; depression, nervousness, brain damage.

Works With: Biotin, pantothenic acid; B_1, B_2, B_3, B_6, B_{12}, C, E, and sex hormones in male and female.

Factors Affecting Need: Illness, intestinal disorders, genetic factors or aging may cause poor absorption; as much as seventy-five percent may be excreted in urine, and even greater urine loss may be caused by high vitamin C intake.

Best Dietary Sources: Yeast, dark green leafy vegetables such as spinach and beet greens; liver; asparagus; dried legumes such as lentils, navy beans; wheat.

Minimum Daily Intake: .4 milligrams.

Overdose Symptoms: None. However, the absence of *either* B_{12} or folic acid in the system can produce pernicious anemia, and if folic acid is taken while B_{12} is not, a patient can have irreversible nervous damage caused by pernicious anemia without having the blood signs of the disease. For that reason, the FDA forbids sale of folic acid in tablets larger than 0.4 mgs.

Where It is Stored: Liver.

How Long It is Stored: Short term storage.

BIOTIN. A water-soluble B vitamin.

Chief Functions: Affects growth; important to health of skin, hair, nerves, bone marrow, and glands, including sex glands.

Deficiency Symptoms: Believed to be rare. Fatigue, depression, muscle pain, hypersensitive skin, other skin disorders.

Works With: B_2, B_6, B_{12}, folic acid, pantothenic acid, and testosterone.

Factors Affecting Need: Most people can manufacture biotin in their intestines, but illness or nutritional deficiencies could interfere with this and cause a deficiency; antibiotics and sulfa drugs destroy intestinal bacteria that produce biotin; raw egg white robs the system of biotin.

Best Dietary Sources: Yeast, lamb and pork liver, grains, dried legumes, cooked eggs, nuts and peanuts.

Minimum Daily Intake: Normally 300 milligrams (made by your own body).

Overdose Symptoms: None known.

Where Stored: Liver.

How Long Stored: Long term storage.

PANTOTHENIC ACID. A water-soluble B vitamin.

Chief Functions: Used in carbohydrate, fat, and protein metabolism. Important in forming adrenal cortical hormones. Useful in fighting stress and developing antibodies against infection; recently found useful in combatting arthritis and aging.

Deficiency Symptoms: Nerve and muscle disturbances; heart trouble; digestive malfunctions; susceptibility to infection; weakness; depression.

Works With: B_1, B_2, B_3, B_{12}, biotin, folic acid, and C.

Factors Affecting Need: Easily destroyed in cooking; used up during stress such as illness, anxiety, or fatigue; more needed to fight aging and arthritis.

Best Dietary Sources: Yeast, brain, liver, heart, kidney, eggs, peanuts, herring.

Minimum Daily Intake: 10–15 milligrams (estimated).
Overdose Symptoms: None known.
Where It is Stored: Liver, heart, kidney.
How Long It is Stored: Short term storage.

VITAMIN C (Ascorbic acid). Water-soluble.

Chief Functions: Aids absorption of iron; important in the manufacture of adrenal cortical hormones; of polysaccharid, and of collagen; used in forming bones, teeth, and cartilage; maintains strength of capillaries; prevents oxidation of nutrients within the body; promotes growth and wound healing; important in forming white blood cells which fight infection; detoxifies drugs and environmental poisons in the system; fights emotional and environmental stress; protects circulatory system from fat deposits.

Deficiency Symptoms: Scurvy; tooth decay, bleeding gums; slow wound healing; abnormal bone development; aching joints; tendency to bruise easily; susceptibility to infection; mental disorders.

Works With: A, E, B_{12}, B_6, K, folic acid, pantothenic acid, and testosterone.

Factors Affecting Need: Stress from tension or fatigue, or from the environment (air pollution, cigarette smoke, food additives, and other toxic elements, drugs, allergies, or illness) will use up reserves of vitamin C; also destroyed by heat of cooking.

Best Dietary Sources: Broccoli; turnip or collard greens; kale, brussels sprouts, cauliflower, cabbage parsley, rose hips, citrus fruits, other fresh fruit.

Minimum Daily Intake: 60 milligrams.

Overdose Symptoms: Rare; possible diarrhea, possible activation of peptic ulcer in ulcer-prone individuals.

Where It is Stored: Adrenal cortex.

How Long It is Stored: Short term storage.

VITAMIN D. Fat-soluble.

Chief Functions: Regulates calcium and phosphorous metabolism; necessary for bone growth; important in nerve excitation.

Deficiency Symptoms: Rickets; poor bone growth; increase in nervous system irritability caused by low blood calcium and phosphorous.

Works With: B_3, A, calcium, phosphorous; sunlight.

Factors Affecting Need: Growing children need more vitamin D; older people may need more to prevent loss of calcium from bones; since vitamin D is made on the skin with sunlight, people whose clothing and life style keep them out of the sun may need more; it is believed that dark-skinned people living in northern climates may not synthesize enough vitamin D; similarly for people who live where the sunlight is cut by smog.

Best Dietary Sources: Fish liver oils; egg yolks; fish.

Minimum Daily Intake: 400 I.U.s.

Overdose Symptoms: Loss of appetite; weakness; nausea; thirst; diarrhea;

joint pains; frequent urination; hardening of arteries; calcium deposits in tissues.
Where It is Stored: Liver, skin.
How Long It is Stored: Long term storage.

VITAMIN E (tocopherol). Fat-soluble.
Chief Functions: Promotes normal growth; aids normal functioning of muscle, vascular, and nerve cells; anti-oxidant (important for protecting essential fatty acids); aids absorption of unsaturated fats; acts as detoxifying agent; fights stress.
Deficiency Symptoms: Diarrhea; anemia; gall bladder disorders; liver diseases; fibrosis of pancreas; muscle weakness; nervous disorders; skin disorders; degeneration of reproductive tissue.
Works With: Vitamins A, B_6, B_{12}, C, K, folic acid; estrogen, testosterone.
Factors Affecting Need: Nervous or environmental stress increases your need for vitamin E; since it is used to protect unsaturated fats in the body, preventing them from turning rancid, a diet high in unsaturated fats will increase your need for vitamin E. Much is lost in heat of cooking and food processing; much is lost when foods are frozen.
Best Dietary Sources: Cold-pressed vegetable oils, especially safflower or sunflower oil; yeast; cabbage, spinach, asparagus.
Minimum Daily Intake: 30 I.U.'s.
Overdose Symptoms: Rare; elevated blood pressure.
Where It is Stored: Muscle, fatty tissue.
How Long It is Stored: Short term storage.

VITAMIN K. Fat-soluble.
Chief Functions: Helps liver to form prothrombin to control normal blood clotting; aids electron transport.
Deficiency Symptoms: Hemorrhaging.
Works With: Vitamins A, C, and E.
Factors Affecting Need: In a normal adult, vitamin K is completely manufactured by healthy bacteria in the intestines. When antibiotics and sulfa drugs kill these bacteria, vitamin K deficiency may result. These bacteria can be restored by taking two capsules of acidophilous, three times daily. Vitamin K might also be needed by someone who had had an overdose of some anticoagulant drug.
Best Sources: Provided by intestine.
Daily Intake: No supplement recommended except in unusual cases such as hemorrhaging in newborn infant, or in woman in labor.
Overdose Symptoms: Possible abnormally fast blood clotting (thrombosis); vomiting.
Where It is Stored: Liver.
How Long It is Stored: Short term storage.

INDEX

A

Academy of Orthomolecular Psychiatry, 40
Academy of Sciences (U.S.S.R.), 131
Acidophilus bacteria, 160–161
Addiction, 44–61
  alcohol, 44–46
  food, 46–61; fasting to cure, 51–54
Addison's disease, 166
Additives, 15
Adenosine triphosphate (ATP), 157, 161
Adrenal cortical extract, 92–96
Adrenal cortical hormones, 80, 201
Adrenal glands, 201; emotions and, 210, 211–212
Afro-Americans, 102
Aging process, 303–321
  cell therapy for, 319–320
  chemistry importance, 305–307
  immunological aspects of, 308–309
  inositol and choline for, 317–318
  liver spots, 316–317
  in older people, 312–315
    niacin needs, 313–315
    nutritional care, 312–313

overfeeding factor, 315–316
PABA and, 318–319
pantothenic acid, 316–317
postponing, 307–308
turning point in, 305
vitamins in, 309–312
Agricultural Research Center (Maryland), 116
Air pollution, 24
Alcoholics, 19, 24, 102, 276
  beginning pattern of, 44–46
  diet and, 219–233
    B_{12} absorption, 229–230
    B_{12b} needs, 229
    calcium pantothenate, 231
    choline and inositol, 228
    desire to drink, 223–225
    dolomite, 226
    fatty acid, 230
    glutamine, 226–228
    proper nutrition, 231–232
    psychiatrists, 232–233
    sex hormones, 231
    thiamin, 228
  DT's, 162
  hypoglycemia and, 77–79; toxic foods, 78–79

349